Progress in Inflammation Research

Series Editor

Prof. Dr. Michael J. Parnham
PLIVA
Research Institute
Prilaz baruna Filipovica 25
10000 Zagreb
Croatia

Forthcoming titles:

Neuroinflammatory Mechanisms in Alzheimer's Disease, J. Rogers (Editor), 2001
Mechanisms and Mediators of Neuropathic Pain, A.B. Malmberg, S.R. Chaplan (Editors), 2001
Disease-modifying Therapy in Vasculitides, C.G.M. Kallenberg, J.W. Cohen Tervaert (Editors), 2001
Inflammation and Stroke, G. Feuerstein (Editor), 2001
NMDA Antagonists as Potential Analgesic Drugs, R.G. Hill, D.J.S. Sirinathsinghji (Editors), 2001

(Already published titles see last page.)

Nitric Oxide and Inflammation

Daniela Salvemini
Timothy R. Billiar
Yoram Vodovotz

Editors

Springer Basel AG

Editors

Daniela Salvemini, Ph.D.
MetaPhore Pharmaceuticals
3655 Vista Avenue
St. Louis, MO 63110
USA

Timothy R. Billiar, M.D.
A1010 Presbyterian University Hospital
Department of Surgery
200 Lothrop Street
Pittsburgh, PA 15213
USA

Yoram Vodovotz, Ph.D.
University of Pittsburgh
Department of Surgery
UPMC Montefiore
NW 653
3459 Fifth Avenue
Pittsburgh, PA 15213
USA

A CIP catalogue record for this book is available from the Library of Congress, Washington D.C., USA

Deutsche Bibliothek Cataloging-in-Publication Data
Nitric oxide and inflammation / Daniela Salvemini, Timothy R. Billiar, Yoram Vodovotz eds..
- Basel ; Boston ; Berlin : Birkhäuser, 2001
    (Progress in inflammation research)
    ISBN 978-3-0348-9488-3   ISBN 978-3-0348-8241-5 (eBook)
    DOI 10.1007/978-3-0348-8241-5

The publisher and editor can give no guarantee for the information on drug dosage and administration contained in this publication. The respective user must check its accuracy by consulting other sources of reference in each individual case.

The use of registered names, trademarks etc. in this publication, even if not identified as such, does not imply that they are exempt from the relevant protective laws and regulations or free for general use.

ISBN 978-3-0348-9488-3

© 2001 Springer Basel AG
Originally published by Birkhäuser Verlag in 2001
Softcover reprint of the hardcover 1st edition 2001

Printed on acid-free paper produced from chlorine-free pulp. TCF ∞
Cover design: Markus Etterich, Basel
Cover illustration: Immunohistochemical analysis for iNOS in lungs collected 4 h following the intrapleural injection of carrageenan in rats. Using a specific anti-iNOS antibody positive brown staining was found localised in the epithelial cell as well as in inflammatory cells. The original magnification is 150x. With the friendly permission of Daniela Salvemini.

ISBN 978-3-0348-9488-3

9 8 7 6 5 4 3 2 1

Contents

List of contributors

Galaleldin E. Abdelkarim, Inotek Corporation, Suite 419E, 100 Cummings Center, Beverly, MA 01915, USA; e-mail: gabdelkarim@mediaone.net

Graciela Andonegui, Immunology Research Group, University of Calgary, Health Sciences Center, 3330 Hospital Drive NW, T2N 4N1, Calgary, Alberta, Canada; e-mail: andonegu@ucalgary.ca

Mary H. Barccellos-Hoff, Life Sciences Division, Lawrence Berkeley Laboratory, Berkeley, CA 94720, USA

Clara Batista Lorigados, Hospital das Clinicas FMUSP Sao Paulo, SP, Brazil

Salvatore Cuzzocrea, Institute of Pharmacology, School of Medicine, University of Messina, Torre Biologica – Policlinico Universitario Via C. Valeria-Gazzi, 98100 Messina, Italy; e-mail: salvator@www.unime.it

Péter Ferdinandy, Department of Biochemistry, Faculty of Medicine, University of Szeged, Dóm tér 9, Szeged, 6720 Hungary; e-mail: peter@bioch.szote.u-szeged.hu

Henri R. Ford, Children's Hospital of Pittsburgh, Department of Surgery, Pittsburgh, PA 15213, USA; e-mail: fordh@chplink.chp.edu

Ferenc Gallyas, Department of Biochemistry, Pécs University Medical School, Pécs, Hungary; e-mail: ferenc.gallyas.jr@aok.pte.hu

Francisco Garcia Soriano, Hospital das Clinicas FMUSP Sao Paulo, SP, Brazil; e-mail: gsoriano@usp.br

David A. Geller, Starzl Transplantation Institute, University of Pittsburgh, Falk Clinic, 4th Floor, 3601 Fifth Avenue, Pittsburgh, PA 15213, USA; e-mail: gellerda@msx.upmc.edu

Laura Gray, Department of Molecular and Cellular Physiology, Louisiana State University Health Sciences Center, 1501 Kings Highway, P.O. Box 33932, Shreveport, LA 71130, USA

Matthew B. Grisham, Department of Molecular and Cellular Physiology, Louisiana State University Health Sciences Center, 1501 Kings Highway, P.O. Box 33932, Shreveport, LA 71130; email: mgrish@lsuhsc.edu

György Haskó, Department of Surgery, University of Medicine and Dentistry New Jersey, 185 South Orange Avenue, Newark, NJ 07103, USA; e-mail: haskoge@umdnj.edu

Jason Hoffman, Department of Molecular and Cellular Physiology, Louisiana State University Health Sciences Center, 1501 Kings Highway, P.O. Box 33932, Shreveport, LA 71130, USA

Rosemary A. Hoffman, University of Pittsburgh, Department of Surgery, W1545 Bioscience Tower, 200 Lothrop Street, Pittsburgh PA 15213, USA; e-mail: hoffmanr3@msx.upmc.edu

Prakash Jagtap, Inotek Corporation, Suite 419E, 100 Cummings Center, Beverly, MA 01915, USA

Shigeyuki Kawachi, Department of Molecular and Cellular Physiology, Louisiana State University Health Sciences Center, 1501 Kings Highway, P.O. Box 33932, Shreveport, LA 71130, USA

Victoria Kolb-Bachofen, Immunobiology Research Group, Heinrich-Heine-Universität, PO Box 101007, 40001 Düsseldorf, Germany; e-mail: bachofen@uni-duesseldorf.de

Paul Kubes, Immunology Research Group, University of Calgary, Health Sciences Center, 3330 Hospital Drive NW, T2N 4N1, Calgary, Alberta, Canada; e-mail:pkubes@ucalgary.ca

F. Stephen Laroux, Department of Molecular and Cellular Physiology, Louisiana State University Health Sciences Center, 1501 Kings Highway, P.O. Box 33932, Shreveport, LA 71130, USA

James K. Liao, Department of Medicine, Brigham & Women's Hospital and Harvard Medical School, 221 Longwood Avenue LMRC322, Boston, MA 02115, USA; e-mail:jliao@rics.bwh.harvard.edu

Lucas Liaudet, Department of Surgery, University of Medicine and Dentistry New Jersey, 185 South Orange Avenue, Newark, NJ 07103, USA; e-mail: lliaudet@usa.net

Charles Lowenstein, Division of Cardiology, Dpt of Medicine, John Hopkins University School of Medicine, 720 Rutland Avenue, Baltimore, Maryland 21205, USA; e-mail: clowenst@jhmi.edu

Jon Mabley, Inotek Corporation, Suite 419E, 100 Cummings Center, Beverly, MA 01915, USA; e-mail: jmabley@inotekcorp.com

Anita Marton, Inotek Corporation, Suite 419E, 100 Cummings Center, Beverly, MA 01915, USA; e-mail: amarton@inotekcorp.com

Carol A. McCloskey, University of Pittsburgh, Department of Surgery, 677 Scaife Hall, 3550 Terrace Street, Pittsburgh, PA 15213, USA; e-mail: mccloskeyc@msx.upmc.edu

Tomokazu Ohnishi, Division of Cardiology, Department of Medicine, John Hopkins University School of Medicine, 720 Rutland Avenue, Baltimore, MD 21205, USA; e-mail: tomton825@aol.com

Daniela Salvemini, MetaPhore Pharmaceuticals, 1910 Innerbelt Business Center Drive, St Louis, MO 63314, USA; e-mail: dsalvemini@metaphore.com

Andrew L. Salzman, Inotek Corporation, Suite 419E, 100 Cummings Center, Beverly, MA 01915, USA; e-mail: alsalzman@aol.com

Wolfram Samlowski, Huntsman Cancer Institute, 2000 Circle of Hope Dr., Salt Lake City, UT 84112, USA; e-mail: wolfram.samlowski@hci.utah.edu

Richard Schulz, Departments of Pediatrics and Pharmacology, University of Alberta, 4-62 Heritage Medical Research Centre, Edmonton, Alberta T6G 2S2, Canada; e-mail: richard.schulz@ualberta.ca

Garry J. Southan, Inotek Corporation, Suite 419E, 100 Cummings Center, Beverly, MA 01915, USA; e-mail: gjsouthan@aol.com

Martin Spiecker, Medizinische Klinik II, St. Josef Hospital, Ruhr-Universität Bochum, Gudrunstrasse 56, 44791 Bochum, Germany; e-mail: martin.spiecker@ruhr-uni-bochum.de

Csaba Szabó, Inotek Corporation, Suite 419E, 100 Cummings Center, Beverly, MA 01915, USA; e-mail: szabocsaba@aol.com

Éva Szabó, Inotek Corporation, Suite 419E, 100 Cummings Center, Beverly, MA 01915, USA; e-mail: eszabo@inotekcorp.com

Bradley S. Taylor, Department of Cardiothoriac Surgery, University of Pittsburgh, C-700 Presbyterian Hospital, 200 Lothrop Street, Pittsburgh, PA 15213, USA; e-mail: taylorb@msx.upmc.edu

Henri van der Heyde, Department of Microbiology and Immunology, Louisiana State University Health Sciences Center, 1501 Kings Highway, P.O. Box 33932, Shreveport, LA 71130, USA

László Virág, Inotek Corporation, Suite 419E, 100 Cummings Center, Beverly, MA 01915, USA; e-mail: viraglaszlo@hotmail.com

Richard Weller, Department of Dermatology, University of Edinburgh, EH3-9YW, UK

Yong Xia, Molecular and Cellular Biophysics Laboratories, Department of Medicine, Division of Cardiology, EPR Center, Johns Hopkins University School of Medicine, 5501 Hopkins Bayview Circle, Baltimore, Maryland, 21224, USA; e-mail: yongxia@jhmi.edu

Jay L. Zweier, Molecular and Cellular Biophysics Laboratories, Department of Medicine, Division of Cardiology and the EPR Center, Johns Hopkins University School of Medicine, 5501 Hopkins Bayview Circle, Baltimore, Maryland, 21224, USA; e-mail:jzweier@welchlink.welch.jhu.edu

Preface

Nitric oxide (NO) and its reaction products (reactive nitrogen oxide species; RNOS) have been found to modulate all facets of physiology and pathology in species as distant evolutionarily as plants and man. Additionally, the chemical literature regarding the role of NO, especially as a pollutant, has been with us for over a century. The naming of NO as "Molecule of the Year" by *Science* magazine in 1992, and the award in 1998 of the Nobel Prize in Medicine for the role of NO in the cardiovascular system reflects the importance given to this molecule by the general scientific community. Clinically useful drugs have often rapidly followed the developments elucidating the basic biology of NO, another testament to the importance of NO to biomedical research. We expect that this side-by-side advance of basic and clinical knowledge involving NO will continue unabated in the 21st century.

These advances will require both a broad and a deep understanding of the biology and chemistry of NO. The voluminous literature regarding the incredible range of chemical and biological effects of NO and RNOS may at first present a tangle of confusing and often contradictory information to the uninitiated researcher. While in the early years of research into the biological roles of NO it was possible to write comprehensive review articles or book chapters, it is quite difficult to do so at this time without great oversimplification.

Accordingly, we have taken on the task of producing a book on a single aspect of NO: its effects on inflammation. Nitric oxide was described very early on in its "modern" history (i.e., the last two decades) as an effector product of activated macrophages. As is often the tendency is science, the ability of NO to cause cytostasis and cytotoxicity in tumor cells and certain pathogens resulted in its initial perception as a beneficial mechanism to the host. Furthermore, the finding that NO derived from the endothelial nitric oxide synthase (eNOS) could block the adhesion of activated neutrophils suggested a beneficial role for NO in ischemia/reperfusion injury.

However, the finding that the massive expression of the inducible nitric oxide synthase (iNOS) in conditions such as sepsis was associated with hypotension led to a change in this perception. Rapidly, data were published which implicated the aberrant expression of iNOS in numerous inflammatory conditions (e.g., inflammatory bowel disease, Crohn's disease, Alzheimer's disease, and hemorrhagic shock, to name a few). This perception was strengthened by the demonstration that NO could lead to apoptosis of certain cell types during inflammatory diseases. These studies and numerous others began to paint a darker picture of NO as a toxic byproduct of inflammation that should be inhibited in order to restore homeostasis.

More recently, however, NO has been "re-invented" as a suppressor of inflammation. Nitric oxide was found to suppress the proliferation of lymphocytes and cause their apoptosis. Simultaneously, NO was described to inhibit apoptosis of various cell types, notably hepatocytes, through mechanisms involving the nitrosative suppression of caspases. This see-sawing between beneficial and detrimental roles of NO has undoubtedly caused consternation to those researchers attempting to wade through the literature. We believe that this volume in the series *Progress in Inflammation Research* will serve to put into perspective the state-of-the-art in research on NO and inflammation. We have gathered together leading authors in the field to present their views on the role of NO in various aspects of inflammation. We hope that the reader will benefit by the balanced overview on the complex way in which NO modulates various inflammatory processes. Moreover, we hope the reader will share some of the same enthusiasm we have for studying this multifunctional molecule and its effects on inflammation.

Daniela Salvemini
Timothy R. Billiar
Yoram Vodovotz

Regulation of the inducible nitric oxide synthase (iNOS) gene

Bradley S. Taylor[1] and David A. Geller[2]

[1]Department of Cardiothoracic Surgery, University of Pittsburgh, C-700 Presbyterian Hospital, 200 Lothrop Street, Pittsburgh, PA 15213, USA; [2]Starzl Transplantation Institute, University of Pittsburgh, Falk Clinic, 4th floor, 3601 Fifth Avenue, Pittsburgh, PA 15213, USA

Introduction

Induced nitric oxide (NO), the end product of the enzyme inducible nitric oxide synthase (iNOS), has been shown to be an important mediator in a number of human diseases and cancers [1–4]. L-arginine is converted to the NO and L-citrulline by the inducible isoform of nitric oxide synthase and produces high levels of NO (Fig. 1). Once produced, NO has a short half-life ($t_{1/2}$ = s) and undergoes spontaneous oxidation to the inactive metabolites nitrite and nitrate (NO_2^- and NO_3^-). Because iNOS is involved in the pathogenesis of the inflammatory response, the characterization of the cis- and trans-activating factors which regulate lipopolysacharide- (LPS) and cytokine-induced iNOS expression have been pursued. This review will summarize and contrast the molecular regulation of the murine and human iNOS genes. The regulation of iNOS is complex and occurs at multiple sites within the signal transduction pathways that lead to iNOS gene expression and includes transcription and post-transcriptional mechanisms of modification.

The inducible nitric oxide synthase gene

Cytokine-induced human iNOS expression was initially described in cultures of primary human hepatocytes [5]. The first human iNOS cDNA was isolated from LPS- and cytokine-stimulated primary human hepatocytes in 1993 [6]. The sequence of the human hepatocyte iNOS clone reveals a 4,145 base pair cDNA containing a 3,459 base pair open reading frame which encodes a polypeptide of 1,153 amino acids with a calculated molecular mass of 131 kDa (Fig. 2). Overall, human iNOS displays an 80% sequence identity to murine macrophage iNOS [7–9] and 50% homology to either human endothelial cNOS [10, 11] or human neuronal cNOS [12]. (For a review on the molecular regulation of all three human NOS genes, see [13]). Similar to other NOS isoforms, hepatocyte iNOS contains consensus recognition sites for the cofactors FMN, FAD, and NADPH in the carboxyl half of the pro-

Nitric Oxide and Inflammation, edited by Daniela Salvemini, Timothy R. Billiar and Yoram Vodovotz
© 2001 Birkhäuser Verlag Basel/Switzerland

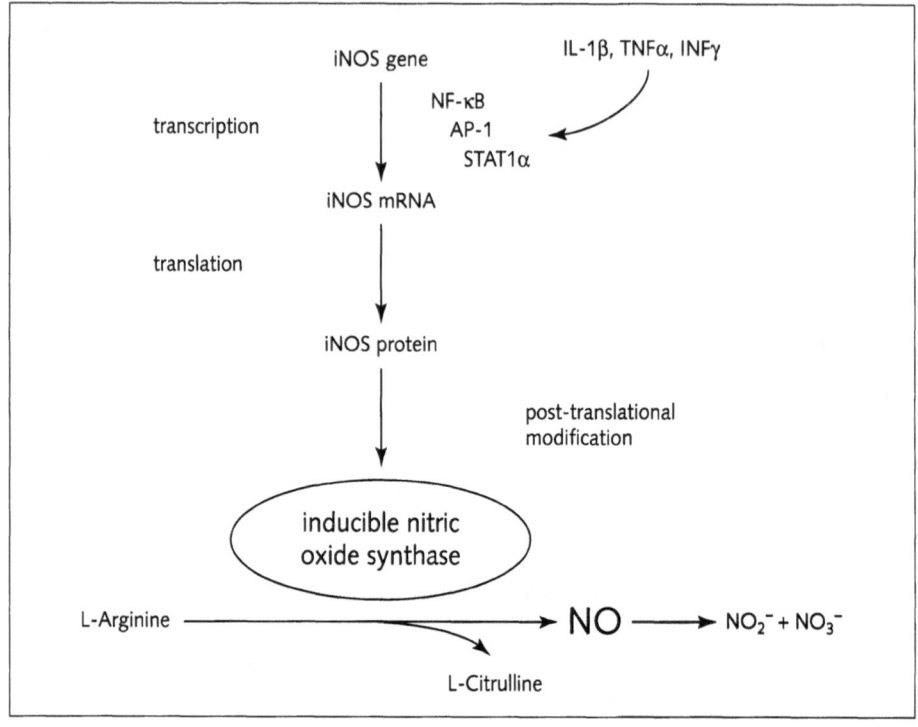

Figure 1

NO biosynthetic pathway. Inducible nitric oxide synthase catalyzes the conversion of L-argi-nine, in the presence of oxygen, to the free radical NO and L-citrulline. NO has a short half-life and is oxidized to the inactive end-products nitrite and nitrate (NO_2^- and NO_3^-). iNOS expression is upregulated by cytokines through the transcription factors NF-κB, AP-1, and STAT1α. Transcriptional and post-transcriptional mechanisms play an important role in iNOS regulation.

tein which have been shown to be important for iNOS enzyme activity. In addition, binding sites for heme, biopterin, and calmodulin are also present. The functional role of the human iNOS cDNA was confirmed by transfection of an iNOS cDNA expression vector into human kidney cells, which resulted in a substantial increase in NOS activity as detected by conversion of radiolabeled arginine to citrulline [6]. Since the initial report, human iNOS cDNA has been cloned from chondrocytes [14, 15], DLD-1 colon carcinoma cell line [16], A-172 glioblastoma cell line [17], and human cardiac myocytes [18]. Each of these cDNAs are identical to the human hepatocyte iNOS cDNA with > 99% sequence homology.

The human iNOS gene was isolated by John S. Mudgett, Ph.D. and subsequent-ly cloned by using the iNOS cDNA to screen a fibroblast genomic library [19]. The

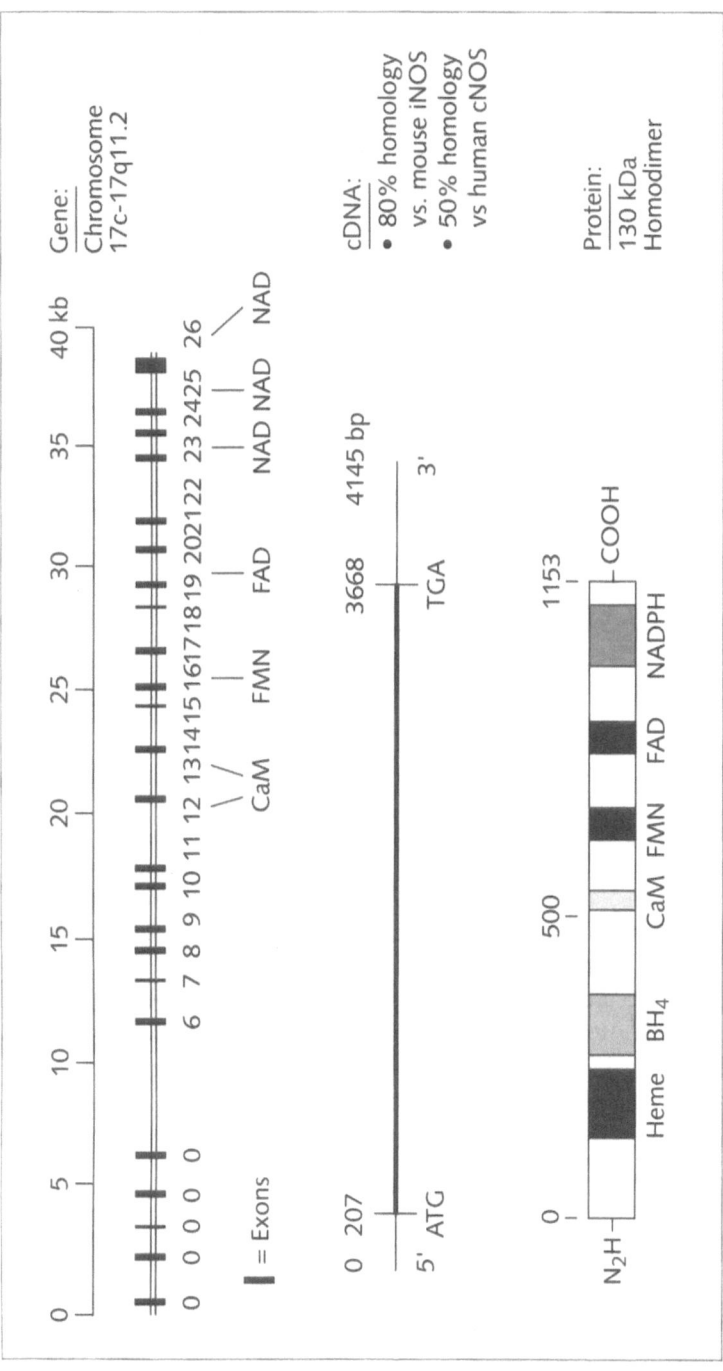

Figure 2
Human iNOS gene, cDNA, and protein. The human iNOS gene is 37 kilobases in length and is composed of 26 exons and 25 introns. It is mapped to chromosome 17 at position 17 cen-q11.2. The cDNA is 4145 basepairs in size with an open reading frame of 3459 base pairs. The polypeptide is 1153 amino acids with a calculated mass of 131 kDa and contains recognition sites for the cofactors FMN, FAD, NADPH, heme, biopterin, and calmodulin.

Table 1 - Cells and tissues that express human inducible nitric oxide synthase

astrocytes	mast cells
chondrocytes	neurons
cardiac myocytes	neutrophils
eosinophils	osteoblasts
endometrium	osteoclasts
fibroblasts	placental trophoblasts
hepatocytes	platelets
islet cells	retinal epithelium
keratinocytes	sertoli cells
Kupffer cells	skeletal muscle
lipocytes	vascular endothelial cells
lung epithelium	vascular smooth muscle cells
monocytes/macrophages	

Cell lines

A-172 glioblastoma	DLD-1 adenocarcinoma
AKN-1 liver epithelium	MG 63 osteosarcoma
A549 lung epithelium	Neuroblastoma NB-39-nu
B cell lymphoma	SW480/SW620 colon carcinoma
CaCO-2 adenocarcinoma	

full-length human iNOS gene is 37 kb in length and is composed of 26 exons and 25 introns (Fig. 2). Primer extension analysis of LPS and cytokine-stimulated human hepatocyte RNA identified the transcriptional initiation site 30 base pairs downstream of the TATA box. By utilizing a somatic cell hybrid mapping panel and flourescent in situ hybridization, the human iNOS gene was mapped to chromosome 17 at position 17 cen-q11.2 [19]. Human eNOS [20] and nNOS [21] reside on chromosome 7 and 12, respectively, confirming that the three NOS genes are distinct. Since its initial identification in primary human hepatocytes [5, 6], a variety of human cell-types, neoplasms and cell lines have been shown to express iNOS [22]. Table 1 is a list of cells and tissues where human iNOS expression has been documented.

Molecular regulation of the murine iNOS gene

Considerable work has been done to elucidate the functional promoter elements within the murine iNOS promoter. Figure 3 illustrates the major differences between

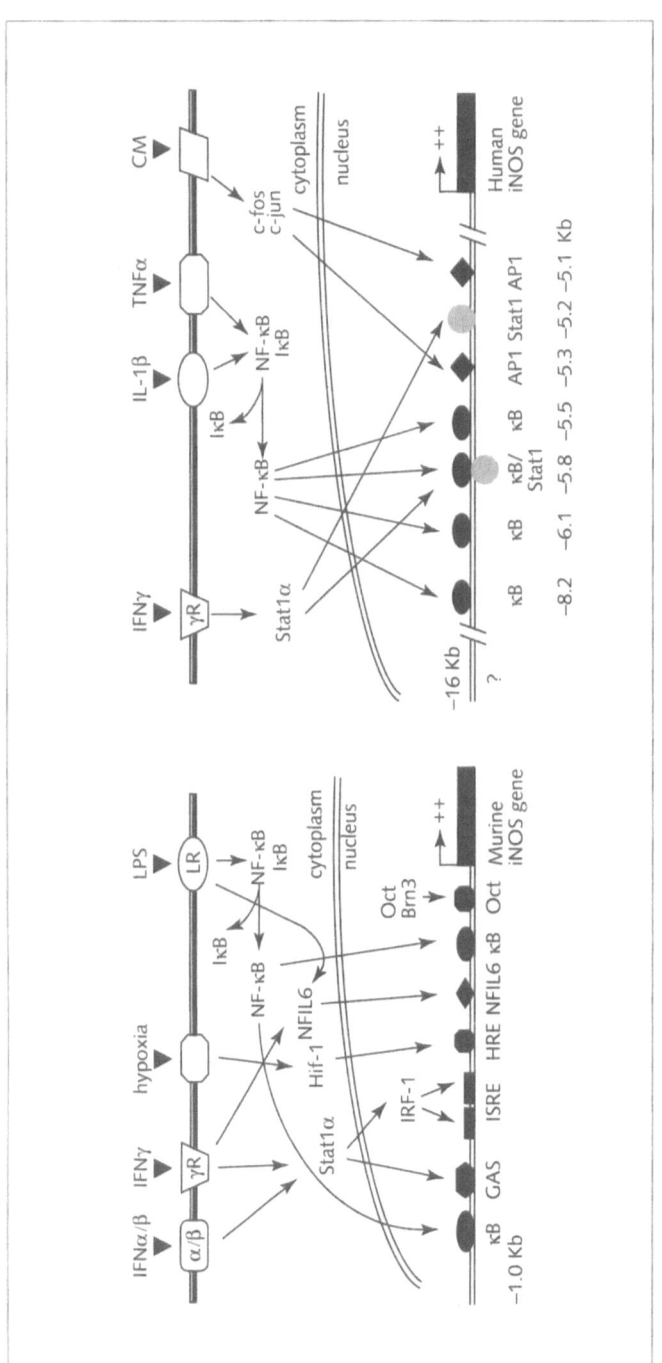

Figure 3

Schematic representation of the 5' flanking region of the murine and human iNOS genes. The figure shows the signal transduction pathways by which cytokines activate the specific transcription factors that translocate to the nucleus and bind to their respective cis-regulatory element that result in iNOS gene expression.

the molecular regulation of the murine and human iNOS genes. The murine iNOS promoter consists of two functionally distinct regulatory regions (region I: -48 to -209, region II: -913 to -1029) [23, 24]. These two regions govern the synergistic effects of LPS and IFNγ on iNOS expression. The proximally located region I has been shown to be LPS-responsive and contains a functional NF-κB and several other cytokine-responsive binding sites. Previous work by Xie determined that the proximal NF-κB at -85 bp in the murine iNOS promoter is functionally important in LPS-stimulated RAW 264.7 cells [25]. Xie also identified a novel LPS response element, which is downstream from the proximal NF-κB and is required for LPS-induced promoter activity [26]. Interestingly, neither deletion nor mutation of the proximal NF-κB site at -115 bp of the human iNOS promoter had a significant effect on cytokine-induced promoter activity, suggesting that this promoter-proximal NF-κB motif is neither necessary nor sufficient for transcriptional activation of the human iNOS gene by cytokines [27].

Additional transcription factors have been shown to play an important role in murine iNOS regulation. *In vivo* footprinting of region I shows occupation of a proximal octamer (Oct) motif [28] and IL-6 induced iNOS expression in murine myeloid cells involves a reciprocal change in Oct-1 and Oct-2 binding to this site [29]. Recent evidence suggests that the POU family transcription factors Brn-3a and Brn-3b also bind to this site in response to LPS and IFNγ [30]. In addition, recent work has identified the binding of NF-IL6, a member of the CCAAT/enhancer binding protein family of transcription factors, that binds to a proximal NF-IL6 response element [31].

The upstream region II responds to IFNγ and IFNα/β and consists of two adjacent IFN-stimulated response elements (ISRE), a NF-κB element, and a GAS site. The upstream IRF-1 binding element at -913 to -923 binds IRF-1 following IFNγ stimulation [32, 33]. The GAS site has been shown to bind STAT1α following IFNα/β stimulation [34]. Work by Murphy's group has shown that the upstream NF-κB at -974 bp is required for maximal iNOS inducibility by LPS [35]. The upstream NF-κB is also responsible for the responsiveness to triple cytokine induction in murine vascular smooth muscle cells [36]. Within the murine iNOS promoter region at position -212 to -226 exists a functional hypoxia response element (HRE) [37], which is lacking within the first 7.2 kb of the human iNOS promoter. IFNγ-treated murine macrophages that were oxygen-depleted expressed iNOS mediated by Hif-1 binding to the HRE.

Also in contrast to the murine iNOS promoter, the human iNOS promoter has been shown to be hyporesponsive to LPS and IFNγ [38, 39]. Two explanations for the hyporesponsiveness of the human iNOS promoter in macrophages were found to be secondary to: (1) multiple inactivating nucleotide substitutions in the human counterpart of the enhancer element have been shown to regulate LPS and IFNγ induced expression of the murine iNOS gene, and (2) an absence of one or more nuclear factors in human macrophages that are required for maximal iNOS expression. Interestingly, transfection of a human monocyte cell line expressing retroviral human iNOS results in iNOS mRNA and iNOS protein expression, without NO release [40]. NO synthesis in this cell line is strictly dependent on exogenous tetrahydrobiopterin, demonstrating the importance of post-transcriptional regulation of iNOS as well.

Molecular regulation of human iNOS

Human iNOS expression is synergistically stimulated by multiple cytokines as shown by Northern blot analysis of RNA from cultured human hepatocytes treated with LPS, TNFα, IL-1β, and IFNγ for 2–48 h demonstrated that no iNOS mRNA was detected in the unstimulated human hepatocytes [5, 6]. However, a single mRNA band at ~4.5 kb first appeared 4 h after cytokine and LPS stimulation, peaked at 8 h, and was barely detectable by 48 h (Fig. 4). Similarly, NO_2^- and NO_3^- levels were measured from the culture supernatants and were found to increase 20- to 30-fold at 24 and 48 h after stimulation. While most cell types require a combination of cytokines to activate iNOS expression, IL-1β alone at high doses can induce iNOS mRNA in cultures of primary human hepatocytes [41] and chondrocytes [14]. In addition, TGFβ has been shown to induce iNOS mRNA expression in human keratinocytes [42].

Because primary human hepatocytes do not undergo mitosis in culture, a human liver epithelial cell line (designated AKN-1) was isolated [43]. These cells are derived from normal human liver and immunohistochemical staining and karotype analysis revealed a transformed liver cell line with both biliary and epithelial cell features. When stimulated with the cytokine mix (CM) of TNFα, IL-1β, and INFγ, a similar pattern of iNOS mRNA was observed. NO release lagged behind the iNOS mRNA expression in a time-dependent fashion. Stimulation with single cytokines revealed that only IFNγ weakly stimulated AKN-1 mRNA expression. Double and triple cytokine combinations had a synergistic effect with CM inducing maximal iNOS mRNA expression [44]. These results are similar to those seen in primary human hepatocytes and indicate that the AKN-1 cell line is useful for studying the regulation of human iNOS.

Transcriptional regulation of human iNOS gene expression

The human iNOS gene is regulated in part by gene transcription. This was demonstrated in nuclear run-on assays performed in the AKN-1 cells. As shown in Figure 5, cytokine-induced transcriptional activity for iNOS was five-fold greater than that in untreated cells [44]. As expected, an iNOS nuclear transcript is only detected when hybridized to the anti-sense (AS) cRNA, and not the sense (S) cRNA, which

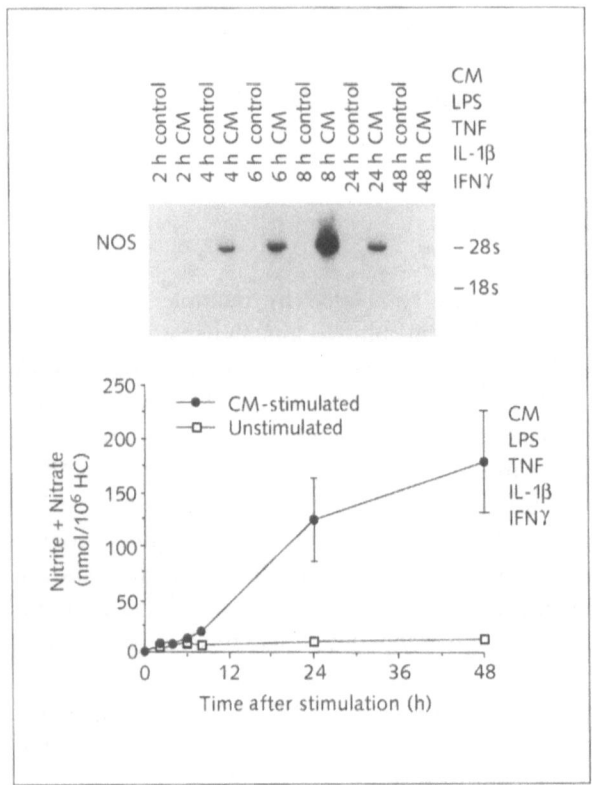

Figure 4

Cytokine-induced iNOS expression in primary human liver cells. Forty-eight h time-course of iNOS mRNA induction (Northern blot, upper) and nitrite and nitrate (NO_2^- and NO_3^-) production in culture supernatants (lower) following stimulation with LPS, TNFα (1000 μ/ml) + IL-1β (100 μ/ml) + IFNγ (250 μ/ml) (cytokine mix, CM). Values for NO_2^- and NO_3^- are expressed as mean ± SEM. (cytokine mix, CM).

serves as a negative control. Interestingly, a basal nuclear transcript was seen in the unstimulated cells (time =0 h) and indicates constitutive, low-level human iNOS transcription. This was unexpected given that we do not see a basal iNOS mRNA on Northern blot analysis in resting primary human cells or most cell lines (Fig. 4). This suggests that the iNOS mRNA transcript is highly labile and is rapidly degraded in the absence of cytokine stimulation. In addition, these experiments demonstrated that iNOS expression is regulated at the level of transcription and prompted further experiments to define the cis- and trans-activating factors important for iNOS expression.

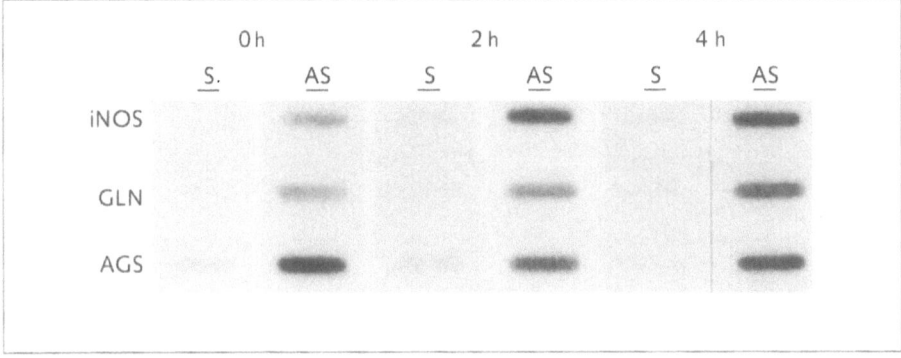

Figure 5
Nuclear run-on analysis of cytokine-induced iNOS message in human liver (AKN-1) cells.
Control cells (0 h) were not exposed to cytokines. Cytokine-stimulation for 2 and 4 h was
conducted with TNFα (1000 μ/ml) + IL-1β (100 μ/ml) + IFNγ (250 μ/ml) (cytokine mix,
CM). Nuclei were isolated and incubated with radiolabelled CTP ^{32}P-labelled nuclear RNA
was hybridized to a GeneScreen membrane containing 5 μg of immobilized sense (S) and
antisense (AS) cRNA probes of iNOS, glutaminase (GLN), and argininosuccinate synthetase
(AGS).

Deletional analysis of the human iNOS promoter

To delineate the cytokine-responsive regions of the human iNOS promoter, ~ 16 kb of the human iNOS gene 5'-flanking region was isolated and deletional iNOS promoter constructs ranging in size from 1.3 to 16 kb were generated [44]. These deletional segments were then ligated in front of the luciferase reporter gene. After liposomal transfection of the iNOS promoter-luciferase reporter constructs into human liver (AKN-1) or lung (A549) epithelial cells, analysis of the first 4.7 kb upstream demonstrated basal promoter activity, but failed to show any cytokine-inducible activity (Fig. 6). However, a three- to four-fold increase in promoter activity was seen in constructs extending up to –5.8 and –7.2 kb, and a nine-fold increase in promoter activity was induced by cytokines after transfection of the –16 kb construct. Therefore, the functional cytokine-responsive promoter elements are located upstream from –4.7 kb. The three- to nine-fold increase in cytokine-stimulated promoter activity with the larger constructs correlated reasonably well with the ~ five-fold induction of transcription that we detected by nuclear run-on (Fig. 5). To further establish that the proximal 5'-flanking region was not a critical component of the human iNOS promoter, 2.6 kb of DNA was deleted from the 5'-flanking region (–2.1 to –4.7 kb) in the context of the 7.2 kb iNOS-Luciferase promoter construct.

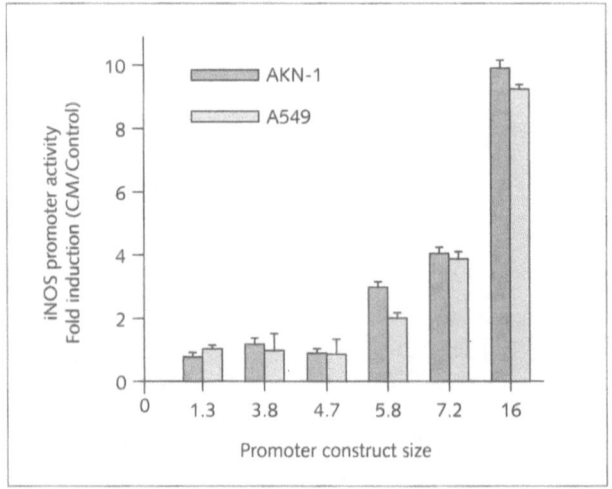

Figure 6
Deletional analysis of the upstream 5'-flanking region of the human iNOS gene. The size of the 5' deletional constructs utilized in the study are shown. Relative luciferase activity was measured from human liver (AKN-1) cells and lung (A549) cells that were stimulated with CM following transient transfections of the constructs and compared to control cells that were not exposed to CM. Fold induction (CM/Control) of iNOS promoter activity was calculated.

Transfection and cytokine-stimulation in either human cell line maintained the same ~ four-fold induction as the full-length 7.2 kb iNOS-Luciferase promoter construct, confirming that this proximal region was dispensable [27, 44]. These results contrast markedly with the murine macrophage iNOS promoter [23, 24] where only 1 kb of the proximal 5'-flanking region is required to confer LPS and cytokine inducibility, indicating that regulation of the human iNOS gene is unique compared to the murine iNOS gene.

Studies by other groups have verified that the upstream regions are required for cytokine-inducible human iNOS promoter activity. Similar to our results in human liver and lung cells, Laubach and Marks were unable to demonstrate any inducible activity with a 3.7 kb iNOS promoter construct in human DLD-1 colon cells [45] and human A549 cells [46]. Kolyada has also demonstrated no LPS and IFNγ-inducibility in human vascular smooth muscle cells transfected with a 1.1 kb human iNOS promoter segment [47]. Recent work by Linn identified an enhancer region from −8.7 to −10.7 kb in the human iNOS promoter which confers IL-1β and IFNγ

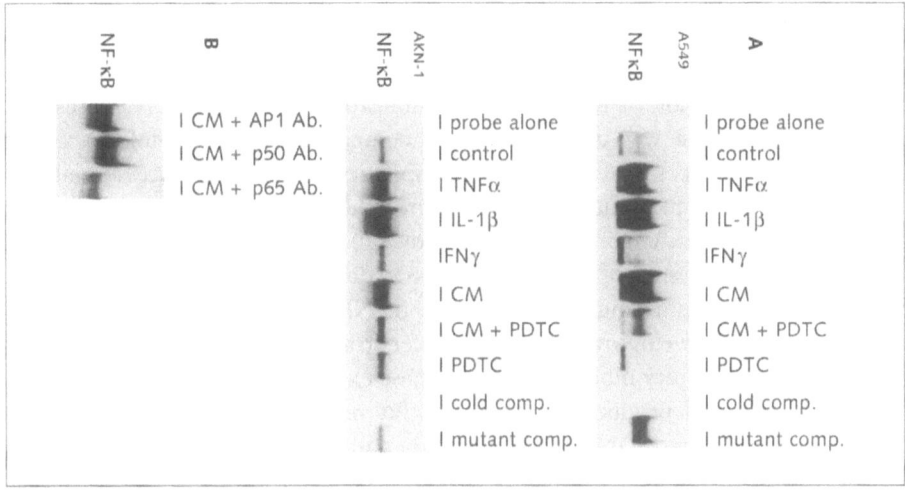

Figure 7
Cytokine-induction of NF-κB DNA binding activity. A.) Gel shift assay performed on 5 μg of nuclear extracts from human liver (AKN-1) and lung (A549) cells after 1 h of treatment with TNFα (1,000 U/ml), IL-1β (100 U/ml), IFNγ (250 U/ml) alone or a cytokine mixture (CM) of all three agents. A consensus labeled oligonucleotide containing a NF-κB response sequence was used. Some groups were pre-treated with PDTC (100 μM) or DDTC (10 mM) for 1 h prior to CM stimulation. Specificity for NF-κB binding was determined by using excess, unlabeled probes as cold and mutant competitors. (B) Supershift experiments using AKN-1 nuclear extracts and antibodies against the AP-1, p50 or p65 subunits of NF-κB.

responsiveness in DLD-1 cells [48]. Further work to characterize the functional promoter elements in that region is needed.

Role of transcription factor NF-κB in regulating cytokine-induced human iNOS expression

Since NF-κB is known to mediate transcriptional induction of many cytokine-responsive genes, (including the murine iNOS gene), we focused first on this transcription factor. In addition, the human iNOS promoter sequence contained numerous putative NF-κB response elements. Pharmacological NF-κB inhibitors significantly suppressed cytokine-stimulated iNOS mRNA expression and NO synthesis, indicating that NF-κB is involved in the induction of the human iNOS gene [27]. Figure 7 is a gel shift assay for NF-κB DNA-binding from human liver (AKN-1) and lung (A549) cells. Basal levels of NF-κB DNA binding were seen in control cells. The addition of cytokines TNFα or IL-1β induced a strong gel shift complex for NF-κB, while IFNγ had no effect. All three agents together (CM) also induced DNA-binding activity for NF-κB, and the appearance of this complex was markedly suppressed by the addition of PDTC, further implicating NF-κB in iNOS expression. Specificity for NF-κB was demonstrated by competition with 100-fold excess of unlabelled oligonucleotide (cold comp). Competition studies with excess unlabeled mutant NF-κB oligonucleotide partially restored the NF-κB DNA complex, further demonstrating specificity for NF-κB. Antibody supershift studies in the A549 lung cells showed the presence of both p50 and p65 subunits of NF-κB in the complex. Further evidence confirming the importance of NF-κB for iNOS gene expression was demonstrated by employing a gene transfer strategy using an adenoviral vector expressing the inhibitory molecule IκBα. In these experiments, adenoviral IκBα was readily infected and produced functional IκBα protein that completely blocked cytokine-induced NF-κB DNA binding activity and iNOS expression [49].

Mutational analysis identifies an upstream NF-κB enhancer region in the human iNOS promoter

To determine whether any of the putative NF-κB elements in the region upstream from −4.7 kb were functional, site-directed mutagenesis was used to generate five additional 7.2 kb constructs, each with a 2 base point mutation in the core sequence of the NF-κB element (Fig. 8). These mutant NF-κB promoter constructs were transfected into human cells and then stimulated with cytokines to detect inducible promoter activity. The mutation at −5.8 kb resulted in loss of both basal and inducible promoter activity, while mutations of the sites at −5.2, −5.5, and −6.1 kb decreased inducible promoter activity by 60%, 45%, and 65%, respectively [27]. The NF-κB mutant at site −6.5 kb retained the full cytokine-inducibility typically seen with the 7.2 kb construct. The results showed that the NF-κB motif at −5.8 kb is required for cytokine-induced promoter activity, while the sites at −5.2, −5.5, and −6.1 kb have a cooperative effect. Gel shifts using the site-specific oligonucleotide sequence from −5.8 kb produced similar results. These data indicate that NF-κB activation is required for cytokine induction of the human iNOS gene and identifies four unique far-upstream NF-κB enhancer element from −5.2 to −6.1 kb in the human iNOS promoter that confer inducibility to TNFα and IL-1β. Some recent data suggests that the sites at −5.2 and −5.8 kb in the human iNOS promoter actually contain overlapping NF-κB and STAT1α response elements, and that STAT1α may be the dominant transcription factor binding at the −5.2 kb site [50]. In addition, a recent report indicated that a NF-κB site at −8.2 kb in the human iNOS promoter is also functional [46].

The fact that NF-κB is required for iNOS gene expression is not surprising if one considers that NF-κB elements are present in the 5'-flanking regions of several

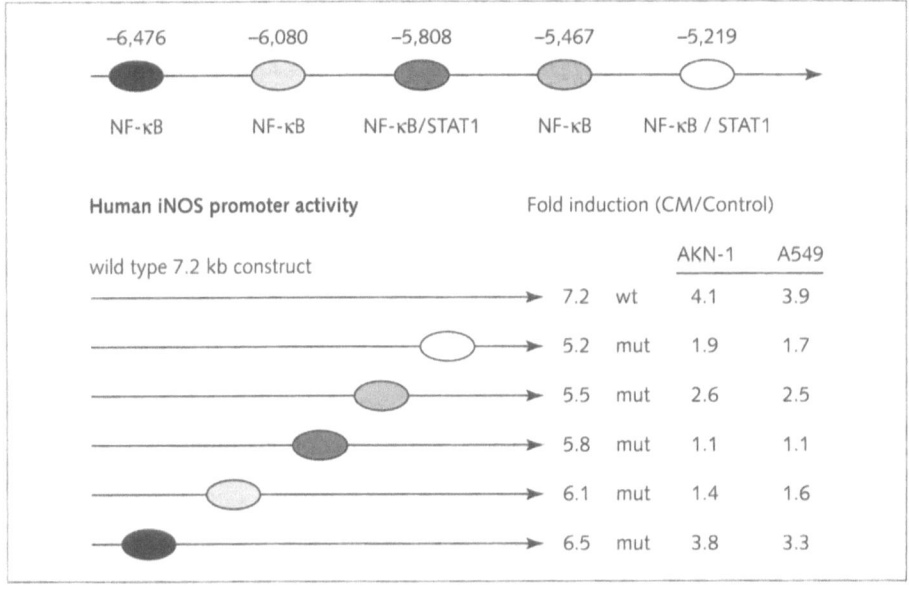

Figure 8

Site-directed mutational analysis of the upstream NF-κB cis-regulatory elements. The site-directed mutational constructs utilized in the study are shown along with their location in the 5' flanking region of the human iNOS promoter. Human liver (AKN-1) and lung (A549) cells were stimulated with CM following transient transfections of the constructs and relative luciferase activity was measured. Values are expressed as fold induction (CM/Control).

inflammatory response genes including cell adhesion molecules [51–53] and cytokines [54–56]. However, each of these promoters has only one or two proximally-located functional NF-κB binding sites compared to the human iNOS promoter which has multiple NF-κB elements localized to a segment of DNA which spans ~ 800 base pairs and is more than 5.2 kb upstream of the TATA box. The NF-κB elements from –5.2 to –6.1 kb in the human iNOS gene are spaced in approximate multiples of nucleosome units (200 bp) and this spacing may contribute to the three-dimensional structure necessary for efficient iNOS transcription. Therefore, the presence of multiple functional NF-κB binding sites so far upstream is unique to the human iNOS promoter.

Because iNOS is expressed in a number of different cell types and under different conditions we speculate that this arrangement may serve as a means for cell-type specificity and tight control in iNOS regulation. For example, the number of binding sites in a promoter may influence the intensity of the response to a given transcription factor depending on the concentration of that factor in that given cell type. In this scenario, low concentrations would be expected to evoke only a minimal response; however, with increasing levels of NF-κB translocating into the nucleus more NF-κB sites would become occupied, resulting in a greater transcriptional response. Another potential mechanism may be that more NF-κB binding sites over a segment of DNA serve to recruit the transcription factor to that portion of the genome and concentrate them toward the active elements.

Role of JAK-STAT and AP-1 signal transduction pathways in human iNOS expression

Although TNFα or IL-1β were sufficient to induce NF-κB activation, these cytokines alone were not adequate to stimulate iNOS expression in the human cell lines. The fact that a combination of cytokines is required to induce iNOS promoter activity (and detectable iNOS mRNA) suggests that activation of additional transcription factors is necessary for iNOS expression. This is supported by the work of Ohmori who demonstrated that IFNγ-activated STAT1α can cooperate with TNFα-induced NF-κB to promote transcription of a number of inflammatory genes [57]. Gao has shown that STAT1α is also involved in mediating IFNγ-inducibility in the murine iNOS promoter [33, 34]. A role for cytokine-induced STAT1α activation in human iNOS expression has been demonstrated by Kleinert using pharmacological inhibitors of the JAK-STAT kinase pathway [58]. In these studies cytokine-induced iNOS mRNA levels and nitrite production were significantly decreased in those groups exposed to the JAK-STAT kinase inhibitors. In addition, the inhibitors demonstrated reduced CM-induced STAT1α DNA binding activity by gel shift assay.

Aside from NF-κB and STAT1α, the 5'-flanking region of the human iNOS promoter contains a number of AP-1 consensus recognition sites and recent studies have identified a role for this transcription factor in human iNOS expression. Kleinert demonstrated that AP-1 appears to be a negative regulator of iNOS expression because its expression is down-regulated by CM in DLD-1 cells [58]. In contradistinction, Marks demonstrated that AP-1 DNA binding activity is increased by CM and, through mutational analysis, that the AP-1 sites at −5.1 and −5.3 are important for iNOS expression [46]. Clearly, further work needs to be done to characterize the 16 kb of 5-flanking region associated with the human iNOS gene which is one of the largest and most complex promoters described to date.

Post-transcriptional regulation of iNOS gene expression

Along with transcriptional control, post-transcriptional mechanisms of regulation play an important role in the regulation of iNOS expression and are only beginning to be understood. The 3'-UTR of the human hepatocyte iNOS cDNA contains several AT-rich sequences that correspond to the AU sequences in the mRNA [6]. These ATTTA sequence motifs have been shown in many labile cytokine and proto-oncogene transcripts and have been shown to destabilize mRNA [59, 60] and inhibit translational effiency [61]. Nunokawa demonstrated a cooperative interaction between the 5'-promoter and the 3'-region using luciferase promoter constructs containing the both the iNOS 5'-flanking region and the 3'-UTR [62]. Transfection of the constructs containing both the 5'- and 3'-region resulted in a decrease in constitutive reporter gene activity and an increase in cytokine-responsiveness. A functional role for the AUUUA motifs in the human iNOS 3-UTR was recently reported by Kleinert and colleagues [63]. In this study, the Elav-like RNA binding protein HuR was shown to bind to the AUUUA motifs and destabilize the human iNOS mRNA, confirming an important post-transcriptional regulation of the human iNOS gene.

Luss cloned and characterized the expression of iNOS in human cardiac myocytes [18]. The human cardiac myocyte iNOS cDNA is > 99% identical to the human hepatocyte iNOS cDNA that was previously cloned. Interestingly, although iNOS mRNA was readily detected in cytokine-stimulated myocytes, they were unable to detect iNOS protein or NO synthesis. These data suggest that a translational defect exists for expression of iNOS in human cardiac myocytes, and implies that cell-specific post-transcriptional mechanisms may be operating here. Whether this observation reflects rapid degradation of iNOS mRNA or a block in translational machinery has not been established.

Chu has identified structural diversity in the 5'-untranslated region of the human iNOS gene. Despite the presence of a TATA box in the promoter [19], multiple transcription initiation sites were observed in ~6% of iNOS mRNAs expressed in cytokine-stimulated human A549 lung epithelial cells [64]. The TATA-independent iNOS mRNAs were also upregulated by cytokines. Alternative splicing in the 5'-untranslated region also accounted for further structural diversity due to the presence of eight partially overlapping open reading frames (ORF's) upstream from the major iNOS ATG. These ORF's may or may not have an important role in the translational regulation of the human iNOS mRNA.

In addition to alternative splicing in the 5'-UTR, Eissa has identified alternative mRNA splicing within the human iNOS mRNA [65]. Four alternative mRNA transcripts were seen with internal deletions of exon 5, exons 8 and 9, exons 9–11, and exons 15 and 16. The deletion of exon 5 resulted in a truncated protein, while the other three variants produced in-frame deletions. Interestingly, expression of the exon 8–9-iNOS cDNA in a human cell line produced iNOS protein that lacked functional NOS activity and did not result in production of NO [66]. The molecular basis for this observation was the lack of iNOS protein dimerization as a result of the deleted exons, indicating a critical role of exon 8–9 region for iNOS protein dimerization.

Additional mechanisms of post-translational modification including protein stabilization, dimerization, phosphorylation, subcellular localization, cofactor binding and substrate availability may play an important role in human iNOS expression. Experiments have been conducted to examine the rate-limiting aspect of BH_4 availability in perfused livers and isolated hepatocytes [67]. Suppression of BH_4 levels markedly reduced the conversion of phenylalanine to tyrosine by phenylalanine hydroxylase but had little impact on iNOS activity. Furthermore, phenylalanine increased BH_4 synthesis as previously described [68] while arginine had no effect. These findings are not entirely unexpected because the iNOS Km for BH_4 is 100-fold lower than the phenylalanine hydroxylase Km for BH_4. Thus, the requirement of iNOS for BH_4 is much lower. While phenylalanine hydroxylase relies on allosteric upregulation of BH_4 synthesis by the substrate, iNOS does not.

Down-regulators of iNOS expression

A number of factors including steriods, cytokines, and NO itself have all been shown to suppress iNOS expression. Glucocorticoids have been shown to inhibit induced NO synthesis in several cell types [69-72] and this effect appears to be tissue- and species-specific. Kleinert demonstrated that dexamethasone inhibits cytokine-induced iNOS mRNA in human A549 epithelial cells by a direct protein-protein interaction between the glucocorticoid receptor and NF-κB without an increase in IκBα mRNA levels [71]. Work in our laboratory showed that dexamethasone decreases iNOS mRNA levels in rat hepatocytes and that this down-regulation occurs at the level of transcription [72]. This effect is a result of increased cytosolic IκBα levels and a concomitant decrease in nuclear p65 translocation in the presence of dexamethasone. In human colon carcinoma DLD-1 cells, Salzman reported that dexamethasone exhibited only a slight decrease in iNOS mRNA expression [73], and Kleinert found no inhibition of iNOS mRNA levels by dexamethasone in the same DLD-1 cells [58]. Perrella found that dexamethasone decreased iNOS mRNA levels in rat aortic vascular smooth muscle cells only when given before IL-1β, but not after [74]. In contrast, Kunz reported that dexamethasone did not alter IL-1β-induced iNOS mRNA in rat mesangial cells. Surprisingly, nuclear run-on experiments showed that dexamethasone markedly attenuated IL-1β-induced iNOS gene transcription and this was counteracted by a prolongation in iNOS mRNA half-life from 1 to 2.5 h [75]. Despite extensive clinical use of glucocorticoids as immunosuppressive agents in patients with autoimmune diseases or after organ transplants, we have only begun to understand the mechanisms by which these drugs elicit their anti-inflammatory actions. Down-regulation of iNOS expression during inflammation is one additional means by which steroids may exert their therapeutic effects.

The end-product NO has been shown to exert a negative regulatory effect on iNOS gene expression [76–79]. Similar feedback regulatory loops have been described for many cellular mediators. The addition of the NO donor nitroprusside, S-nitroso-N-acetyl-D,L-penicillamine (SNAP), and even the overexpression of NO *via* infection with the adenoviral iNOS gene, resulted in decreased iNOS mRNA and protein levels in rat and human hepatocytes [76]. Nuclear run-on analysis revealed that SNAP inhibited CM-stimulated iNOS gene transcription, and gel shift assays of the nuclear extracts revealed that this effect is secondary to decreased CM-induced DNA binding activity for NF-κB. This work identifies a negative feedback loop whereby NO down-regulates iNOS gene expression, possibly to limit over production during pathophysiologic conditions. Others have shown that NO can also inhibit iNOS enzyme activity [78], indicating another level of negative feedback regulation for post-translational control of induced NO synthesis.

NO has been implicated in carcinogenesis because it has been shown to cause DNA strand breaks as well as mutations in human cells. The tumor suppressor gene p53 is well characterized due to the fact that mutations in p53 result in loss of tumor suppressor activity and is seen in about half of all human cancers [80]. Since p53 plays an important role in cellular response to DNA damage from exogenous mutagens, Forrester et al. hypothesized that p53 may perform a similar role in regulating iNOS expression. Exposure of human cells to a NO donor resulted in wild-type p53 accumulation [81]. Over-expression of wild-type, but not mutant, p53 resulted in a down-regulation of iNOS transcription in a variety of human and rodent cells. These data imply a negative feedback loop where NO-induced DNA damage activates p53 expression which then trans-represses iNOS transcription, functioning as a safeguard against NO-induced DNA damage. As a follow-up to this *in vitro* study, the relationship between iNOS and p53 was examined *in vivo* in cancer-prone p53 knockout (KO) mice [82]. Untreated p53 KO mice excreted 70% more urinary nitrate than wild-type controls and iNOS protein expression was constitutively detected in the spleens of the KO mice, but not in the spleens of the wild-type mice. Following *C. parvum* injection, urinary nitrate excretion in the KO mice exceeded that of the wild-type controls by 200%. These data corroborate the *in vitro* findings and indicate that p53 is an important trans-repressor of basal and stimulated iNOS expression *in vivo*.

Studies have demonstrated that the induction of the heat shock response by hyperthermia or sodium arsenite exposure blocked subsequent iNOS expression in AKN-1 human liver cells [83]. The inhibitory effect of heat shock on iNOS expression was observed in promoter transfection experiments, however there was no effect of heat shock response on iNOS enzyme activity in AKN-1 cells transduced to express iNOS. These results indicate that prior induction of the heat shock response inhibits iNOS gene transcription, but not iNOS translation or enzyme activity. These findings underscore the complex array of phenotypic responses in the liver during stress conditions. Similarly, Feinstein has shown that heat shock protein

70 mediates suppresssion of iNOS expression in brain astroglial cells by inhibiting NF-κB-DNA-binding activity [84]. The induction of the heat shock response appears to be an adaptive response to prevent over-expression of iNOS during certain inflammatory conditions. This is supported by the observation that increased NO exposure stimulates the heat shock response [85].

TGFβ also partially prevents induced NO synthesis. Suppression of iNOS expression by TGFβ has been shown in macrophages [86], mesangial cells [87], and cardiac myocytes [88]. In rat aortic smooth muscle cells, TGFβ decreased IL-1β-stimulated iNOS mRNA by decreasing iNOS transcription [89] and promoter activity [90]. In primary murine macrophages this inhibition occurs at the post-transcriptional level and not by a direct effect on transcription [91]. TGFβ inhibited induced NO synthesis in murine hepatocytes (77%), rat hepatocytes (17%), and human hepatocytes (10%), highlighting the significant variation between species [92]. Interestingly, TGFβ actually enhances induction of iNOS mRNA in Swiss 3T3 fibroblasts [93, 94] and human keratinocytes [42]. These results underscore the complexity of iNOS regulation and lend support to the notion that species-, tissue-, and cell-specific mechanisms are likely to be important in controlling iNOS expression.

In other studies, the effects of hepatocellular mitogens on cytokine-induced iNOS expression in cultures of primary human hepatocytes were examined. Hepatocyte growth factor (HGF), epidermal growth factor (EGF), and transforming growth factor TGFβ all down-regulated LPS and cytokine-induced human iNOS mRNA, iNOS enzyme activity, and NO release [95]. Interestingly, the cytokine-stimulated NO release caused a decrease in hepatocyte protein and DNA synthesis, and this effect was partially reversed by the liver growth factors. These mitogens are known to directly trigger hepatic DNA and protein synthesis; however, our results raise the possibility that these hepatic growth factors may also promote protein and DNA synthesis during inflammatory conditions, in part, by suppressing iNOS expression. The precise mechanism by which these growth factors exert their effects on iNOS expression is unknown. Finally, certain protein phosphatase inhibitors were shown to also inhibit iNOS expression, indicating a role for specific phosphatases in regulating cytokine-stimulated iNOS expression [96].

Conclusions

The regulation of human iNOS gene expression is complex and is unique from its murine counterpart. Research to date indicates that human iNOS gene expression is primarily under transcriptional control mechanisms and that the transcription factors NF-κB, AP-1, and STAT1α function synergistically by binding to far upstream enhancer elements. Translational and post-transcriptional regulatory mechanisms also play a role in NO expression. Because iNOS is expressed in so many conditions which affect human disease understanding, the molecular mechanisms that govern NO synthesis can potentially lead to novel therapeutic strategies.

Acknowledgments
National Institutes of Health Grant GM-52021 (D.A.G.) supported this work. Dr. Geller is a recipient of the George H.A. Clowes, Jr., MD, FACS, Memorial Research Career Development Award of the American College of Surgeons.

References

1   Moncada S, Higgs EA (1991) Endogenous nitric oxide: physiology, pathology and clinical relevance. *Eur J Clin Invest* 21: 361–374

2   Szabo C, Thiemermann C (1994) Invited opinion: role of nitric oxide in hemorrhagic, traumatic, and anaphylactic shock and thermal injury. *Shock* 2 (2): 145–155

3   Kolb H, Kolb-Bachofen V (1998) Nitric oxide in autoimmune disease: cytotoxic or regulatory mediator? *Immunol Today* 19: 556–561

4   Kronke KD, Fehsel K, Kolb-Bachofen V (1998) Inducible nitric oxide synthase in human diseases. *Clin Exp Immunol* 113: 147–156

5   Nussler A, Di Silvio M, Billiar TR, Hoffman RA, Geller DA, Selby R, Madriaga J, Simmons RL (1992) Stimulation of the nitric oxide synthase pathway in human hepatocytes by cytokines and endotoxin. *J Exp Med* 176: 261–264

6   Geller DA, Lowenstein CJ, Shapiro RA, Nussler AK, Di Silvio M, Wang SC, Nakayama DK, Simmons RL, Snyder SH, Billiar TR (1993) Molecular cloning and expression of inducible nitric oxide synthase from human hepatocytes. *Proc Natl Acad Sci USA* 90: 3491–3495

7   Lowenstein CJ, Glatt CS, Bredt DS, Snyder SH (1992) Cloned and expressed macrophage nitric oxide synthase contrasts with the brain enzyme. *Proc Natl Acad Sci USA* 89: 6711–6715

8   Xie Q, Cho HJ, Calaycay J, Mumford RA, Swiderek KM, Lee TD, Ding A, Troso T, Nathan C (1992) Cloning and characterization of inducible nitric oxide synthase from mouse macrophages. *Science* 256: 225–28

9   Lyons CR, Orloff GJ, Cunningham JM (1992) Molecular cloning and functional expression of an inducible nitric oxide synthase from a murine macrophage cell line. *J Biol Chem* 267: 6370–6374

10   Marsden PA, Schappert KT, Chen HS, Flowers M, Sundell CL, Wilcox JN, Lamas S, Michel T (1992) Molecular cloning and characterization of human endothelial nitric oxide synthase. *FEBS Lett* 307: 287–293

11   Janssens SP, Shimouchi A, Quertermous T, Bloch DB (1992) Cloning and expression of a cDNA encoding human endothelium-derived relaxing factor/nitric oxide synthase. *J Biol Chem* 267 (21): 14519–14522

12 Nakane M, Schmidt HHHW, Pollock JS, Forstermann U, Murad F (1993) Cloned human brain nitric oxide synthase is highly expressed in skeletal muscle. *FEBS Lett* 316: 175–180

13 Geller DA, Billiar TR (1998) Molecular biology of nitric oxide synthases. *Cancer Metast Rev* 17: 7–23

14 Charles IG, Palmer RMJ, Hickery MS, Bayliss MT, Chubb AP, Hall VS, Moss DW, Moncada S (1993) Cloning, characterization, and expression of a cDNA encoding an inducible nitric oxide synthase from the human chondrocyte. *Proc Natl Acad Sci USA* 90: 11419–11423

15 Maier R, Bilbe G, Rediske J, Cotz M (1994) Inducible nitric oxide synthase from articular human chondrocytes: cDNA, cloning and analysis of mRNA expression. *Biochem Biophys Acta* 1208: 145–150

16 Sherman PA, Laubach VE, Reep BR, Wood ER (1993) Purification and cDNA sequence of an inducible nitric oxide synthase (NOS) from a human tumor cell line. *Biochem* 32: 11600–11605

17 Hokari A, Zeniya M, Esumi H (1994) Cloning and functional expression of human inducible nitric oxide synthase (NOS) from a glioblastoma cell line A-172. *J Biochem* 116: 575–581

18 Luss H, Watkins SC, Freeswick PD, Imro AK, Nussler AK, Billiar TR, Simmons RL, del Nido PJ, McGowan FX Jr (1996) Characterization of inducible nitric oxide synthase expression in endotoxemic rat cardiac myocytes *in vivo* and following cytokine exposure *in vitro*. *J Mol Cell Cardiol* 27: 2015–2029

19 Chartrain N, Geller DA, Koty PP, Sitrin NF, Nussler AK, Hoffman EP, Billiar TR, Hutchinson NI, Mudgett JS (1994) Molecular cloning, structure, chromosomal localization of the human inducible nitric oxide synthase gene. *J Biol Chem* 269: 6765–6772

20 Marsden PA, Heab HHQ, Scherer SW, Stewart RJ, Hall AV et al (1993) Structural and chromosomal localization of the human constituitive endothelial nitric oxide synthase. *J Biol Chem* 268: 17478–17488

21 Kishimoto J, Spurr N, Liao M, Lizhi L, Emsonp Xu W (1992) Localization of brain nitric oxide synthase (NOS) to human chromosome 12. *Genomics* 14: 802–804

22 Taylor BS, Geller DA (2000) Molecular regulation of the human inducible nitric oxide synthase (iNOS) gene (Review). *Shock* 13: 413–424

23 Xie QW, Whisnant R, Nathan C (1993) Promoter of the mouse gene encoding calcium-independent nitric oxide synthase confrs inducibility by interferon-γ and bacterial LPS. *J Exp Med* 177: 1779–1785

24 Lowenstein CJ, Alley EW, Raval P, Snowman AM, Snyder SH, Russell SW, Murphy WJ: Macrophage nitric oxide synthase gene (1993) two upstream regions mediate induction by interferon gamma and lipopolysaccharide. *Proc Natl Acad Sci USA* 90: 9730–9738

25 Xie Q-w, Kashiwabara Y, Nathan C (1994) Role of transcription factor NF-kappa B/Rel in induction of nitric oxide synthase. *J Biol Chem* 269: 4705–4708

26 Xie Q-w (1997) A novel lipopolysaccharide-response element contributes to induction of nitric oxide synthase. *J Biol Chem* 272 (23): 14867–14872

27   Taylor, BS, de Vera, ME, Ganster, RW, Wang, Q, Shapiro, RA, Morris, SM, Billiar TR, Geller DA (1998) Multiple NFκB enhancer elements regulate cytokine induction of the human inducible nitric oxide synthase gene. *J Biol Chem* 273: 15148–15156

28   Goldring CE, Reveneau S, Algarte M, Jeannin JF 1996) *In vivo* footprinting of the mouse inducible nitric oxide synthase gene: inducible protein occupation of numerous sites including Oct and NF-IL6. *Nucleic Acids Research* 24 (9): 1682–1687

29   Sawada T, Falk LA, Padmini R, Murphy WJ, Pluznik DV (1997) IL-6 induction of protein-DNA complexes *via* a novel regulatory region of the inducible nitric oxide synthase gene promoter: Role of octamer binding proteins. *J Immunol* 158: 5267–5276

30   Gay RD, Dawson SJ, Murphy WJ, Russell SW, Latchman DS (1998) Activation of the iNOS gene promoter by Brn-3 POU family transcription factors is dependent upon the octamer motif in the promoter. *Bioch Biophy Acta-Gene Structure and Expression* 1443 (3): 315–322

31   Dlaska M, Weiss G (1999) Central role of transcription factor NF-IL6 for cytokine and iron-mediated regulation of murine inducible nitric oxide synthase expression. *J Immunol* 162: 6171–6177

32   Martin E, Nathan C, Xie QW (1994) Role of interferon regulatory factor 1 in inducton of nitric oxide synthase. *J Exp Med* 180 (3): 977–984

33   Gao J, Morrison DC, Parmely TJ, Russell SW, Murphy WJ (1997) An interferon-g-activated site (GAS) is necessary for full expression of the mouse iNOS gene in response to interferon-γ and LPS. *J Biol Chem* 272: 1226–1230

34   Gao JJ, Filla MB, Fultz MJ, Vogel SN, Russell SW, Murphy WJ (1998) Autocrine/paracrine IFN-αβ mediates the lipopolysaccharide-induced activation of transcription factor Stat1α in mouse macrophages: Pivotal role of Stat1a in induction of the inducible nitric oxide synthase gene. *J Immunol* 161: 4803–4810

35   Murphy WJ, Muroi M, Zhang CX, Suzuki T, Russell SW (1996) Both basal and enhancer elements are required for full induction of the mouse inducible nitric oxide synthase gene. *J Endotoxin Res* 3: 381–393

36   Spink, J, Cohen J, Evans TJ (1995) The cytokine responsive vascular smooth musle cell enhancer of inducible nitric oxide synthase. *J Biol Chem* 270: 29541–29547

37   Melillo G, Musso T, Sica A, Taylor LS, Cox GW, Varesio L (1995) A hypoxia responsive element mediates a novel pathway of activation of the inducible nitric oxide synthase promoter. *J Exp Med* 182: 1683–1693

38   Zhang X, Laubach VE, Alley EW, Edwards KA, Sherman PA, Russell SW, Murphy WJ (1996) Transcriptional basis for hyporesponsiveness of human inducible nitric oxide synthase gene to lipopolysaccharide/interferon-γ. *J Leukocyte Biol* 59: 575–585

39   Spitsin SV, Farber JL, Bertovich M, Moehren G, Koprowski H, Michaels FH (1997) Human- and mouse-inducible nitric oxide synthase gene promoters require activation of phosphatidylcholine-specific phospholipase C and NF-κB. *Mol Med* 3: 315–326

40   Bertholet S, Tzeng E, Felley-Bosco E, Mauel J (1999) Expression of the induciible nitric oxide synthase in human monocytic U937 cells allows high output nitric oxide production. *J Leukoc Biol* 65: 50–58

41 Geller DA, de Vera ME, Russell DA, Shapiro RA, Nussler AK, Simmons RL, Billiar TR 1995) A central role for interleukin-1β in the *in vitro* and *in vivo* regulation of hepatic inducible nitric oxide synthase. *J Immunol* 155: 4890–4898

42 Arany I, Brysk MM, Brysk H, Tyring SK (1996) Regulation of inducible nitric oxide synthase mRNA levels by differentiation and cytokines in human keratinocytes. *Biochem Biophys Res Commun* 220: 618–622

43 Nussler AK, Vergani G, Gollin SM, Dorko K, Morris SM Jr, Demetris AJ, Nomoto M, Beger HG, Strom SC (1999) Isolation and characterization of a human hepatic epithelial-like cell line (AKN-1) from a normal liver. *In vitro Cellular & Developmental Biology* 35: 190–197

44 de Vera ME, Shapiro RA, Nussler AK, Mudgett JS., Simmons RL, Morris SM, Billiar TR, Geller DA 1996) Transcriptional regulation of human inducible nitric oxide synthase (iNOS) gene by cytokines: Initial analysis of the human iNOS promoter. *Proc Natl Acad Sci USA* 93: 1054–1059

45 Laubach, VE, Zhang CX, Russell SW, Murphy WJ, Sherman PA (1997) Analysis of expression and promoter function of the human inducible nitric oxide synthase gene in DLD-1 cells and monkey hepatocytes. *Biochim Biophys Acta* 1351: 287–295

46 Marks-Konczalik J, Chu SC, Moss J (1998) Cytokine-mediated transcriptional induction of the human inducible nitric oxide synthase gene requires both activator protein 1 and nuclear factor-κB-binding sites. *J Biol Chem* 273: 22201–22208

47 Kolyada AY, Savikovsky N, Madias NE (1996) Transcriptional regulation of the human iNOS gene in vascular-smooth-muscle cells and macrophages: evidence for tissue specificity. *Biochem Biophys Res Commun* 220: 600–605

48 Linn, SC, Morelli PJ, Edry I, Cottongim SE, Szabo C, Salzman AL (1997) Transcriptional regulation of human inducible nitric oxide synthase in an intestinal epithelial cell line. *Am J Physiol* 35: G1499–G1508

49 Taylor, BS, Shao, LF, Gambotto, A, Ganster, RW, Geller, DA (1999) Inhibition of cytokine-induced nitric oxide synthase (iNOS) expression by gene transfer of adenoviral IκBα. *Surgery* 126: 142–147

50 Ganster RW, Geller DA (2000) Molecular regulation of inducible nitric oxide synthase. In: L Ignarro (ed): *Nitric oxide*. Academic Press, San Diego, 129–156

51 Montgomery KF, Osborn, L, Hession C, Tizard R, Goff D, Vassallo C, Tarr PI, Bomsztyk K, Lobb R, Harlan JM, Pohlman TH (1991) Activation of endothelial-leukocyte adhesion molecule 1 (ELAM-1) gene transcription. *Proc Natl Acad Sci USA* 88: 6523–6527

52 Neish AS, Williams AJ, Palmer HJ, Whitley MZ, Collins T (1992) Functional analysis of the human vascular cell adhesion molecule 1 promoter. *J Exp Med* 176: 1583–1593

53 Voraberger G, Schafer R, Stratowa, C (1991) Cloning of the human gene for intracellular adhesion molecule 1 and analysis of its 5'-regulatory region. Induction by cytokines and phobol ester. *J Immunol* 147: 2777–27786

54 Mukaida N, Mahe Y, Matsushima K (1990) Cooperative interaction of nuclear factor-kappa B- and cis regulatory enhancer binding protein-like factor binding elements in

activating the interleukin-8 gene by pro-inflammatory cytokines. *J Biol Chem* 265: 21128–21133

55 Cogswell JP, Godlevski MM, Wisely GB, Clay WC, Leesnitzer LM, Ways JP, Gray JG (1994) NF-kappa B regulates IL-1 beta transcription through a consensus NF-kappa B binding site and a non-consensus CRE-like site. *J Immunol* 153 (2): 712–723

56 Zhang L, Nabel GJ (1994) Positive and negative regulation of IL-2 gene expression: role of multiple regulatory sites. *Cytokines* 6 (3): 221–228

57 Ohmori Y, Schreiber RD, Hamilton TA (1997) Synergy between interferon-gamma and tumor necrosis factor-alpha in transcriptional activation is mediated by cooperation between signal transducer and activator of transcription 1 and nuclear factor kappaB. *J Biol Chem* 272: 14899–14907

58 Kleinert H, Wallerath T, Fritz G, Ihrig-Biedert I, Geller D, Forstermann U (1998) Cytokine induction of NO synthase II in human DLD-1 cells: roles of the JAK-STAT, AP-1, and NF-kB-signaling pathways. *Br J Pharmacol* 125 (1): 193–201

59 Shaw G, Kamen R (1986) A conserved AU sequence from the 3' untranslated region of GM-CSF mRNA mediates selective mRNA degradation. *Cell* 46: 659–667

60 Caput D, Beutler B, Hartog K, Thayer R, Brown-Shimer S, Serami A (1986) Identification of a common nucleotide sequence in the 3'-untranslated region of mRNA molecules specifying inflammatory mediators. *Proc Natl Acad Sci USA* 83: 1670–1674

61 Han J, Brown T, Beutler B (1990) Endotoxin-reponsive sequences control cachectin/tumor necrosis factor biosynthesis at the translational level. *J Exp Med* 171: 465–475

62 Nunokawa, Y, Oikawa, S, Tanaka, S (1996) Expression of human inducible nitric oxide synthase is regulated by both promoter and 3'-regions. *Biochem Biophys Res Commun* 223, 347–352

63 Kleinert H, Rodriguez-Pascual F, Hausding M, Furneaux H, Levy AP, Forstermann U (2000) Regulation of the expression of the human inducible nitric oxide synthase gene by the RNA-binding protein HuR. *Nitric Oxide: Biology and Chemistry* 4: 258

64 Chu SC, Wu HP, Banks TC, Eissa NT, Moss J (1995) Structural diversity in the 5'-untranslated region of cytokine-stimulated human inducible nitric oxide synthase mRNA. *J Biol Chem* 270: 10625–10630

65 Eissa NT, Strauss AJ, Haggerty CM, Choo EK, Chu SC, Moss J (1996) Alternative splicing of human inducible nitric oxide synthase mRNA: tissue specific regulation and induction by cytokines. *J Biol Chem* 271 (43): 27184–27187

66 Eissa NT, Yuan JW, Haggerty CM, Choo EK, Palmer CD, Moss J (1998) Cloning and characterizaion of human inducible nitric oxide synthase splic variant: A domain, encoded by exons 8 and 9, is critical for dimerization. *Proc Natl Acad Sci USA* 95: 7625–7630

67 Pastor CM, Williams D, Yoneyama T, Hatakeyama K, Singleton, Naylor E, Billiar TR (1996) Competition for tetrahydrobiopterin between phenylalanine hydroxylase and nitric oxide synthase in rat liver. *J Biol Chem* 271: 24534–24538

68 Harada T, Kagamiyama H, Hatakeyama K (1993) Feedback regulation mechanisms for the control of GTP cyclohydrolase I activity. *Science* 260: 1507–1510

69 Knowles RG, Salter M, Brooks SL, Moncada S (1990) Anti-inflammatory glucocorticoids inhibit the induction by endotoxin of nitric oxide synthase. *Biochem Biophys Res Commun* 172: 1042–1048

70 Geller DA, Nussler AK, Di Silvio M, Lowenstein CL, Shapiro RA, Wang SC, Simmons RL, Billiar TR (1993) Cytokines, endotoxin, and glucocorticoids regulate the expression of inducible nitric oxide synthase in hepatocytes. *Proc Natl Acad Sci USA* 90: 522–526

71 Kleinert H, Euchenhofer C, Ihrig-Biedert I, Forstermann U (1996) Glucocorticoids inhibit the induction of nitric oxide synthase II by down-regulating cytokine-induced activity of transcription factor NF-κB. *Mol Pharmacol* 49: 15–21

72 de Vera ME, Taylor BS, Wang Q, Shapiro RA, Billiar TR, Geller DA (1997) Dexamethasone suppresses inducible nitric oxide synthase gene expression by upregulating I-κBα and inhibiting NF-κB. *Am J Physiol* 273: G1290–96

73 Salzman AL, Denenberg AG, Ueta I, O'Connor M, Linn SC, Szabo C (1996) Induction and activity of nitric oxide synthase in cultured human intestinal epithelial monolayers. *Am J Physiol* 270: G565–G573

74 Perrella MA, Yoshizumi M, Fen Z, Tsai J-C, Hsieh C-M, Kourembanas S, Lee M-E (1994) Transforming growth factor-ß1, but not dexamethasone, down-regulates nitric-oxide synthase mRNA after its induction by interleukin-1β in rat smooth muscle cells. *J Biol Chem* 269: 14595–14600

75 Kunz D, Walker G, Eberhardt W, Pfeilschifter J (1996) Molecular mechanisms of dexamethasone inhibition of nitric oxide synthase expression in interleukin 1β-stimulated mesangial cells: evidence for the involvement of transcriptional and posttranscriptional regulation. *Proc Natl Acad Sci USA* 93: 255–259

76 Taylor BS, Kim YM, Wang Q, Shapiro RA, Billiar TR, Geller DA (1997) Nitric oxide down-regulates hepatocyte-inducible nitric oxide synthase gene expression. *Arch of Surgery* 132: 1177–1183

77 Park SK, Lin HL, Murphy S (1997) Nitric oxide regulates nitric oxide syntase-2 gene expression by inhibiting NF-κB binding to DNA. *Biochem J* 322: 609–613

78 Griscavage JM, Rogers NE, Sherman MP, Ignarro LJ (1993) Inducible nitric oxide synthase from a rat alveolar macrophage cell line is inhibited by nitric oxide. *J Immunol* 151 (11): 6329–6337

79 Colasanti M, Persichini T, Menegazzi M, Mariotto S, Giordano E Caldarera CM (1995) Induction of nitric oxide synthase mRNA expression. Suppression by nitric oxide. *J Biol Chem* 270 (45): 26731–26733

80 Ambs S, Hussain SP, Harris C (1997) Interactive effects of nitric oxide and the p53 tumor suppressor gene in carcinogenesis and tumor progression. *FASEB J* 11: 443–448

81 Forrester K, Ambs S, Lupold SE, Kapust RB, Spillare EA, Weinberg WC, Felley-Bosco E, Wang XW, Geller DA, Tzeng E, Billiar TR, Harris CC (1996) Nitric oxide-induced p53 accumulation and regulation of inducible nitric oxide synthase expression by wild-type p53. *Proc Natl Acad Sci USA* 93: 2442–2447

82 Ambs S, Ogunfusika M, Merriam W, Bennett WP, Billiar TR, Harris CC (1998) Up-reg-

ulation of inducible nitric oxide synthase expression in cancer-prone p53 knockout mice. *Proc Natl Acad Sci USA* 95 (15): 8823–8828

83 de Vera ME, Wong J, Zhou JY, Tzeng E, Wong H, Billiar TR, Geller DA (1996) Cytokine-induced nitric oxide synthesis in human liver cells is inhibited by the heat shock response. *Surgery* 120: 144–149

84 Feinstein DL, Galea E, Aquino DA, Li GC, Xu H, Reis DJ (1996) Heat shock protein 70 suppresses astroglial-inducible nitric oxide synthase expression by decreasing NF-κB activation. *J Biol Chem* 271: 17724–17732

85 Kim YM, de Vera ME Watkins SC, Billiar TR (1997) Nitric oxide protects cultured rat hepatocytes from TNFα-induced apoptsosis by inducing heat shock protein 70 expression. *J Biol Chem* 272: 1402–1411

86 Ding A, Nathan CF, Graycar J, Derynck R, Stuehr DJ, Srimal S (1990) Macrophage deactivating factor and transforming growth factors-β1, -β2, and -β3 inhibit induction of macrophage nitrogen oxide synthesis by IFN-γ. *J Immunol* 145: 940–946

87 Pfeilschifter J, Vosbeck K (1991) Transforming growth factor-β2 inihibits interleukin-1β and tumor necrosis factor -α induction of nitric oxide synthase in rat renal mesangial cells. *Biochem Biophys Res Commun* 175: 372–375

88 Roberts AB, Vodovotz Y, Roche NS, Sporn MB, Nathan CF (1992) Role of nitric oxide in antagonists effects of transforming growth factor-β and interleukin-1β on the beating rate of cultured cardiac myocytes. *Mol Endocrinol* 6: 1921–1928

89 Perrella MA, Yoshizumi M, Fen Z, Tsai JC, Hseih CM, Kourembanas S, Lee ME (1994) Transforming growth factor-b1, but not dexamethasone, down regulates nitric oxide synthase mRNA after its induction by interleukin-1β in rat smooth muscle cells. *J Biol Chem* 269: 14595–14600

90 Perrella MA, Patterson C, Tan L, Yet SF, Hseih CM, Yoshizumi M , Lee ME (1996) Suppression of interleukin 1-b induced nitric oxide synthase promoter/enhancer activity by transforming growth-b in vascular smooth muscle cells. *J Biol Chem* 271: 13776–13780

91 Vodovotz Y, Bogdan C, Paik J, Xie QW, Nathan C (1993) Mechanisms of suppression of macrophage nitric oxide release by transforming growth factor-β. *J Exp Med* 178: 605–613

92 Nussler AK, Di Silvio M, Liu Z-Z, Geller DA, Freeswick PD, Dorko K, Bartoli F, Billiar T (1995) Further characterization and comparison of inducible nitric oxide synthase in mouse, rat and human hepatocytes. *Hepatology* 21: 1552–1560

93 Gilbert RS, Herschman HR (1993) Transforming growth factor beta differentially modulates the inducible nitric oxide synthase gene in distinct cell types. *Biochem Biophys Res Commun* 195: 380–384

94 Kleinert, H, Euchenhofer C, Ihrig-Biedert I, Forstermann U (1996) In murine 3T3 fibroblasts, different second messenger pathways resulting in the induction of NO synthase II (iNOS) converge in the activation of transcription factor NF-kappaB. *J Biol Chem* 271: 6039–6044

95 Liu ZZ, Cui S, Billiar TR, Dorko K, Halfter W, Geller DA, Michalopoulos G, Beger HG,

Albina J, Nussler AK (1996) Effects of hepatocellular mitogens on cytokine-induced nitric oxide synthesis in human hepatocytes. *J Leuk Biol* 60: 382–388

96 Taylor BS, Liu S, Villavicencio RT, Ganster RW, Geller DA (1999) The role of protein of phosphatases in the expression of inducible nitric oxide synthase in the rat hepatocyte. *Hepatology* 29: 1199–1207

Superoxide anion release from inducible nitric oxide synthase

Yong Xia and Jay L. Zweier

Molecular and Cellular Biophysics Laboratories, Department of Medicine, Division of Cardiology and the EPR Center, Johns Hopkins University School of Medicine, 5501 Hopkins Bayview Circle, Baltimore, MD 21224, USA

Introduction

Nitric oxide (NO), a gaseous free radical, plays a central regulatory role in a variety of physiological and pathological processes including inflammation and host defense [1]. In biological systems, NO is primarily derived from a cationic amino acid L-arginine and oxygen in a reaction catalyzed by a family of NO synthases (NOS). To date, three NOS isoforms have been identified as neuronal NOS (nNOS, type I), inducible NOS (iNOS, type II), and endothelial NOS (eNOS, type III) [2]. nNOS and eNOS constitutively exist in cells and their activity is mainly regulated by the levels of intracellular free Ca^{2+}. Upon external stimulation, such as from neurotransmitters, elevated cytosolic Ca^{2+} combines with calmodulin to form the Ca^{2+}/calmodulin complex, which subsequently activates eNOS and nNOS. Recently, it was also shown that phosporylation of serine-threonine or tyrosine residues on eNOS modulates enzyme activity and this does not require increase of cytosolic Ca^{2+} [3]. NO generated by eNOS and nNOS serves as a signaling molecule participating in various physiological processes ranging from regulation of vascular tone to development of learning and memory. Abnormal NO production in cells and tissues, either too much or too little, has been implicated in the pathogenesis of a number of diseases including stroke, hypertension, atherosclerosis and heart attack [4]. In contrast to the two constitutive NOS isoforms, iNOS is generally not present in quiescent cells. Its expression is often induced by inflammatory substances such as cytokines and microbial endotoxin. Though most of the original studies on iNOS expression were performed in murine macrophages, it is clear now that with proper stimulation iNOS expression can be induced in almost any type of cell and tissue. Calmodulin is also an essential cofactor for the catalytic function of iNOS; however, activation of iNOS does not require elevation of intracellular Ca^{2+}. With a tightly bound calmodulin, iNOS is fully active under basal cytosolic Ca^{2+} concentration [5]. The quantity of NO production from iNOS is therefore primarily determined by the amounts of enzyme transcribed. iNOS is also a more potent enzyme with higher L-arginine to NO turnover as compared with eNOS or nNOS. The constant

Nitric Oxide and Inflammation, edited by Daniela Salvemini, Timothy R. Billiar and Yoram Vodovotz

catalytic activity along with high output enzymatic efficacy makes iNOS ideal to serve its role in host defense and inflammation.

In addition to NO, NOSs have recently been shown to also generate superoxide anion ($^{\bullet}O_2^-$) [6, 7]. Compared with the well established NO synthesis process, $^{\bullet}O_2^-$ formation from NOSs was understood in less detail. In the early studies, there were only clues that purified nNOS may produce hydrogen peroxide (H_2O_2) or $^{\bullet}O_2^-$ in the absence of L-arginine. While these observations were intriguing, not much attention was focused on this probably due to the overwhelming interest in the process of NO synthesis as well as NO associated biological effects. In fact, there was an array of important questions associated with this interesting phenomenon. For example, it was not clear whether $^{\bullet}O_2^-$ production is a general property of all NOS isoforms or just a unique feature of nNOS. Little was known about the catalytic details of $^{\bullet}O_2^-$ synthesis from NOS and how this is regulated. Moreover, it was not known whether NOS-mediated $^{\bullet}O_2^-$ formation occurs in cells or tissues and what roles this $^{\bullet}O_2^-$ may play in physiological or pathological processes. One of the obstacles hampering the initial efforts to tackle these questions was the limited ability to obtain sufficient pure enzyme to conduct definitive oxygen free radical measurements. Largely owing to the various protein expression systems which enable the preparation of recombinant NOS holoenzyme or certain domains on a large scale, the mechanisms and potential biological significance of the $^{\bullet}O_2^-$ formation by NOSs begin to be unveiled. It is now clear that $^{\bullet}O_2^-$ generation occurs from all NOS isoforms. Among them, iNOS is distinct in its primarily release of $^{\bullet}O_2^-$ from the flavin sites of its reductase domain. In L-arginine-depleted macrophages, iNOS-derived $^{\bullet}O_2^-$ and NO further interact to form another potent oxidant peroxynitrite ($ONOO^-$). iNOS-mediated $^{\bullet}O_2^-$ and $ONOO^-$ may contribute to the cytotoxic actions of macrophages in inflammation and immune defense.

NO synthases and superoxide

While derived from separate genes, all NOSs have considerable similarity in their structure and function [8]. Structure analysis reveals a 50–60% homology in amino acid sequence among any two of the three isoforms. Sequences of substrate and cofactor binding regions are highly conserved in these enzymes. Three NOSs are all bi-domain enzymes comprising a C-terminal reductase domain and N-terminal oxygenase domain. The reductase domain structurally resembles cytochrome P_{450} reductase and contains similar NADPH, FAD, and FMN binding sites. The sites of heme, L-arginine, as well as tetrahydrobiopterin (BH_4) are located on the oxygenase domain. Calmodulin binds a consensus region and serves a critical role to facilitate the electron transfer from reductase to oxygenase domain, where the molecular oxygen is incorporated into the guanidino group of L-arginine giving rise to NO and L-citrulline. A five electron transfer from NADPH to the heme is involved in the catalytic process and L-arginine is converted to NO and L-citrulline through an intermediate product N-hydroxyl-L-arginine. FAD, FMN, and BH_4 are the essential cofactors in these enzymatic reactions.

The first report suggesting that NOS may produce reactive oxygen species in addition to NO was based on studies conducted on purified nNOS. With the enzyme isolated from pork brain, Heinzel et al. reported that purified nNOS produced H_2O_2 at low concentrations of L-arginine or BH_4 [6]. They showed that nNOS was switched from NO to H_2O_2 production when L-arginine concentration was under 100 µM. Like the process of NO and L-citrulline production, H_2O_2 formation from nNOS also requires Ca^{2+} and calmodulin. However, this H_2O_2 formation exhibited distinct responses to different types of NOS blockers. The N-nitro L-arginine analogues such as N-nitro-L-arginine (L-NNA) and N-nitro-L-arginine methyl ester (L-NAME) inhibit H_2O_2 generation from nNOS, whereas the N-methyl compounds such as N-monomethyl-L-arginine (L-NMMA) do not. Though in this study H_2O_2 was measured from nNOS under the conditions of low L-arginine or BH_4, it remained uncertain whether H_2O_2 was the primary product of nNOS or secondarily derived from other oxygen free radicals such as $\cdot O_2^-$. To answer this question, an unambiguous measurement of oxygen free radicals on nNOS is needed. Direct evidence demonstrating nNOS mediated production of oxygen free radicals came from electron paramagnetic resonance (EPR) spin-trapping measurements. While many assays have been used in the detection of oxygen free radicals, EPR remains the most definitive technique to directly measure free radicals *per se*. With the well-characterized spin trap 5,5-dimethyl-1-pyrroline-N-oxide (DMPO), Pou and colleagues carried out direct measurements of $\cdot O_2^-$ generation from rat nNOS purified from stably transfected cells [7]. In the absence of L-arginine, strong $\cdot O_2^-$ signals were detected from nNOS. These signals were totally abolished by superoxide dismutase (SOD) but not affected by catalase, reconfirming that $\cdot O_2^-$ is the primary product of nNOS when the enzyme is not coupled with L-arginine. Hence, the previously reported H_2O_2 formation by nNOS likely arises from the dismutation of $\cdot O_2^-$. Indeed, the later studies demonstrated that $\cdot O_2^-$ is also the primary reactive oxygen species generated by eNOS and iNOS. Consistent with the prior results, $\cdot O_2^-$ generation from nNOS also required Ca^{2+}/calmodulin and was blocked by L-NAME, but not by L-NMMA.

Though these *in vitro* experiments showed that activated nNOS produces $\cdot O_2^-$ under low concentrations of L-arginine, major concerns still remained that this $\cdot O_2^-$ generation might stem from alterations in the properties or conformation of this enzyme after isolation. Therefore it was critical to investigate whether nNOS produces $\cdot O_2^-$ inside cells. To address this issue, we applied EPR spin trapping to study oxygen radical formation from nNOS in the stably transfected HEK 293 cells [9]. Normally, activation of nNOS with Ca^{2+} ionophore A23187 only resulted in NO production from these cells. However, with the cells subjected to L-arginine depletion by incubating cells in L-arginine free medium, A23187 triggered prominent oxygen radical formation. This oxygen radical formation was quenched by SOD, but not affected by catalase, indicating that $^{\bullet}O_2^-$ was the primary radical formed in these cells. L-NAME, but not D-NAME, prevented $^{\bullet}O_2^-$ generation from these cells, demonstrating that $^{\bullet}O_2^-$ was derived from nNOS. These results demonstrated that nNOS-catalyzed $^{\bullet}O_2^-$ formation does occur in intact cells. nNOS-mediated $^{\bullet}O_2^-$ formation was also observed in cultured cerebellar granule neurons upon the stimulation of N-methyl-D-asparate under conditions of L-arginine depletion [10]. A detailed analysis by correlating cytosolic L-arginine levels with the intensity of NO and $^{\bullet}O_2^-$ production from nNOS showed that L-arginine concentration was the controlling factor that determined whether nNOS produces either NO or $^{\bullet}O_2^-$. A putative mechanism has been proposed to illustrate how the presence or absence of L-arginine may lead activated nNOS to produce either NO or $^{\bullet}O_2^-$ (Fig. 1). When adequate L-arginine is present, nNOS is coupled with both L-arginine and molecular oxygen, the electrons donated from NADPH are therefore integrated into oxygen and the guanidino group of L-arginine giving rise to NO and L-citrulline. When L-arginine is absent as happened in L-arginine-depleted cells, the electrons received by the heme will be delivered to molecular oxygen leading to $^{\bullet}O_2^-$ formation.

Since the availability of L-arginine determines whether nNOS produces either NO or $^{\bullet}O_2^-$, suboptimal levels of L-arginine may result in simultaneous NO and $^{\bullet}O_2^-$ production. This prediction has been proven to be true as both $^{\bullet}O_2^-$ and NO signals were detected by EPR spectroscopy in nNOS-transfected cells under L-arginine depletion. In these cells, decreased L-arginine content only permits some nNOS to have both L-arginine and oxygen to generate NO as usual. Those nNOS molecules uncoupled with L-arginine will catalyze $^{\bullet}O_2^-$ formation. This immediately raised another question if these two radicals combine to form $ONOO^-$. It has been well established that NO reacts with $^{\bullet}O_2^-$ at diffusion-limited rate to form $ONOO^-$, a highly reactive oxidant that causes lipid peroxidation, thiol oxidation, and nitration of the functional groups of amino acids including tyrosine [11, 4]. In most of the previous reports, $ONOO^-$ was thought to be formed when NO generated from NOS reacts with $^{\bullet}O_2^-$, derived from different enzymes or pathways such as xanthine oxidase, mitochondria, or leukocyte NADPH oxidase. However, under conditions of L-arginine depletion, concurrent NO and $^{\bullet}O_2^-$ production from nNOS may make this enzyme a sole $ONOO^-$ generating source. Indeed, immunocytochemical staining of nitrotyrosine was found when nNOS was activated in L-arginine-depleted cells, but not in normally cultured cells [9]. As a result of this $^{\bullet}O_2^-$ and $ONOO^-$ formation, severe cell damage was seen in L-arginine-depleted cells. Thus, nNOS generates $^{\bullet}O_2^-$ and $ONOO^-$ in cells depleted of L-arginine and this leads to cellular injury.

It is interesting to note that the other constitutive NOS, eNOS, also produces $^{\bullet}O_2^-$ in a Ca^{2+}/calmodulin dependent manner [12, 13]. However, there is a clear difference in the regulatory mechanism between these two isoforms. Unlike nNOS, eNOS-mediated $^{\bullet}O_2^-$ formation was little affected by L-arginine and was primarily triggered by the absence of BH_4. It is still not clear why these two constitutive NOS

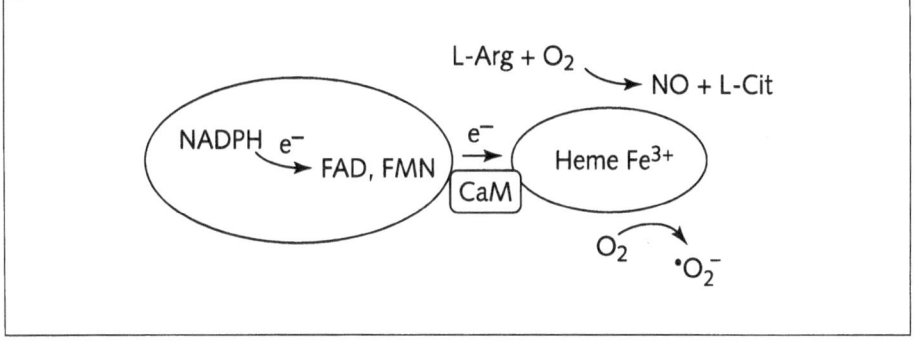

Figure 1

Model illustrating $^{\bullet}O_2^-$ and NO generation from nNOS. nNOS consists of one reductase domain containing NADPH, FAD, and FMN binding sites, and one oxygenase domain containing heme, L-arginine, and tetrahydrobiopterin sites (only heme is shown). Calmodulin (CaM) binding facilitates the electron shuttling from NADPH to FAD, then FMN, finally to the heme. In the presence of L-arginine (L-Arg) and oxygen, electrons are passed to these two substrates giving rise to NO and L-citrulline (L-Cit). In the absence of L-arginine, electrons are delivered to molecular oxygen leading to $^{\bullet}O_2^-$ formation.

isoforms exhibit distinct characteristics regarding the control of $^{\bullet}O_2^-$ production. Nevertheless, the existence of the difference in their $^{\bullet}O_2^-$ production suggests that the previous perspective that an identical catalytic process occurs for these two isoforms is oversimplified and must be reconsidered.

iNOS-mediated superoxide production

In the view of the structural and functional similarity among the NOS isoforms, it would not be surprising for iNOS to also produce $^{\bullet}O_2^-$. However, in initial studies demonstration of $^{\bullet}O_2^-$ production iNOS remained elusive. With iNOS purified from the mouse macrophage cell line RAW 264.7, it was reported that iNOS caused much less NADPH oxidation in the absence of L-arginine as compared with nNOS [14]. Since molecular oxygen would be the putative acceptor of the electrons from NADPH when L-arginine is not present, these results suggested that iNOS produces little if any $^{\bullet}O_2^-$. In fact, there was a perspective that $^{\bullet}O_2^-$ generation is just a unique property of nNOS and does not happen with iNOS [6]. A highly limited $^{\bullet}O_2^-$-generating capacity for iNOS was proposed to be critical for its biological function since $^{\bullet}O_2^-$ could in turn react with and scavenge NO, which was hypothesized to perturb iNOS-mediated immune defense actions [15]. However, this hypothesis was based on indirect evidence and no efforts to directly measure $^{\bullet}O_2^-$ production were made. Though these initial indirect observations have provided interesting clues, the question of whether iNOS generates $^{\bullet}O_2^-$ remained unanswered until direct measurements were performed.

The first clear evidence showing that iNOS does produce significant amounts of $^{\bullet}O_2^-$ came from EPR spin trapping experiments on RAW 264.7 cells [16]. This mouse macrophage cell line has been used as a classical system in iNOS studies. To determine if iNOS produces $^{\bullet}O_2^-$, iNOS expression was induced by the stimulation of bacterial lipopolysaccharide and recombinant mouse interferon γ (IFNγ). Oxygen radical signals were not seen in either non-stimulated or stimulated cells, whereas abundant NO generation occurs after iNOS induction as previously reported. However, with cells stimulated in L-arginine free medium in the presence of the spin trap DMPO, prominent 1:2:2:1 quartet radical signals of the DMPO-OH adduct were detected (Fig. 2). These signals were totally quenched by SOD but not affected by catalase, demonstrating that the signals were derived from $^{\bullet}O_2^-$. iNOS was demonstrated to be responsible for this $^{\bullet}O_2^-$ formation because this $^{\bullet}O_2^-$ production was prevented by the specific NOS blocker L-NAME, but not by D-NAME, the non-inhibitory enantiomer of L-NAME. The fact that the $^{\bullet}O_2^-$ formation was specifically inhibited by L-NAME or L-NMMA also excluded the potential involvement of NADPH oxidase, another potent $^{\bullet}O_2^-$-generating pathway in these cells. Control experiments confirmed that $^{\bullet}O_2^-$ generated by NADPH oxidase was not altered by L-NAME. Further examination of the relationship of $^{\bullet}O_2^-$ production and cytosolic L-arginine content showed that L-arginine depletion was required for iNOS-mediated $^{\bullet}O_2^-$ generation. Together, these findings indicated that iNOS catalyzes $^{\bullet}O_2^-$ formation in L-arginine-depleted macrophages.

Unequivocal evidence demonstrating that iNOS generates $^{\bullet}O_2^-$ was further provided by EPR measurements of free radical generation carried out on purified iNOS [17]. With the recombinant mouse iNOS isolated from an *E. coli* expression system, strong $^{\bullet}O_2^-$ formation was seen using nitrone spin traps including the commonly used spin trap DMPO; or the recently developed trap DEPMPO, a phosphorylated derivative of DMPO which gives rise to a more stable $^{\bullet}O_2^-$ spin adduct. In either case, the characteristic $^{\bullet}O_2^-$-spin trap adduct was seen. This $^{\bullet}O_2^-$ detection was further confirmed by the fact that SOD totally quenched the $^{\bullet}O_2^-$ signals, whereas catalase had no effect (Fig. 3). Together with the experiments on macrophages, all lines of evidence demonstrate that iNOS does produce $^{\bullet}O_2^-$.

Since the studies on macrophages showed that L-arginine depletion was required for iNOS-mediated $^{\bullet}O_2^-$ formation, the effect of L-arginine on the $^{\bullet}O_2^-$ formation from purified iNOS was also examined. The results from these experiments turned out to be rather unexpected. The $^{\bullet}O_2^-$ production from iNOS was not affected by low levels of L-arginine. With 100 μM L-arginine present, the concentration that prevented $^{\bullet}O_2^-$ formation from nNOS, iNOS-mediated $^{\bullet}O_2^-$ generation was essentially unchanged. However, L-arginine at high concentrations (1~5 mM) markedly

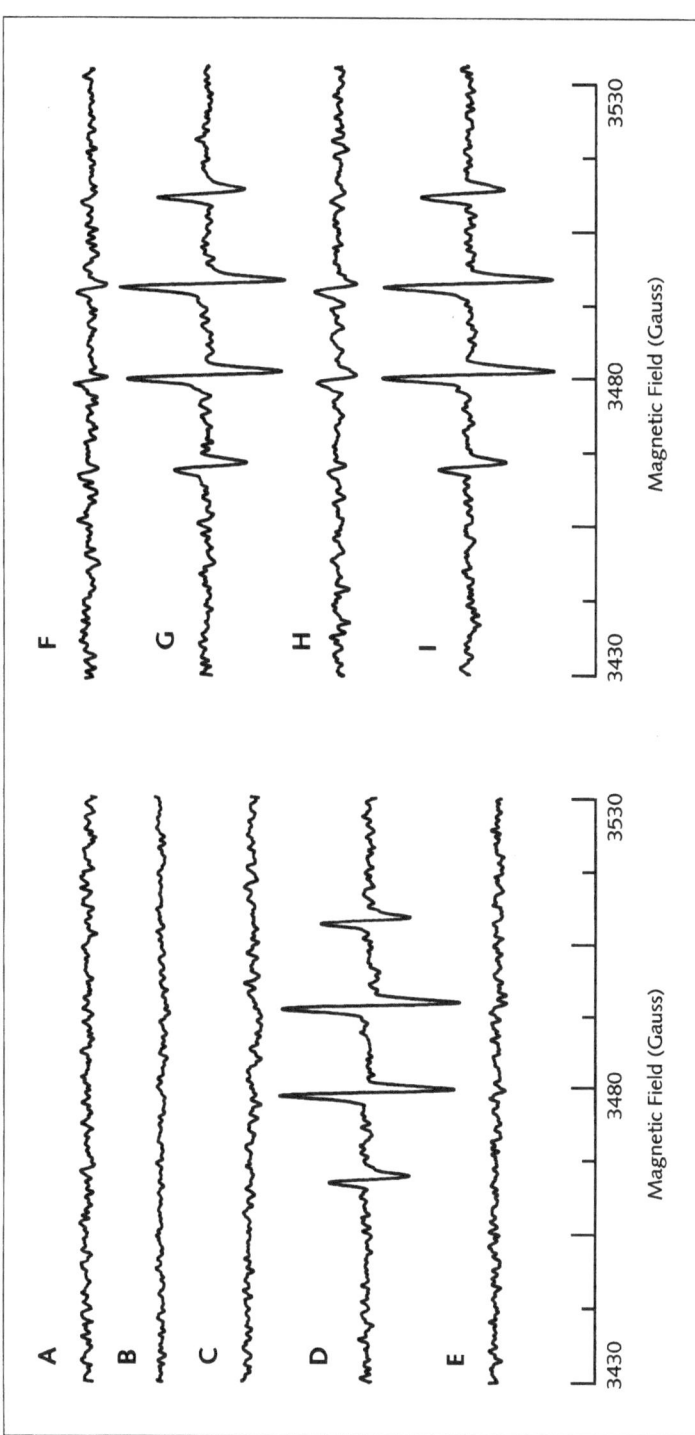

Figure 2

iNOS-mediated oxygen radical generation in macrophages measured by EPR spin trapping. EPR spectra were obtained in the presence of 50 mM DMPO from: (A) Normal cultured cells. (B) Cells after 24 h activation with LPS and IFNγ in DMEM. (C) Cells incubated in L-Arg-free medium for 24 h. (D) Cells after 24 h activation with LPS and IFNγ in L-Arg-free medium (L-Arg-depleted cells). (E) L-Arg-depleted cells with SOD (200 units/ml). (F) L-Arg-depleted cells with 1 mM L-NAME. (G) L-Arg-depleted cells with 1 mM D-NAME. (H) L-Arg-depleted cells with 1 mM L-NMMA. (I) L-Arg-depleted cells with catalase (300 units/ml) [16].

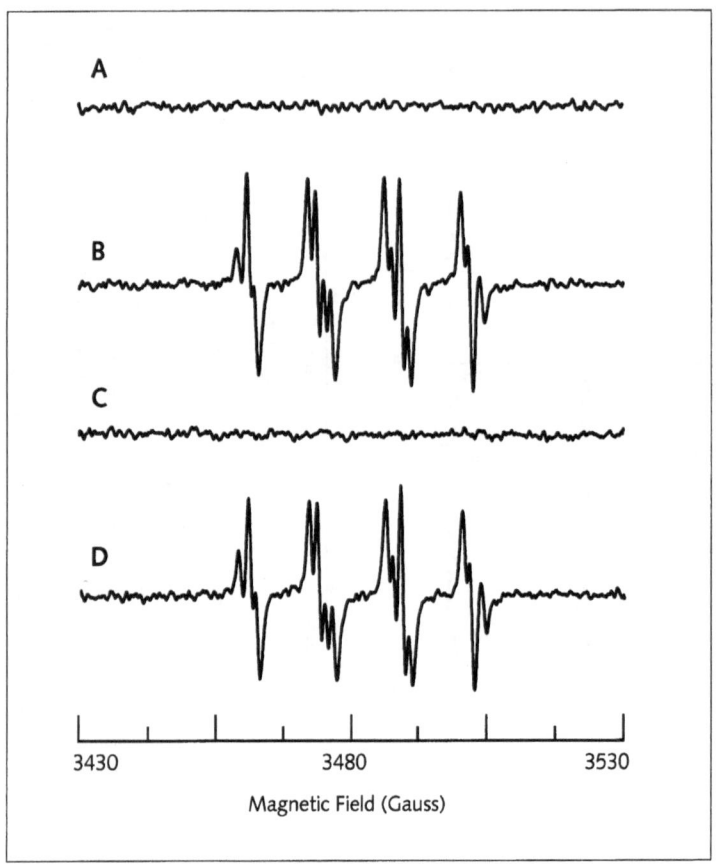

Figure 3

iNOS-catalyzed $^{\bullet}O_2^-$ generation. Inset A: EPR spectra of oxygen free radicals generated from iNOS. The reaction system consisted of 0.5 mM NADPH, 0.5 mM Ca^{2+}, 10 μg/ml calmodulin, and 50 mM DMPO in 50 mM Tris-HCl buffer (pH 7.4). While no signal was observed in the reaction system without enzyme (trace A), a prominent spectrum of the DMPO-OOH adduct was seen after adding 7.3 μg/ml iNOS (trace B). These signals were totally abolished by SOD (200 units/ml, trace C) but not affected by catalase (300 units/ml, trace D) (17).

decreased the $^{\bullet}O_2^-$ production. This inhibition was specifically elicited by L-arginine because its enantiomer, D-arginine, at the same concentration (5 mM) had no effect. Since higher levels of L-arginine were needed to inhibit $^{\bullet}O_2^-$ production from iNOS, iNOS appears to be more prone to produce $^{\bullet}O_2^-$ *in vitro* than *in vivo*. The fact that iNOS continued to catalyze $^{\bullet}O_2^-$ formation even in the presence of significant amount of L-arginine (over 100 μM) raised the question of whether $^{\bullet}O_2^-$ was syn-

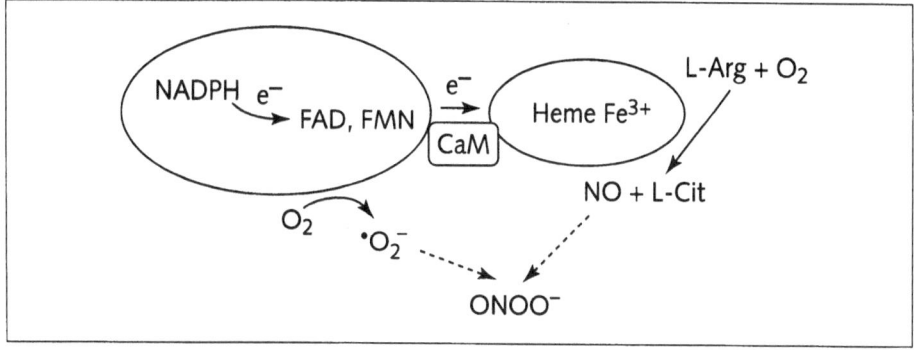

Figure 4
Schematic diagram illustrating the $\cdot O_2^-$ generation from the flavin sites of the reductase domain of iNOS. Solid arrows indicate electron flow. In the presence of certain concentrations of L-arginine, simultaneous $\cdot O_2^-$ and NO generation occur at the reductase and oxygenase domain. These two radicals may further combine to form ONOO$^-$ (shown in the dashed arrows).

thesized at the heme center of the oxygenase domain or the flavins bound at the reductase domain. Further studies using the flavoprotein inhibitor diphenylene iodonium (DPI) and heme blocker sodium cyanide (NaCN) showed that $\cdot O_2^-$ generation from iNOS was completely blocked by DPI but not affected by NaCN. The effects of DPI and NaCN strongly suggest that iNOS-catalyzed $\cdot O_2^-$ synthesis primarily occurs at the flavin-binding sites of its reductase domain, not the heme center of its oxygenase domain (Fig. 4). Further studies using expressed iNOS construct (residues 499–1144) demonstrated that the isolated iNOS reductase domain alone was indeed able to catalyze $\cdot O_2^-$ formation. Like the $\cdot O_2^-$ production from the holoenzyme, the $\cdot O_2^-$ generated by the reductase domain was also sensitive to DPI, but not affected by NaCN.

These findings reveal an important difference between iNOS and nNOS mediated $\cdot O_2^-$ generation with respect to the enzyme sites where $\cdot O_2^-$ is synthesized as well as L-arginine-dependent inhibition. nNOS produces $\cdot O_2^-$ from the heme of its oxygenase domain when L-arginine is not present. iNOS-mediated $\cdot O_2^-$ formation primarily occurs at the flavins of its reductase domain. The $\cdot O_2^-$ generation from nNOS is more sensitive to L-arginine than that from iNOS. While 100 μM L-arginine can totally block $\cdot O_2^-$ generation from nNOS [6], iNOS-mediated $\cdot O_2^-$ formation was essentially unaltered by 100 μM L-arginine. Inhibition of $\cdot O_2^-$ generation from iNOS was seen only at high L-arginine concentrations. It remains puzzling why large amounts of L-arginine are required to quench the $\cdot O_2^-$ generated from the reductase domain, especially in light of the low K_m value for L-arginine with iNOS (1–10 μM). A non-specific effect of the amino acid is unlikely since identical concentration of D-arginine had no effect. It is speculated that higher concentrations of L-arginine may suppress the $^{\bullet}O_2^-$ generation from iNOS either by altering the conformation of the protein and accessibility of the flavin, or by rendering the flavins in a more oxidized state due to more rapid electron transfer to the heme.

Cytotoxicity of iNOS-derived $^{\bullet}O_2^-$ and ONOO$^-$

The fact that substantial $^{\bullet}O_2^-$ generation is sustained even in the presence of 100 μM L-arginine strongly suggests that $^{\bullet}O_2^-$ and NO synthesis may occur simultaneously within iNOS. These will create a situation favoring ONOO$^-$ formation. Indeed, two lines of evidence demonstrated that $^{\bullet}O_2^-$ and NO generated by iNOS combine to from ONOO$^-$ in L-arginine-depleted macrophages [16]. With luminol, ONOO$^-$-mediated chemiluminescence was measured in L-arginine-depleted macrophages and this was demonstrated to arise from iNOS. Also, the ONOO$^-$ specific nitration product nitrotyrosine was found in L-arginine-depleted macrophages and this was prevented by iNOS blockade. These findings reveal a new ONOO$^-$ forming mechanism in biological systems. Conventionally, ONOO$^-$ is shown to arise from the combination of NO and $^{\bullet}O_2^-$ generated from distinct enzymatic pathways. Here, NO and $^{\bullet}O_2^-$ are all produced by the same enzyme iNOS, but stem from different domains. Figure 2 illustrates that under certain levels of L-arginine $^{\bullet}O_2^-$ and NO generated from the reductase and oxygenase domain combine to form ONOO$^-$.

There is evidence suggesting that $^{\bullet}O_2^-$ and ONOO$^-$ production from iNOS may participate in the immune function of macrophages. Both $^{\bullet}O_2^-$ and NO have been individually shown to be cytotoxic and play roles in the antimicrobial action of macrophages [15, 18]. NO is produced by iNOS and $^{\bullet}O_2^-$ is believed to be solely synthesized from NADPH oxidase. These two pathways were thought to be differentially regulated to avoid simultaneous activation. However, there were also reports showing that NO alone exerted minimal activity to kill bacteria, but NO markedly potentiated the toxicity of other oxidants such as H_2O_2 [19]. NO reacts with $^{\bullet}O_2^-$ to form ONOO$^-$ which is a more potent oxidant and possesses strong bactericidal effect [20]. With cytokine-treated human neutrophils, abundant nitrotyrosine was detected around phagocytosed bacteria, indicating that ONOO$^-$ likely conveyed the killing activity in these cells instead of NO *per se* [21]. All these suggest that ONOO$^-$ formation from iNOS may enhance the immune function of macrophages. To explore the functional significance of iNOS–mediated $^{\bullet}O_2^-$ and ONOO$^-$ in the antibacterial action of macrophages, experiments were performed to compare the effects of macrophages activated in normal medium with those activated in L-arginine free medium on the growth of *E. coli*. The macrophages activated in L-arginine free medium, which generated $^{\bullet}O_2^-$ and ONOO$^-$, exhibited more than two-fold increased inhibitory effect than the cells activated in normal medium, which only produced NO. These data suggested that $\cdot O_2^-$ and $ONOO^-$ from iNOS contribute to the immune defense function of macrophages.

In summary, $\cdot O_2^-$ generation appears to be another important function of iNOS. By comparing the processes of $\cdot O_2^-$ formation from NOSs, it may help to better understand why evolution favors the existence of different isoforms. For example, while iNOS and nNOS structurally resemble each other and both produce $\cdot O_2^-$, there are significant differences between the mechanism and regulation of their $\cdot O_2^-$ formation. nNOS produces $\cdot O_2^-$ primarily from the oxygenase domain and is sensitive to L-arginine inhibition, whereas iNOS releases $\cdot O_2^-$ from its reductase domain and is not inhibited by higher levels of L-arginine. These different properties appear tailored to satisfy their biological missions. nNOS mainly generates NO that serves as a neurotransmitter. Because of the relatively high L-arginine levels in cytosol (200–800 μM), under physiological conditions $\cdot O_2^-$ generation would rarely occur. This will ensure that nNOS only produces NO and operates properly in signal transduction in neurons. On the other hand, host defense is the main role of iNOS. Simultaneous NO and $\cdot O_2^-$ generation may be more beneficial than NO formation alone, because these two free radicals interact to form the more toxic $ONOO^-$. Moreover, the cross reaction of $\cdot O_2^-$ and NO prevents the feedback inhibition on iNOS caused by NO or $\cdot O_2^-$, promoting sustained NO and $\cdot O_2^-$ generation which eventually enhances the killing activity of iNOS. It is noted that both $\cdot O_2^-$ and $ONOO^-$ are toxic oxidants without specificity to invaders or host cells. It remains a mystery how macrophages produce these oxidants to destroy invaders, while limiting self-toxicity. It is conceivable that there may be an intrinsic mechanism existing in macrophages to prevent potential self-destruction by these oxidants.

The production of $\cdot O_2^-$ by macrophages is critical for host defense. The cytotoxic nature of $\cdot O_2^-$ and its associated oxidants not only contributes to the killing of invading microbes, but also causes tissue damage in inflammation [15, 18]. iNOS appears to be another important $\cdot O_2^-$ generating source besides NADPH oxidase in phagocytic cells. The elucidation of $\cdot O_2^-$ production from iNOS has provided new insight into understanding how macrophages function in inflammation and host defense. Though L-arginine has been shown to be critical in the antimicrobial actions of macrophages, there is also evidence that the cytotoxicity of macrophages can be enhanced by L-arginine depletion. For example, it has long been recognized that tumoricidal actions of activated macrophages are dependent on depletion of environmental L-arginine [22]. L-arginine depletion was also reported in inflammatory sites during macrophage infiltration and wound healing [23]. Under these circumstances, iNOS-mediated $\cdot O_2^-$ and $ONOO^-$ could participate in the cytostatic and cytotoxic actions of macrophages. Modulating the $\cdot O_2^-$ and $ONOO^-$ formation from iNOS may provide new approaches to regulate macrophage function in inflammatory process and host defense.

Acknowledgments

This work was supported by National Institutes of Health Grants HL38324, HL65608 and HL63744 (to J.L.Z.) and AG00835 (to Y.X.); and Grant-in-Aid awards from the American Heart Association.

References

1   Moncada S, Palmer RM, Higgs EA (1991) Nitric oxide: physiology, pathophysiology, and pharmacology. *Pharmac Rev* 43: 109–142

2   Nathan C, Xie QW (1994) Nitric oxide synthases: roles, tolls, and controls. Cell 78: 915–918

3   Fulton D, Gratton JP, McCabe TJ, Fontana J, Fujio Y, Walsh K, Franke TF, Papapetropoulso A, Sessa WC (1999) Regulation of endothelium derived nitric oxide production by the protein kinase Akt. *Nature* 399: 597–601

4   Gross SS, Wolin MS (1995) Nitric oxide: pathophysiological mechanisms. *Annu Rev Physiol* 57: 737–769

5   Cho HJ, Xie QW, Calaycay J, Mumford RA, Swiderek KM, Lee TD, Nathan C (1992) Calmodulin is a subunit of nitric oxide synthase from macrophages. *J Exp Med* 176: 599–604

6   Heinzel B, John M, Klatt P, Bohme E, Mayer B (1992) Ca^{2+}/Calmodulin-dependent formation of hydrogen peroxide by brain nitric oxide synthase. *Biochem J* 281: 627–630

7   Pou S, Pou WS, Bredt DS, Snyder SH, Rosen GM (1992) Generation of superoxide by purified brain nitric oxide synthase. *J Biol Chem* 267: 24173–24176

8   Griffith OW, Stuehr DJ (1995) Nitric oxide synthase: properties and catalytic mechanism. *Annu Rev Physiol* 57: 707–736

9   Xia Y, Dawson VL, Dawson TM, Snyder SH, Zweier JL (1996) Nitric oxide synthase generates superoxide and nitric oxide in arginine-depleted cells leading to peroxynitrite-mediated cellular injury. *Proc Natl Acad Sci USA* 93: 6770–6774

10 Culcasi M, Lafon-Cazal M, Pietri S, Bockaert J (1994) Glutamate receptors induce a burst of superoxide *via* activation of nitric oxide synthase in arginine-depleted neurons. *J Biol Chem* 269: 12589–12593

11 Beckman JS, Beckman TW, Chen J, Marshall PA, Freeman BA (1990) Apparent hydroxyl radical production by peroxynitrite: implications for endothelial injury from nitric oxide and superoxide. *Proc Natl Acad Sci USA* 87: 1620–1624

12 Xia Y, Tsai AL, Berka V, Zweier JL (1998) Superoxide generation from endothelial nitric-oxide synthase: a Ca^{2+}/calmodulin-dependent and tetrahydrobiopterin regulatory process. *J Biol Chem* 273: 25804–25808

13 Vasquez-Vivar J, Kalyanaraman B, Martasek P, Hogg N, Masters BSS, Karoui H, Tordo P, Pritchard KA Jr (1998) Superoxide generation by endothelial nitric oxide synthase: the influence of cofactors. *Proc Natl Acad Sci USA* 95: 9220–9225

14 Abu-Soud HM, Stuehr DJ (1993) Nitric oxide synthase reveals a role for calmodulin in controlling electron transfer. *Proc Natl Acad Sci USA* 90: 10769–10772

15 Bastian NR, Hibbs JB Jr (1994) Assembly and regulation of NADPH oxidase and nitric oxide synthase. *Curr Opin Immunol* 6; 131–139

16 Xia Y, Zweier JL (1997) Superoxide and peroxynitrite generation from inducible nitric oxide synthase in macrophages. *Proc Natl Acad Sci USA* 94: 6954–6958

17 Xia Y, Roman LJ, Masters BSS, Zweier JL (1998) Inducible nitric-oxide synthase generates superoxide from the reductase domain. *J Biol Chem* 273: 22635–22639

18 Rosen GM, Pou S, Ramos CL, Cohen MS, Britigan BE (1995) Free radicals and phagocytic cells. *FASEB J* 9:200–209

19 Pacelli R, Wink DA, Cook JA, Krishna MC, DeGraff W, Friedman N, Tsokos M, Samuni A, Mitchell JB (1995) Nitric oxide potentiates hydrogen peroxide-induced killing of *Escherichia coli. J Exp Med* 182: 1469–1479

20 Zhu L, Gunn C, Beckman JS (1992) Batericidal activity of peroxynitrite. *Arch Biochem Biophys* 298: 452–457

21 Evans TJ, Buttery LDK, Carpenter A, Springall DR, Polak JM, Cohn J (1996) Cytokine-treated human neutrophils contain inducible nitric oxide synthase that produces nitration of ingested bacteria. *Proc Natl Acad Sci USA* 93: 9553–9558

22 Currie GA (1978) Activated macrophages kill tumor cells by releasing arginase. *Nature* 273: 758–759

23 Albina JE, Mills CD, Barbul A, Thirkill CE, Henry WL Jr, Mastrofrancesco B, Caldwell MD (1988) Arginine metabolism in wounds. *Am J Physiol* 254: E459–E467

Direct and indirect modulation of the inducible nitric oxide synthase by nitric oxide: feedback mechanisms in inflammation

Yoram Vodovotz[1] and Mary H. Barccellos-Hoff[2]

[1]University of Pittsburgh, Department of Surgery, UPMC Montefiore, NW 653, 3459 Fifth Avenue, Pittsburgh, PA 15213, USA; [2]Life Sciences Division, Lawrence Berkeley Laboratory, Berkeley, CA 94720, USA

Introduction

Cytokines are peptide hormones with a vast array of effects on growth, development, immunity, and disease that are regulated in complex ways at the transcriptional, post-transcriptional, translational, and post-translational levels. Cytokine activities interact with one another, regulate each other's expression and activity, and baffle investigators with their often-overlapping spectra of action [1]. Cytokines are required to mediate many cellular functions and thereby affect physiology and pathology. One target of many cytokines is regulation of reactive oxygen species (ROS) and reactive nitrogen oxide species (RNOS). In turn, ROS such as superoxide and RNOS such as nitric oxide (NO) and its reaction products can modulate the expression and function of numerous cytokines. Nitric oxide is of particular biological interest because its rapid and wide-ranging effects on physiological responses pose a central problem to determine how the system is ramped up quickly, and furthermore, due to its toxicity, what controls are in place to modulate its activity.

Studies over the last decade have demonstrated that all nitric oxide synthases (NOS), whether initially thought to be constitutive or inducible, are regulated at the transcriptional, post-transcriptional, translational, and post-translational levels [2–6]. What has been more recently appreciated is that the expression and activity of each isoform of NOS can be regulated by their end product(s), NO, or as yet not fully defined RNOS [7]. This chapter is specifically concerned with the regulation of the inducible isoform of NOS, NOS2. This isoform of NOS – which may be central to numerous physiological and pathological processes due to its high output of NO – is regulated primarily by cytokines, both positively and negatively [2]. In turn, NO and/or RNOS can regulate the expression and activity of some of these cytokines.

Nitric Oxide and Inflammation, edited by Daniela Salvemini, Timothy R. Billiar and Yoram Vodovotz
© 2001 Birkhäuser Verlag Basel/Switzerland

Our working hypothesis regarding the role of NO in the modulation of NOS2 has been that elevated levels of NO engender a broad-spectrum negative feedback response. This response involves *direct* post-translational effects on NOS2 protein, effects on transcription and translation of NOS2 mRNA, and *indirect* effects on cytokines that induce or suppress the expression of NOS2. The positive modulation of cytokines that induce the expression of NOS2 may serve as a feed-forward loop to enhance NO production in the early stages of inflammation. We place particular emphasis on the interactions between the high levels of NO derived from NOS2 and the cytokine transforming growth factor-β_1 (TGF-β_1), which we have suggested is the most potent physiological negative regulator of NOS2 [6]. We hypothesize that these interactions form a feedback loop for control of high-output NO production as part of the suppression of the inflammatory process. We also discuss the effect of NO on the cytokines interleukin-6 (IL-6), interleukin-18 (IL-18), and monocyte chemoattractant protein-1 (MCP-1), which in and of themselves do not modulate the expression of NOS2, but which do control the activation status of inflammatory cells and therefore may affect the expression of NOS2 indirectly.

Direct effects of NO on NOS2

Few enzymes have undergone the intense scrutiny that NOS2 has, due to the numerous modulatory roles of NO in species as diverse as insects and man. In the course of these studies, investigators found numerous control points on the expression and activity of this enzyme. A relatively small subset of these studies was directed at defining the role of the end product(s) of NOS2 in feedback or feed-forward control of the enzyme. As discussed below, NOS2 can be regulated at the transcriptional, translational, and post-translational levels by NO or RNOS. We have chosen to discuss these effects from the most immediate (post-translational effects) to the least immediate (transcriptional effects).

Post-translational effects of NO on NOS2 protein

While much of the research into inducible NO production was initially directed towards defining the inducing stimuli for NOS2, it quickly became apparent that this enzyme could be modified post-translationally [8, 9]. Some studies suggested that the enzyme could be modified as a consequence of high enzymatic activity [10, 11]. This control point is a very powerful one, since the speed at which NOS2 activity can be reduced in response to its own end-product(s) is theoretically much faster than that required to suppress the expression of the enzyme through modulation of transcription or translation.

Studies on NOS2 in lysates from peritoneal mouse inflammatory macrophages demonstrated that the enzyme was phosphorylated as well as ubiquitinated, though these modifications did not appear to be associated with modulation of enzyme activity [8]. A study in the macrophage-like cell line RAW264.7 demonstrated that NOS2 was phosphorylated on tyrosine residues; these workers found that the enzymatic activity of NOS2 was increased upon treatment with an inhibitor of tyrosine phosphorylation [9].

Similarly to the studies on phosphorylation, different groups found different results regarding end-product inhibition of NOS2. The purified enzyme from a rat bone marrow-derived macrophages cell line appeared to be downregulated by NO itself [10]. However, in intact mouse thioglycollate-elicited macrophages, the enzymatic shutdown of NOS2 after prolonged *in vitro* production of NO appeared to be due to undefined post-translational mechanisms, but not to NO itself [11]. Evidence in support of this concept was presented by Albakri and Stuehr, who found that the dimerization of NOS2 in RAW264.7 cells was inhibited by NO indirectly by interfering with the availability of free heme (a cofactor for the enzyme) [12]. This effect may be due to expression of heme oxygenase, since the two enzymes are often co-induced [13–15]. A recent study demonstrated that heme oxygenase could be induced by NO in mesangial cells [16].

Furthermore, a link between systemic NO levels and the capacity of macrophages to produce NO may depend on the presence of endogenous TGF-β_1, as suggested from recent studies using peritoneal macrophages from TGF-β_1 null mice [17]. This hypothesis is based on the finding that the IFNγ-inducible NO production of macrophages from wild-type mice whose systemic NO levels were high was depressed as compared to the NO production of macrophages from wild-type mice with low systemic NO production. In contrast, the NO production of macrophages from null or null heterozygote mice was not inversely proportional to the systemic NO levels of those mice [17]. It is highly speculative, but interesting nonetheless, to suggest that TGF-β_1 carries out this effect through modulation of heme oxygenase [18, 19] (see [13–16] and discussion above).

Modulation of NOS2 mRNA

The next most immediate control points for the regulation of NOS2 by NO are at the transcriptional, post-transcriptional, and translational levels. Indeed, Assreuy et al. [20] and Sheffler et al. [21] demonstrated that NO gas or chemical NO donors could bring about the reduction of NOS2 mRNA and protein. Borgending and Murphy have reported that the expression and activity of NOS2 in endothelial cells are suppressed following treatment with the chemical NO donor spermine-NONOate (SPERNO [22]), or in co-culture with astrocytes activated to produce NO with IL-1 + IFNγ or LPS + IFNγ [23]. Other studies demonstrated that inhibition of NO production resulted in increased expression of NOS2 in hepatocytes in an *in vivo* model of liver injury [24], which again suggests that elevated NO production is in some way associated with reduced expression of NOS2.

These studies did not examine the mechanism(s) by which these profound effects were mediated; one hypothesis is that NO can modulate certain transcription factors involved in the expression of NOS2. The upstream sequences of NOS2 contain numerous consensus sites for transcription factors, including *Fos*, *Jun*, and NF-κB [25, 26]. Several groups reported an increase in the expression and function of Fos and Jun by NO [27–30]. Additionally, NO can increase the activity of the transcription factor NF-κB in some instances [31]. These studies suggest that NO can drive further expression of NOS2. However, NO can also decrease the activity of NF-κB [32, 33] and can increase the activity of the inhibitor of NF-κB (IκB) [34], which suggests that a negative feedback effect may also occur at this level. Taylor et al. found that treatment with the NO donor SNAP of hepatocytes induced by cytokines to express NOS2 resulted in decreased expression of NOS2 mRNA and protein; this effect was associated with a reduction in the binding of NF-κB to its cognate DNA element [33].

Indirect effects of NO on NOS2

The earliest studies on the control of NOS2 suggested that numerous cytokines can modulate the expression of this enzyme [2, 5, 6, 35]. As summarized above, there is clear evidence, at least *in vitro*, for direct effects of NO or RNOS on NOS2. As discussed below, NO can also modulate the expression of cytokines that control the expression of NOS2. We have chosen to discuss these effects of NO or RNOS on cytokines which induce NOS2 *versus* effect on cytokines which suppress NOS2. Note that we do not use the more traditional designation of "pro-inflammatory" and "anti-inflammatory" cytokines, respectively, since some of the agents that suppress the expression the expression of NOS2 (e.g. IL-8) are generally considered pro-inflammatory. We can hypothesize that these "anti-inflammatory" effects of "pro-inflammatory" cytokines represent negative feedback mechanisms by which to control over-abundant NO production at sites of inflammation. As mentioned above, we have focused the majority of this section on the modulation by NO of cytokines that suppress the expression of NOS2, most notably TGF-β_1.

Modulation of NOS2-inducing cytokines by NO

A survey of the literature suggests that NO production may lead to further induction of NOS2 by modulation of the cytokines that induce this enzyme. One of the cytokines considered to be key for full induction of NOS2 *in vitro*, especially in cells stimulated with LPS, is tumor necrosis factor α (TNFα). Magrinat et al. were the first to report that NO induced TNFα mRNA expression in the undifferentiated human leukemia cell line HL-60 [36]. Eigler et al. demonstrated that the NO donor 3-morpholino-syndonimine increased the production of TNFα in human peripheral blood mononuclear cells [37] as well as in a mouse macrophage cell line [38]. Nitric oxide was found to affect the expression of TNFα directly in human peripheral blood mononuclear cells, through a cyclic GMP-independent mechanism [39]. The authors found that the expression of the transcription factor NF-κB was enhanced by NO in these cells, and suggested that this was the mechanism by which TNFα was modulated [39]. Later studies demonstrated that the expression of NOS2 could be induced through modulation of NF-κB [31]. Deakin et al reported that inhibition of NO production by a cytokine-stimulated mouse macrophage cell line suppressed the production of TNFα; conversely, treatment with the NO donor S-nitroso-N-acetylpenicillamine (SNAP) potentiated the production of TNFα by these cells [40]. Similar results were obtained by Marcinkiewicz et al. in cytokine-stimulated mouse peritoneal macrophages [41], and by Zinetti et al. in cytokine-stimulated human peripheral blood mononuclear cells [42].

Interleukin-1 is another potent inducer of NOS2, generally in combination with other cytokines or microbial inflammatory mediators [43]. Several groups have demonstrated that the expression and bioactivity of IL-1 is modulated by NO [41, 44, 45]. Marcinkiewicz et al. found that both the NO donor S-nitrosoglutathione (GSNO), as well as mouse macrophage-derived NO, increased the production of IL-1 [41]. Hill et al. demonstrated that inhibition of NO production reduced IL-1 bioactivity in a cytokine-activated mouse macrophage cell line, and that this effect is inhibited by a cyclic GMP donor [45]. Vallette et al. examined the effects on IL-1 production of NO *versus* the nitrosonium (NO$^+$) ion in a human colonic epithelial cell line, and found that NO$^+$ alone induced IL-1 production [44]. In contrast, Kim et al. have demonstrated that NO can inhibit the IL-1 converting enzyme (ICE; caspase-1), and thereby inhibit the production of IL-1 [46].

A more recently described NOS2-inducing cytokine is IL-12 [47, 48], and its gene expression is likewise increased by NO *in vitro* in a mouse macrophage cell line [49]. Interestingly, IL-12 signal transduction requires the functional expression of NOS2 in NK cells, which may impact the course of numerous parasitic diseases [48]. However, it is not clear what effects some of the other NOS2-inducing cytokines have *in vivo*. We have recently demonstrated that endotoxemic TGF-β_1 transgenic mice exhibited greatly increased production of TNFα as compared to wild-type controls while their production of NO was greatly diminished [50]. Other *in vivo* studies have suggested that elevated NO production may engender a negative feedback response at the level of expression of TNFα, since animals producing high levels of NO systemically have been reported to express lower levels of TNFα [51–53]. Additionally, antibodies to TNFα do not block the induction of NOS2 in a model of sepsis [54].

Modulation of NOS2-suppressing cytokines by NO

Among the negative regulators of the expression NOS2 are IL-4, IL-8, IL-10, EGF, FGF [35], and the TGF-β's [5, 6]. Of these cytokines, the two that have been reported to be modulated by NO are IL-8 and TGF-β_1. Both of these cytokines are potent immune modulators, with a variety of both pro- and anti-inflammatory functions.

Several studies have described the increased expression of IL-8, a cytokine which suppresses the expression of NOS2 [55], by NO [56–59]. Villarette and Remick demonstrated that inhibition of NO production suppressed TNFα-induced IL-8 production in a human endothelial cell line [56]. De Caterina et al. demonstrated that GSNO suppressed the production of IL-8 in cytokine-stimulated human saphenous vein endothelial cells [59]. Andrew and Lindley demonstrated the effect of NO on the promoter of the IL-8 gene by transient transfection in a human melanoma cell line [58]. The mechanism(s) for this effect are not known. The reduction of IL-8, a potent chemokine[60], by NO would be expected to act as part of a negative feedback loop to inhibit inflammation.

We have concentrated our studies on the effects of NO on the activity and expression of TGF-β_1, which suppresses the expression of NOS2 both *in vitro* and *in vivo* [5, 6]. The TGF-β's comprise a family of three mammalian cytokines with pleiotropic effects on different cell types [61, 62]. TGF-β_1 suppresses the inducible production of NO by affecting the expression of NOS2 at several levels [5, 6]; in fact, TGF-β_1 null mice exhibit spontaneously elevated expression of NOS2 mRNA and protein accompanied by increased systemic NO production [63].

The TGF-β's are generally secreted in a latent form and are activated by various stimuli. Activation of TGF-β_1 generates the latency-associated peptide (LAP) along with active TGF-β; LAP reassociates and inactivates TGF-β [64]. In macrophages, activation of TGF-β_1 follows exposure to inflammatory cytokines such as IFNγ and IL-1 [65–67] and LPS [68, 69]. In several cell types, ionizing radiation can active latent TGF-β_1 [70]. Recently, we found that co-cultures consisting of mouse macrophages stimulated with IFNγ and LPS and human adenocarcinoma (A549) cells converted latent TGF-β_1 to active TGF-β_1 [71]. This phenomenon led us to hypothesize that NO derived from the activated macrophages caused this effect. Indeed, treatment of A549 cells with the chemical NO donors DEANO or SPERNO caused a dose-dependent activation of latent TGF-β_1 [71]. *In vitro* experiments demonstrated that NO could not activate latent TGF-β_1 directly, but instead inactivated LAP *via* nitrosylation [71]. Since free LAP is an efficient means of neutralizing TGF-β [72], nitrosylation of LAP could prevent reassociation and ensure that TGF-β_1 reaches its ubiquitous receptors. Thus, treatment of A549 cells with NO likely mediates latent TGF-β activation indirectly, perhaps by inducing proteins necessary for activation.

TGF-β_1 may function as a cellular sensor for oxygen free radical stress, as well. In studies of mouse mammary gland, we have demonstrated activation of latent

TGF-β following shortly after exposure to ionizing radiation [70, 73]. The rapidity of this effect led us to evaluate the contribution of radiation generated ROS, since ROS modulate numerous genes [60]. Recent studies demonstrating that TGF-β itself induces a pro-oxidant state [74], including the generation of hydrogen peroxide during signaling events [75], suggest the novel possibility that this type of activation is self-amplifying. Furthermore, these properties of TGF-β_1 may intersect with a complex set of regulatory events since NO can react with oxygen and ROS [76].

Other, more circumstantial data also support our findings. As discussed previously, two groups have demonstrated that NO or chemical NO donors could bring about inhibition of NOS2 mRNA and protein in macrophages [20, 21], while others observed that endogenous activation of latent TGF-β_1 suppresses NO production in activated macrophages [77]. Furthermore, the expression of NOS2 and the capacity of endothelial cells to produce NO are suppressed following treatment with SPER-NO or in co-culture with astrocytes activated to produce NO with cytokines and LPS [23].

Among the RNOS is the nitroxyl anion (NO$^-$), an oxidant which may be produced by NOS [78] and which can be quite cytotoxic [79]. We found that NO-activated latent TGF-β_1 directly *in vitro* (Y. Vodovotz, M.H. Barcellos-Hoff, and D. Wink, manuscript in preparation), unlike NO, which may activate latent TGF-β_1 by inhibiting the neutralizing capacity of LAP [71]. The pro-oxidant hemin also activated latent TGF-β_1 directly (Y. Vodovotz, M.H. Barcellos-Hoff, and D. Wink, manuscript in preparation). We hypothesize that TGF-β_1 may function as a sensor for increased extracellular levels of ROS and ROS by being activated, and thereby suppress the expression of NOS2.

These studies in cell culture systems shed interesting insights on novel biological interactions between NO and TGF-β_1, but raise the issue of whether the two agents are present in sufficient proximity to interact *in vivo*. Nitric oxide is a lipophilic, freely diffusible radical, which can at least theoretically become much more concentrated in lipid bilayers such as those that make up biological membranes [80]. Numerous studies have suggested that NO can diffuse into the mitochondria and subsequently modulate the activity of mitochondrial enzymes [81]. Previous studies demonstrated a membranous subcellular location for as much as 50% of total cellular NOS2 [8, 82], and a recent study demonstrated that a NOS2-like enzyme is present in mitochondria [83]. Interestingly, latent TGF-β_1 has also been localized to the mitochondria [84]. These localizations raise the possibility that high level, localized NO production could occur site-specifically in an organelle in which latent TGF-β_1 is present, and thereby lead to activation of the cytokine. It is not known if this process can occur, and if it did it is not clear what the effect of the presence of active TGF-β_1 in the mitochondria would be. However, studies in TGF-β_1 null mice suggest that TGF-β_1 may be involved functionally in this organelle. The number of mitochondria is increased in hepatocytes of these mice; this finding suggests that an increased number of mitochondria is a compensatory reaction for reduced mitochondrial function [85].

Some of the earliest studies on the role of macrophage-derived inducible NO production were set in the context of infectious diseases [86]. These and numerous other studies suggested that NO was essential to the host's anti-microbial response; thus, modulation of NOS2 inducing cytokines by NO could have either a beneficial or a detrimental effect on the resolution of these infectious diseases, depending on the particular set of temporal and/or spatial circumstances. Active TGF-β_1 is part of the arsenal of immunosuppressive agents employed by intracellular parasites [87–90]. This role of TGF-β_1 appears to be closely related to the suppression of NO, since inhibition of NO production by TGF-β_1 enhances the growth of macrophage intracellular parasites [91–96].

Both NOS2 [97] and TGF-β_1 [98] have multiple roles in the anti-tumor inflammatory response. These interactions are especially interesting in solid tumors, which consist not only of tumor cells, but also of infiltrating host leukocytes whose effector functions are often suppressed [99]. Interestingly, many malignant cells predominantly express active TGF-β_1 [100–107], which in one study was associated with their invasive potential [108]. Additionally, some tumor cells can activate latent TGF-β_1 in neighboring cells [109, 110]. Other studies have demonstrated that activation of latent TGF-β_1 by tumor cells suppresses the NO-dependent cytotoxic capacity of macrophages [107, 111–113].

We found that levels of NO_2^- in co-cultures of A549 cells and activated macrophages, in which latent TGF-β_1 was activated, were lower than in cultures of macrophages alone [71]. Interestingly, A549 cells treated with DEANO are not deficient in their clonogenic potential (W. DeGraff, D.A. Wink, and J. Mitchell, unpublished observations). Although epithelial cells are growth inhibited by TGF-β, many tumor cells are not [114]. Thus the selection of resistant tumor cells may be facilitated by activation of latent TGF-β_1 following exposure of cells to NO, which may also preferentially deactivate infiltrating macrophages, providing a favorable environment for tumor cell growth.

Effects of NO on other cytokines

In addition to the cytokines described above, NO can also modulate the "proinflammatory" cytokines IL-6, IL-18, and MCP-1. De Caterina et al. demonstrated that GSNO suppresses the expression of IL-6 in cytokine-stimulated human saphenous vein endothelial cells [59]. Deakin et al. reported that inhibition of NO production potentiated IL-6 release in a cytokine-stimulated mouse macrophage cell line; conversely, treatment with SNAP suppressed IL-6 production in these cells [40]. Kim et al. demonstrated that the production of functional IL-18 is inhibited by NO both in mouse peritoneal macrophages and in a mouse macrophage cell line [46].

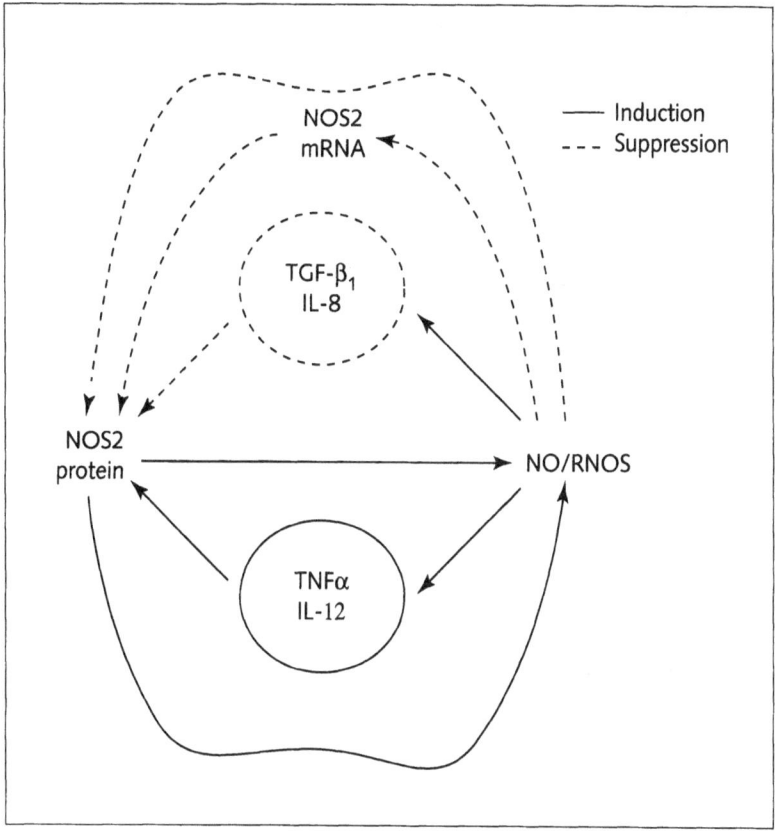

Figure 1

*Direct and indirect modulation of NOS2 by NO. High level production of NO and subse-
quent reactions to form RNOS by NOS2 can modulate the expression and activity of NOS2
either directly, through post-translational modification or modulation of NOS2 mRNA, or
indirectly, through modulation of cytokines which either induce (e.g. TNFα, IL-12) or suppress (TGF-β₁, IL-8) the expression of NOS2. Solid lines represent induction; dashed lines
represent suppression.*

Taken together, these observations suggest that NO can have a complex array of
effects on "pro-inflammatory" and "anti-inflammatory" cytokines. Since the whole
spectrum of actions of these cytokines is yet to be elucidated, the role of NO may
differ from the exact inflammatory condition; however, it may be hypothesized that
NO is central to the signal transduction required to enhance or suppress inflammation.

Conclusions

Intercellular interactions often involve both cytokines and free radicals such as ROS and RNOS, which mediate signals that allow cells to decipher their environment. Much attention has been focused on both cytokines and NO in normal physiology as well as in disease states. Herein, we have attempted to discuss the modulation of NO production by cytokines, as well the reciprocal or possible feedback effects that NO has on the expression and activity of various cytokines (Fig. 1). The findings described above suggest NO can control NOS2, both directly and indirectly, in numerous ways. These findings also suggest the obvious conclusion of multiple negative feedback mechanisms by which to control NOS2. Due to the ubiquity of both NOS2 and the cytokines discussed above, numerous physiological and pathological processes may be affected. While these studies are still in their infancy, they provide the tantalizing possibility that harnessing this complex interplay between cytokines and NO may yield clinically beneficial results.

Acknowledgments
The authors would like to acknowledge the help of Louis Chesler and Seong Jin Kim (Laboratory of Cell Regulation and Carcinogenesis, National Cancer Institute, Bethesda, MD), Honkyong Chong (Life Sciences Division, Lawrence Berkeley Laboratory, Berkeley, CA), and David Wink, John Cook, and Sungmee Kim (Radiation Biology Branch, National Cancer Institute, Bethesda, MD) for their help with experiments described in this chapter.

References

1   Nathan C, Sporn M (1991) Cytokines in context. *J Cell Biol* 113: 981–981
2   Nathan C, Xie Q-W (1994) Regulation of biosynthesis of nitric oxide. *J Biol Chem* 269: 13725–13728
3   Knowles RG. Brain nitric oxide synthesis and neurodegeneration (1994) In: G Racagni, N Brunello, SZ Langer (eds): *Recent advances in the treatment of neurodegenerative disorders and cognitive dysfunction*. Int Acad Biomed Drug Res, Basel, 112–118
4   Sessa WC (1994) The nitric oxide synthase family of proteins. *J Vasc Res* 31: 131–143
5   Vodovotz Y, Bogdan C (1994) Control of nitric oxide synthase expression by transforming growth factor-β: Implications for homeostasis. *Prog Growth Factor Res* 5: 341–351
6   Vodovotz Y (1997) Control of nitric oxide production by transforming growth factor-β1: Mechanistic insights and potential relevance to human disease. *Nitric Oxide: Biol and Chem* 1: 3–17

7   Griscavage JM, Hobbs AJ, Ignarro LJ (1995) Negative modulation of nitric oxide synthase by nitric oxide and nitroso compounds. *Adv Pharmacol* 34: 215–234

8   Vodovotz Y, Russell D, Xie Q-W, Bogdan C, Nathan C (1995) Vesicle association of nitric oxide synthase from primary mouse macrophages. *J Immunol* 154: 2914–2925

9   Pan J, Burgher KL, Sczczepanik AM, Ringeim GE (1996) Tyrosine phosphorylation of inducible nitric oxide synthase: implications for potential post-translational regulation. *Biochem J* 314: 889–894

10   Griscavage JM, Rogers NE, Sherman MP, Ignarro LJ (1993) Inducible nitric oxide synthase from a rat alveolar macrophage cell line in inhibited by nitric oxide. *J Immunol* 151: 6329–6337

11   Vodovotz Y, Kwon N-S, Popischil M, Manning J, Paik J, Nathan C (1994) Inactivation of nitric oxide synthase following prolonged incubation of mouse macrophages with interferon-gamma and bacterial lipopolysaccharide. *J Immunol* 152: 4110–4118

12   Albakri QA, Stuehr DJ (1996) Intracellular assembly of inducible NO synthase is limited by nitric oxide-mediated changes in heme insertion and availability. *J Biol Chem* 271: 5414–5421

13   Hara E, Takahashi K, Tominaga T, Kumabe T, Kayama T, Suzuki H, Fujita H, Yoshimoto T, Shirato K, Shibahara S (1996) Expression of heme oxygenase and inducible nitric oxide synthase mRNA in human brain tumors. *Biochem Biophys Res Commun* 224: 153–158

14   Kurata S, Matsumoto M, Yamashita U (1996) Concomitant transcriptional activation of nitric oxide synthase and heme oxygenase genes during nitric oxide-mediated macrophage cytostasis. *J Biochem* 120: 49–52

15   Yet S-F, Pellacani A, Patterson C, Tan L, Folta SC, Foster L, Lee W-S, Hsieh C-M, Perrella MA (1997) Induction of heme oxygenase-1 expression in vascular smooth muscle cells: A link to endotoxic shock. *J Biol Chem* 272: 4295–4301

16   Datta PK, Lianos EA (1999) Nitric oxide induces heme oxygenase-1 gene expression in mesangial cells. *Kidney Int* 55: 1734–1739

17   Vodovotz Y, Letterio JJ, Geiser AG, Chesler L, Roberts AB, Sparrow J (1996) Control of nitric oxide production by endogenous transforming growth factor-β1 and systemic nitric oxide in retinal pigment epithelial cells and peritoneal macrophages. *J Leukoc Biol* 60: 261–270

18   Kutty RK, Nagineni CN, Kutty G, Hooks JJ, Chader GJ, Wiggert B (1994) Increased expression of heme oxygenase-1 in human retinal pigment epithelial cells by transforming growth factor-β. *J Cell Physiol* 159: 371–378

19   Pellacani A (1998) Induction of heme oxygenase-1 during endotoxemia is downregulated by transforming growth factor-beta1. *Circ Res* 83: 396–403

20   Assreuy J, Cunha FQ, Liew FY, Moncada S (1993) Feedback inhibition of nitric oxide synthase activity by nitric oxide. *Br J Pharmacol* 108: 833–837

21   Sheffler LA, Wink DA, Melillo G, Cox GW (1995) Exogenous nitric oxide regulates IFN-γ plus lipopolysaccharide-induced nitric oxide synthase expression in mouse macrophages. *J Immunol* 155: 886–894

22 Keefer LK, Nims RW, Davies KM, Wink DA (1996) "NONOates" (1-substituted diazen-1-ium-1,2-diolates) as nitric oxide donors: convenient nitric oxide dosage forms. *Methods Enzymol* 268: 281–293

23 Borgerding RA, Murphy S (1995) Expression of inducible nitric oxide synthase in cerebral endothelial cells is regulated by cytokine-activated astrocytes. *J Neurochem* 65: 1342–1347

24 Luss H, DiSilvio M, Litton AL, Molina y Vedia L, Nussler AK, Billiar TR (1994) Inhibition of nitric oxide synthesis enhances the expression of inducible nitric oxide synthase mRNA and protein in a model of chronic liver inflammation. *Biochem Biophys Res Commun* 204: 635–640

25 Xie QW, Cho HJ, Calaycay J, Mumford RA, Swiderek KM, Lee TD, Ding A, Troso T, Nathan C (1992) Cloning and characterization of inducible nitric oxide synthase from mouse macrophages. *Science* 256: 225–228

26 Chartrain NA, Geller DA, Koty PP, Sitrin NF, Nussler AK, Hoffman EP, Billiar TR, Hutchinson NI, Mudgett JS (1994) Molecular cloning, structure, and chromosomal localization of the human inducible nitric oxide synthase gene. *J Biol Chem* 269: 6765–6772

27 Lee J-H, Wilcox GL, Beitz AJ (1992) Nitric oxide mediates Fos expression in the spinal cord induced by mechanical noxious stimulation. *NeuroReport* 3: 841–844

28 Felley-Bosco E, Ambs S, Lowenstein CJ, Keefer LK, Harris CC (1994) Constitutive expression of inducible nitric oxide synthase in human bronchial epithelial cells induces c-fos and stimulates the cGMP pathway. *Am J Respir Cell Mol Biol* 11: 159–164

29 Lo YYC, Cruz TF (1995) Involvement of reactive oxygen species in cytokine and growth factor induction of c-fos expression in chondrocytes. *J Biol Chem* 270: 11727–11730

30 Tabuchi A, Sano K, Oh E, Tsuchiya T, Tsuda M (1994) Modulation of AP-1 by nitric oxide (NO) *in vitro*: NO-mediated modulation of AP-1. *FEBS Lett* 351: 123–127

31 Xie Q-W, Kashiwabara Y, Nathan C (1994) Role of transcription factor NF-kappaB/Rel in induction of nitric oxide synthase. *J Biol Chem* 269: 4705–4708

32 Katsuyama K, Shichiri M, Marumo F, Hirata Y (1998) NO inhibits cytokine-induced iNOS expression and NF-kappaB activation by interfering with phosphorylation and degradation of IkappaB-alpha. *Arterioscler Thromb Vasc Biol* 18: 1796–1802

33 Taylor BS, Kim YM, Wang Q, Shapiro RA, Billiar TR, Geller DA (1997) Nitric oxide down-regulates hepatocyte-inducible nitric oxide synthase gene expression. *Arch Surg* 132: 1177–1183

34 Peng H-B, Libby P, Liao JK (1995) Induction and stabilization of IkappaBa by nitric oxide mediates inhibition of NF-kappaB. *J Biol Chem* 270: 14214–14219

35 Bogdan C, Vodovotz Y, Xie Q-W, Nathan C, Röllinghoff M (1994) Regulation of inducible nitric oxide synthase in macrophages by cytokines and microbial products. In: N Masihi (ed): *Immunotherapy of infections*. Marcel Dekker, New York, 37–54

36 Magrinat G, Mason SN, Shami PJ, Weinberg JB (1992) Nitric oxide modulation of human leukemia cell differentiation and gene expression. *Blood* 80: 1880–1884

37 Eigler A, Sinha B, Endres S (1993) Nitric oxide-releasing agents enhance cytokine-

induced tumor necrosis factor synthesis in human mononuclear cells. *Biochem Biophys Res Commun* 196: 494–501

38   Eigler A, Moeller J, Endres S (1995) Exogenous and endogenous nitric oxide attenuates tumor necrosis factor synthesis in the murine macrophage cell line RAW 264.7. *J Immunol* 154: 4048–4054

39   Lander HM, Sehajpal P, Levine DM, Novogrodsky A (1993) Activation of human peripheral blood mononuclear cells by nitric oxide-generating compounds. *J Immunol* 150: 1509–1516

40   Deakin AM, Payne AN, Whittle BJR, Moncada S (1995) The modulation of IL-6 and TNF-α release by nitric oxide following stimulation of J774 cells with LPS and IFN-γ. *Cytokine* 7: 408–416

41   Marcinkiewicz J, Grabowska A, Chain B (1995) Nitric oxide up-regulates the release of inflammatory mediators by mouse macrophages. *Eur J Immunol* 25: 947–951

42   Zinetti M, Fantuzzi G, Delgado R, Di Santo E, Ghezzi P, Fratelli M (1995) Endogenous nitic oxide production by human monocytic cells regulates LPS-induced TNF production. *Eur Cyt Netw* 6: 45–48

43   Xie Q-W, Nathan C (1994) The high-output nitric oxide pathway: role and regulation. *J Leukoc Biol* 56: 576–582

44   Vallette G, Jarry A, Branka J-E, Laboisse CL (1996) A redox-based mechanism for induction of interleukin-1 production by nitric oxide in a human colonic epithelial cell line (HT29-C1.16E). *Biochem J* 313: 35–38

45   Hill JR, Corbett JA, Kwon G, Marshall CA, McDaniel ML (1996) Nitric oxide regulates interleukin 1 bioactivity released from murine macrophages. *J Biol Chem* 271: 22672–22678

46   Kim YM, Talanian RV, Li J, Billiar TR (1998) Nitric oxide prevents IL-1beta and IFN-gamma-inducing factor (IL-18) release from macrophages by inhibiting caspase-1 (IL-1beta-converting enzyme). *J Immunol* 161: 4122–4128

47   Yu W-G, Ogawa M, Mu J, Umehara K, Tsujimura T, Fujiwara H, Hamaoka T (1997) IL-12-induced tumor regression correlates with *in situ* activity of IFN-γ produced by tumor-infiltrating cells and its secondary induction of anti-tumor pathways. *J Leukoc Biol* 62: 450–457

48   Diefenbach A, Schindler H, Rollinghoff M, Yokoyama WM, Bogdan C (1999) Requirement for type 2 NO synthase for IL-12 signaling in innate immunity. *Science* 284: 951–955

49   Rothe H, Hartmann B, Geerlings P, Kolb H (1996) Interleukin-12 gene-expression of macrophages is regulated by nitric oxide. *Biochem Biophys Res Commun* 224: 159–163

50   Vodovotz Y, Kopp JB, Takeguchi H, Shrivastav S, Coffin D, Lucia MS, Mitchell JB, Webber R, Letterio J, Wink D et al (1998) Increased mortality, blunted production of nitric oxide, and increased production of tumor necrosis factor-a in endotoxemic transforming growth factor-β1 transgenic mice. *J Leukoc Biol* 63: 31–39

51   Florquin S, Amraoui Z, Dubois C, Decuyper J, Goldman M (1994) The protective role

of endogenously synthesized nitric oxide in staphylococcal enterotoxin B-induced shock in mice. *J Exp Med* 180: 1153–1158

52 Fukatsu K, Saito H, Fukushima R, Inoue T, Lin M-T, Inaba T, Muto T (1995) Detrimental effects of a nitric oxide synthase inhibitor (N-omega-nitro-L-arginine-methyl-ester) in a murine sepsis model. *Arch Surg* 130: 410–414

53 Pheng LH, Francoeur C, Denis M (1995) The involvement of nitric oxide in a mouse model of adult respiratory distress syndrome. *Inflammation* 19: 599–610

54 Evans T, Carpenter A, Silva A, Cohen J (1992) Differential effects of monoclonal antibodies to tumor necrosis factor alpha and gamma interferon on induction of hepatic nitric oxide synthase in experimental gram-negative sepsis. *Infect Immun* 60: 4133–4139

55 McCall TB, Palmer RMJ, Moncada S (1992) Interleukin-8 inhibits the induction of nitric oxide synthase in rat peritoneal neutrophils. *Biochem Biophys Res Commun* 186: 680–685

56 Villarete LH, Remick DG (1995) Nitric oxide regulation of IL-8 expression in human endothelial cells. *Biochem Biophys Res Commun* 211: 671–676

57 Brown Z, Robson RL, Westwick J (1993) L-arginine/nitric oxide pathway: a possible signal transduction mechanism for the regulation of the chemokine IL-8 in human mesangial cells. *Adv Exp Med Biol* 351: 65–75

58 Andrew PJ, Harant H, Lindley JD (1995) Nitric oxide regulates IL-8 expression in melanoma cells at the transcriptional level. *Biochem Biophys Res Commun* 214: 949–956

59 De Caterina R, Libby P, Peng H-B, Thannickal VJ, Rajavashisth TB, Gimbrone MA Jr, Shin WS, Liao JK (1995) Nitric oxide decreases cytokine-induced endothelial activation: Nitric oxide selectively reduces endothelial expression of adhesion molecules and proinflammatory cytokines. *J Clin Invest* 96: 60–68

60 Remick DG, Villarete L (1996) Regulation of cytokine gene expression by reactive oxygen and reactive nitrogen intermediates. *J Leukoc Biol* 59: 471–475

61 Roberts AB, Sporn MB. The transforming growth factor-betas (1990) In: MB Sporn, AB Roberts (eds): *Peptide growth factors and their receptors.* Springer-Verlag, Berlin, 419–472

62 Massagué J (1990) The transforming growth factor-β family. *Annu Rev Cell Biol* 6: 597–641

63 Vodovotz Y, Geiser AG, Chesler L, Letterio JJ, Campbell A, Lucia MS, Sporn MB, Roberts AB (1996) Spontaneously increased production of nitric oxide and aberrant expression of the inducible nitric oxide synthase *in vivo* in the transforming growth factor-β1 null mouse. *J Exp Med* 183: 2337–2342

64 Flaumenhaft R, Kojima S, Abe M, Rifkin DB (1993) Activation of latent transforming growth factor β. *Advances Pharmacol* 24: 51–76

65 Assoian RK, Fleurdelys BE, Stevenson HC, Miller PJ, Madtes DK, Raines EW, Ross R, Sporn MB (1987) Expression and secretion of type β transforming growth factor by activated human macrophages. *Proc Natl Acad Sci USA* 84: 6020–6024

66   Twardzik DR, Mikovits JA, Ranchalis JE, Purchio AF, Ellingsworth L, Ruscetti FW (1990) τ-Interferon-induced activation of latent transforming growth factor-Beta by human monocytes. *Ann NY Acad Sci* 593: 276–284

67   Bristol LA, Ruscetti FW, Brody DT, Durum SK (1990) IL-1α induces expression of active transforming growth factor-Beta in nonproliferating T cells *via* a post-transcriptional mechanism. *J Immunol* 145: 4108–4114

68   Grotendorst GR, Smale G, Pencev D (1989) Production of transforming growth factor β by human peripheral blood monocytes and neutrophils. *J Cell Physiol* 140: 396–402

69   Chong H, Vodovotz Y, Cox GW, Barcellos-Hoff MH (1999) Immunocytochemical detection of latent TGF-β activation in cultured macrophages. *J Cell Physiol* 178: 275–283

70   Barcellos-Hoff MH (1993) Radiation-induced transforming growth factor β and subsequent extracellular matrix reorganization in murine mammary gland. *Cancer Res* 53: 3880–3886

71   Vodovotz Y, Chesler L, Chong H, Kim SJ, Simpson JT, DeGraff W, Cox GW, Roberts AB, Wink DA, Barcellos-Hoff MH (1999) Regulation of transforming growth factor-β1 by nitric oxide. Cancer Res 59: 2142–2149

72   Böttinger EP, Factor VM, Tsang ML-S, Weatherbee JA, Kopp JB, Qian SW, Wakefield LM, Roberts AB, Thorgeirsson SS, Sporn MB (1996) The recombinant proregion of transforming growth factor β1 (latency-associated peptide) inhibits active transforming growth factor β1 in transgenic mice. *Proc Natl Acad Sci USA* 93: 5877–5882

73   Ehrhart EJ, Carroll A, Segarini P, Tsang ML-S, Barcellos-Hoff MH (1997) Latent transforming growth factor-β activation *in situ*: Quantitative and functional evidence following low dose irradiation. *FASEB J* 11: 991–1002

74   Das SK, Fanburg BL (1991) TGF-β1 produces a "prooxidant" effect on bovine pulmonary artery endothelial cells in culture. *Am J Physiol* 261: L249–L254

75   Ohba M, Shibanuma M, Kuroki T, Nose K (1994) Production of hydrogen peroxide by transforming growth factor-β1 and its involvement in induction of egr-1 in mouse osteoblastic cells. *J Cell Biol* 126: 1079–1088

76   Wink DA, Vodovotz Y, Grisham MB, DeGraff W, Cook JA, Pacelli R, Krishna M, Mitchell JB (2001) Antioxidant effects of nitric oxide. *Meth Enzymol; in press*

77   Seyler I, Appel M, Devissaguet J-P, Legrand P, Barratt G (1997) Modulation of nitric oxide production in RAW 264.7 cells by transforming factor-beta and interleukin-10: differential effects on free and encapsulated immunomodulator. *J Leukoc Biol* 62: 374–380

78   Schmidt HHHW, Hofmann H, Schindler U, Shutenko ZS, Cunningham DD, Feelisch M (1996) No ˙NO from NO synthase. *Proc Natl Acad Sci USA* 93: 14492–14497

79   Wink DA, Feelisch M, Fukuto J, Christodoulou D, Jourd'heuil D, Grisham MB, Vodovotz Y, Cook JA, Krishna M, DeGraff W et al (1998) Investigation of cytotoxic mechanism of nitroxyl. Implication in pathophysiological mechanisms of NO. *Arch Biochem Biophys* 351: 66–74

80   Lancaster J (1994) Simulation of the diffusion and reaction of endogenously produced nitric oxide. *Proc Natl Acad Sci USA* 91: 8137–8141

81   Drapier J-C, Hibbs JB, Jr. (1988) Differentiation of murine macrophages to express nonspecific cytotoxicity for tumor cells results in L-arginine-dependent inhibition of mitochondrial iron-sulfur enzymes in the macrophage effector cells. *J Immunol* 140: 2829–2838

82   Förstermann U, Schmidt HHW, Kohlhaas KL, Murad F (1992) Induced RAW 264.7 macrophages express soluble and particulate nitric oxide synthase: inhibition by transforming growth factor-β. *Eur J Pharmacol* 225: 161–165

83   Tatoyan A, Giulivi C (1998) Purification and characterization of a nitric-oxide synthase from rat liver mitochondria. *J Biol Chem* 273: 11044–11048

84   Heine UI, Burmester JK, Flanders KC, Danielpour D, Munoz EF, Roberts AB, Sporn MB (1991) Localization of transforming growth factor-β1 in mitochondria of murine heart and liver. *Cell Regul* 2: 467–477

85   Williams AO, Knapton AD, Geiser A, Letterio JJ, Roberts AB (1996) The liver in transforming growth factor-Beta-1 (TGF-beta 1) null mutant mice. *Ultrastruct Pathol* 20: 477–490

86   Nathan CF, Hibbs JB, Jr. (1991) Role of nitric oxide synthesis in macrophage antimicrobial activity. *Curr Opin Immunol* 3: 65–70

87   Silva JS, Twardzik DR, Reed SG (1991) Regulation of Trypanosoma cruzi infections *in vitro* and *in vivo* by transforming growth factor β. *J Exp Med* 174: 539

88   Barral-Netto M, Barral A, Brownell CE, Skeiky YAW, Ellingsworth LR, Twardzik DR, Reed SG (1992) Transforming growth factor-β in leishmanial infection: A parasite escape mechanism. *Science* 257: 545–548

89   Barral A, Barral-Netto M, Yong EC, Brownell CE, Twardzik DR, Reed SG (1993) Transforming growth factor β as a virulence mechanism for Leishmania braziliensis. *Proc Natl Acad Sci USA* 90: 3442–3446

90   Barral A, Teixeira M, Reis P, Vinhas V, Costa J, Lessa H, Bittencourt AL, Reed S, Carvalho EM, Barral-Netto M (1995) Transforming growth factor-β in human cutaneous leishmaniasis. *Am J Pathol* 147: 947–954

91   Nelson BJ, Ralph P, Green SJ, Nacy CA (1991) Differential susceptibility of activated macrophage cytotoxic effector reactions to the suppressive effects of transforming growth factor-β1. *J Immunol* 146: 1849–1857

92   Gazzinelli RT, Oswald IP, Hieny S, James SL, Sher A (1992) The microbicidal activity of interferon-τ-treated macrophages against Trypanosoma cruzi involves an L-arginine-dependent, nitrogen-oxide-mediated mechanism inhibitable by interleukin 10 and transforming growth factor-β. *Eur J Immunol* 22: 2501–2506

93   Oswald IP, Gazzinelli RT, Sher A, James SL (1992) IL-10 synergizes with IL-4 and transforming growth factor-β to inhibit macrophage cytotoxic activity. *J Immunol* 148: 3578–3582

94   Green SJ, Scheller LF, Marletta MA, Seguin MC, Klotz FW, Slayter M, Nelson BJ, Nacy

CA (1994) Nitric oxide: Cytokine-regulation of nitric oxide in host resistance to intracellular pathogens. *Immunol Lett* 43: 87–94

95   Bläuer F, Groscurth P, Schneeman M, Schoedon G, Schaffner A (1995) Modulation of the antilisterial activity of human blood-derived macrophages by activating and deactivating cytokines. *J Interferon Cytokine Res* 15: 105–114

96   Tomioka H, Sato K, Maw WW, Saito H (1995) The role of tumor necrosis factor, interferon-γ, transforming growth factor-β, and nitric oxide in the expression of immunosuppressive functions of splenic macrophages induced by Mycobacterium avium complex infection. *J Leukoc Biol* 58: 704–712

97   Xie K, Dong Z, Fidler IJ (1996) Activation of nitric oxide synthase gene for inhibition of cancer metastasis. *J Leukoc Biol* 59: 797–803

98   Reiss M (1997) Transforming growth factor-beta and cancer: a love-hate relationship? *Oncol Res* 9: 447–457

99   Elgert KD, Alleva DG, Mullins DW (1998) Tumor-induced immune dysfunction: the macrophage connection. *J Leukoc Biol* 64: 275–290

100 Anzano MA, Roberts AB, De Larco JE, Wakefield LM, Assoian RK, Roche NS, Smith JM, Lazarus JE, Sporn MB (1985) Increased secretion of type β transforming growth factor accompanies viral transformation of cells. *Mol Cel Biol* 5: 242–247

101 Coffey RJ, Jr., Shipley GD, Moses HL (1986) Production of transforming growth factors by human colon cancer lines. Cancer Res 46: 1164–1169

102 Coffey RJ, Jr., Goustin AS, Mangelsdorf Soderquist A, Shipley GD, Wolfshohl J, Carpenter G, Moses HL (1987) Transforming growth factor α and β expression in human colon cancer lines: Implications for an autocrine model. *Cancer Res* 47: 4590–4594

103 Derynck R, Goeddel DV, Ullrich A, Gutterman JU, Williams RD, Bringmann TS, Berger WH (1987) Synthesis of messenger RNAs for transforming growth factors α and β and the epidermal growth factor receptor by human tumors. *Cancer Res* 47: 707–712

104 Niitsu Y, Urushizaki Y, Terui K, Mahara K, Kohgo Y, Urushizaki I (1988) Expression of TGF-beta in adult T cell leukemia. *Blood* 71: 263–266

105 Schwarz LC, Wright JA, Gingras M-C, Kondiah P, Danielpour D, Pimentel M, Sporn MB, Greenberg AH (1990) Aberrant TGF-β production and regulation in metastatic malignancy. *Growth Factors* 3: 115–127

106 Terui T, Niitsu Y, Mahara K, Fujisaki Y, Urushizaki Y, Mogi Y, Kohgo Y, Watanabe N, Ogura M, Saito H (1990) The production of transforming growth factor-β in acute megakaryoblastic leukemia and its possible implications in myelofibrosis. *Blood* 75: 1540–1548

107 Murata J, Corradin SB, Felley-Bosco E, Juillerat-Jeanneret L (1995) Involvement of a transforming-growth-factor-β-like molecule in tumor-cell-derived inhibition of nitric-oxide synthesis in cerebral endothelial cells. *Int J Cancer* 62: 743–748

108 Samuel SK, Hurta RAR, Kondaiah P, Khalil N, Turley EA, Wright JA, Greenberg AH (1992) Autocrine induction of tumor protease production and invasion by a metallothionein-regulated TGF-β$_1$ (Ser223, 225). *EMBO J* 11: 1599–1605

109 Takiuchi H, Tada T, Li X-F, Ogata M, Ikeda T, Fujimoto S, Fujiwara H, Hamaoka T

(1992) Particular types of tumor cells have the capacity to convert transforming growth factor β from a latent to an active form. *Cancer Res* 52: 5641–5646

110 Horimoto M, Kato J, Takimoto R, Terui T, Mogi Y, Nitsu Y (1995) Identification of a transforming growth factor beta-1 activator derived from a human gastric cancer cell line. *Br J Cancer* 72: 676–862

111 Alleva DG, Burger CJ, Elgert KD (1994) Tumor-induced regulation of suppressor macrophage nitric oxide and TNF-α production: Role of tumor derived IL-10, TGF-β, and prostaglandin E2. *J Immunol* 153: 1674–1686

112 Maeda H, Tsuru S, Shiraishi A (1994) Improvement of macrophage dysfunction by administration of anti-transforming growth factor-β antibody in EL4-bearing hosts. *Jpn J Cancer Res* 85: 1137–1143

113 Lagadec P, Raynal S, Lieubeau B, Onier N, Arnould L, Saint-Giorgio V, Lawrence DA, Jeannin JF (1999) Evidence for control of nitric oxide synthesis by intracellular transforming growth factor-beta1 in tumor cells. Implications for tumor development. *Am J Pathol* 154: 1867–1876

114 Reiss M, Barcellos-Hoff MH (1997) Transforming growth factor-β in breast cancer: A working hypothesis. *Br Cancer Res Treat* 45: 81–95

Nitric oxide regulation of eicosanoid production

Daniela Salvemini

MetaPhore Pharmaceuticals, 1910 Innerbelt Business Center Drive, St Louis, MO 63114, USA

Introduction

The nitric oxide and cyclooxygenase pathways share a number of similarities. NO is the mediator generated from the nitric oxide synthase (NOS) pathway. Cyclooxygenase (COX), converts arachidonic acid to the prostaglandins (PG), prostacyclin (PGI$_2$) and thromboxane A$_2$ (TXA$_2$). Two major forms of NOS and COX have been identified to date. Under normal circumstances, the constitutive isoforms of these enzymes are found in virtually all organs. Their presence accounts for the regulation of several important physiological effects (e.g. antiplatelet activity, vasodilation, cytoprotection). On the other hand, in an inflammatory setting, these enzymes are induced in a variety of cells resulting in the production of large amounts of pro-inflammatory and cytotoxic NO and PG. Release of NO and PG by these enzymes has been associated with the pathological roles of these mediators in several disease states. An important link between the NOS and COX pathways was made in 1993 by Salvemini and coworkers [1]. They demonstrated that nitric oxide activated the COX enzymes, leading to overt production of PGs. This in turn exacerbated the inflammatory response. Such studies raised the possibility that COX enzymes might represent important endogenous "receptor" targets for the multifaceted roles of NO [1].

Since then, numerous papers have been published extending the observation across various cellular systems and disease states. More importantly, mechanistic studies of how NO activates these enzymes have been undertaken and additional pathways through which NO modulates PG production unraveled. Finally, evidence has been presented to suggest that peroxynitrite, the reaction product of NO with superoxide anions may be the responsible mediator of COX activation. The purpose of this chapter, is to summarize experimental data pertinent to this topic and to outline (due to space restriction) how this discovery has impacted and extended our understanding of these two systems in physiopathological events.

Nitric Oxide and Inflammation, edited by Daniela Salvemini, Timothy R. Billiar and Yoram Vodovotz
© 2001 Birkhäuser Verlag Basel/Switzerland

Biosynthesis of nitric oxide and prostaglandins

Nitric oxide (NO) is generated *via* the oxidation of the terminal guanidino nitrogen atom of L-arginine by NOS. Three major isoforms of nitric oxide synthase (NOS) have been identified. The three isoforms are distinct from each other based on their primary amino acid sequence (only 50–60% identity), tissue and cellular distribution, and mode of regulation. Two expressed constitutively are calcium/calmodulin-dependent and are classified together as constitutive NOS isoforms (cNOS): endothelial-derived NOS (eNOS) and neuronal-derived NOS (nNOS). The third is a cytokine-inducible, calcium/calmodulin-independent isoform of NOS (iNOS) [2]. The distinct properties of each of the NOS isoforms have important implications since, it is the magnitude, the duration, and the cellular sites of NO production which determine the overall physiological or pathophysiological effect of NO. For example, release of NO from cNOS occurs in small amounts and for a short period of time. NO released under these circumstances plays a crucial role in the cardiovascular system where it controls organ blood flow distribution, inhibits the aggregation and adhesion of platelets to the vascular wall, inhibits leukocyte adhesion and smooth muscle cell proliferation [2]. In contrast, the inducible NOS isoform is not continuously present but is expressed in a wide variety of cells in response to inflammatory stimuli such as cytokines and lipopolysaccharide (LPS). The net result is a delayed (typically 4–6 h), but very prolonged synthesis of high levels of NO. NO released from iNOS is thus involved in several pathological events [2–4].

It is now well recognized that most of the actions of NO are mediated by peroxynitrite ($ONOO^-$) [2–6]. Peroxynitrite is a potent pro-inflammatory and cytotoxic molecule [7-10] generated by the combination of NO with superoxide anions (O_2^-) [11].

The prostaglandins (PGs) are formed by the action of the prostaglandin synthase in a two-step conversion of arachidonic acid. First, the enzyme converts arachidonic acid to a cyclic endoperoxide (PGG_2) by the action of cyclooxygenase (COX) activity, which is then followed by a peroxidase that cleaves the peroxide to yield the endoperoxide (PGH_2) [12]. These unstable intermediate products of arachidonic acid metabolism by COX are then rapidly converted to the prostaglandins (e.g. PGE_2, PGF_2, TXA_2, PGI_2) by specific isomerase enzymes [12]. COX was first purified from the sheep seminal vesicle, a prodigious source of the protein [13–16] as a homodimer of approximate molecular mass of 140 kDa and subsequently cloned from the same tissue [15, 16]. With the availability of the cDNA encoding the protein and specific antibodies, numerous studies were performed to evaluate the distribution, expression, and regulation of COX both *in vitro* and *in vivo*.

Initially, it was thought that COX was a single enzyme that produced prostaglandins in most tissues and cell types. However, a number of studies have illustrated that COX activity is increased in certain inflammatory states and is induced in cells by pro-inflammatory cytokines and growth factors *in vitro* [17–19].

Following these observations, extensive research in this field led to the discovery that two forms of COX exist. The constitutive isoform (COX-1) is present in tissues such as the stomach, gut or kidney, where PG production plays a cytoprotective role in maintaining normal physiological processes [20]. In inflammatory processes, the inducible isoform of cyclooxygenase (COX-2) is expressed in many cells including fibroblasts and macrophages and accounts for the release of large quantities of proinflammatory PG at the site of inflammation [20]. Selective inhibition of COX-2 is anti-inflammatory and inhibits nociception [21, 22].

The nitric oxide synthase and cyclooxygenase systems are often present together, share a number of similarities and play fundamental roles in similar physiopathological conditions [20]. An additional feature that links the NOS and COX pathways is that NO can markedly enhance the production of PG by either activating the enzyme of inducing its expression.

Nitric oxide regulates COX enzymes: direct activation and induction of the enzyme

The discovery that NO regulates COX activity was originally made using cellular systems and purified enzymes. Microsomal sheep vesicles are a rich source of COX-1 and can thus be used to explore whether the exogenous application of NO can augment further COX-1 activity [23]. NO gas directly increases COX-1 activity of microsomal sheep seminal vesicles as well as murine recombinant COX-1; this leads to a remarkable seven-fold increase in PGE_2 formation [1, 24]. COX-2 is also activated by NO. COX-2 but not iNOS is induced in human fetal fibroblast by IL-1β. Therefore IL-1β stimulated fibroblasts can be used as a cellular model to investigate the effects of exogenous NO on COX-2 activity [1]. Exposure of IL-1β stimulated fibroblasts to either NO gas or two NO-donors sodium nitroprusside (SNP) and glyceryl trinitrate (GTN) increased COX-2 activity by at least four-fold; this resulted in increased production of PG. The ability of NO to directly activate COX-2 was supported by the findings that NO increases the activity of purified recombinant COX-2 enzymes. Having observed that NO activates COX-1 and COX-2 enzymes, we then asked the question if COX-2 activity was affected by endogenously produced NO. In this respect, the mouse macrophage cell line RAW-264.7 was stimulated with endotoxin to induce iNOS and COX-2 enzymes. This results in the production of large amounts of NO and PG. Inhibition of iNOS activity by non-selective NOS inhibitors such as N^G-monomethyl-l-arginine methyl ester (L-NMMA) or N^G-nitro-L-arginine (NO_2Arg) or more selective iNOS inhibitors such as L-N^6-(1-iminoethyl)lysine (L-NIL) or aminoguanidine (AG) [25–28] attenuates, as expected, the release of NO from these cells. The remarkable finding was that when NO release was inhibited, there was a simultaneous inhibition of PG release [1]. The NOS inhibitors do not behave as non steroidal anti-inflammatory drugs (NSAIDs) for they do not inhibit COX activity [1, 29, 30]. These results suggested that endogenously released NO from the macrophages exerted a stimulatory action on COX-2 activity enhancing the production of PG. Activation of the enzyme has been observed in various cellular systems [31–36] and is independent of the known effects of NO on the soluble guanylate cyclase. Thus, methylene blue, an inhibitor of the soluble guanylate cyclase inhibited the increase in cGMP by NO in the fibroblast, but did not prevent its ability to stimulate COX activity and hence PG production.

The molecular mechanism by which NO activates COX remains to be identified, but it is unlikely to combine with the ferric heme in COX [37]. A few possibilities can be put forward; these are depicted in Figure 1. (First possibility = antioxidant effect) O_2^- is generated during COX activation and has been postulated to be involved in the auto-inactivation of the COX enzyme [38]. NO interacts with O_2^- and limits the amounts of the radical necessary for auto-inactivation [39]. One possibility could therefore be that NO augments COX activity by acting as an antioxidant (removal of O_2^-) preventing the auto-inactivation of COX. (Second possibility = formation of nitrosothiols) NO nitrosylates cysteine residues in the catalytic domain of COX enzymes leading to the formation of nitrosothiols; these can produce changes in the structure of the enzyme which results in increased catalytic efficiency [40]. (Third possibility = generation of peroxynitrite ONOO⁻, the coupling product of superoxide and nitric oxide). Using purified COX-1 and COX-2 enzymes as well as sheep seminal vesicles, Landino and coworkers reported that ONOO⁻ increased COX-1 and COX-2 activity [41]. Peroxynitrite stimulated COX-1 activity in aortic smooth muscle cells [42]. The mechanisms of action by which PN can activate the enzymes remain to be defined, but could involve either oxidative inactivation [43] or modification of key amino acids residues in the polypetide backbone [44]. At this stage, the relative roles of NO or ONOO⁻ on COX activation remain to be defined, although there is no doubt that both species are involved at least *in vitro*. The relevance for ONOO⁻ as an activator of the COX enzymes *in vivo* has not yet been addressed, mainly because selective inhibitors for peroxynitrite have not been available.

In addition to effects on COX-2 enzyme activity, NO, has been shown to increase the production of PGs from macrophages by acting at a post-transcriptional or translational level to increase COX-2 protein [36]. Subsequent studies using human OA chrondrocytes, NO released from sodium nitroprusside induced cell death, an event associated associated with DNA fragmentation, caspace-3 activation, down-regulation of Bcl-2, overexpression of COX-2 and increased release of PGE_2. These events were abolished by blocking the mitogen-activated protein kinase pathway with the mitogen-activated protein kinase inhibitor PD98059, the p38 kinase inhibitor SB202190 and the COX-2 selective inhibitor NS-398. Interestingly, although, PGE_2 alone had no effect on death, it did sensitize SNP-mediated death. These results suggest that NO activates the extracellular signal-related protein kinase and P38 kinase pathway which in turn induce COX-2 and subsequent

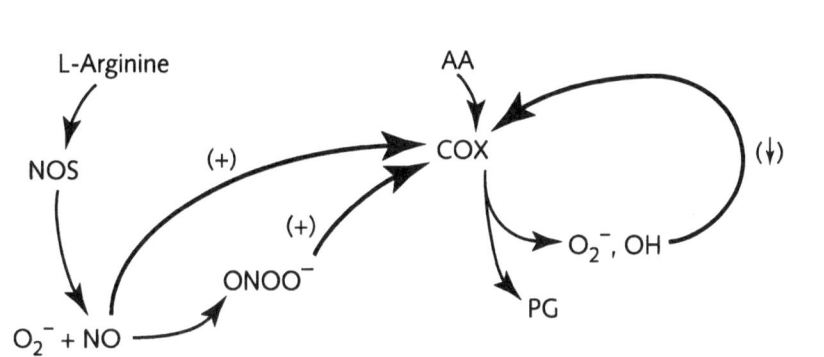

- Inhibition of COX autoinactivation *via* antioxidant property
- Direct activation (e.g., nitrosylation of cysteine residue in catalytic domain)
- Formation of ONOO$^-$

Figure 1
Cyclooxygenase enzymes as potential "receptor" targets for nitric oxide. For simplicity the nitric oxide synthase and cyclooxygenase isoforms are not shown. COX enzymes can be activated through several mechanisms to increase the production of prostaglandins.

PGE_2 release. The latter in turn may sensitize human OA chondrocytes to the cell death induced by NO [45].

NO is also necessary for maintaining prolonged COX-2 gene expression [30] and sustained PGE_2 biosythesis. The NO induced alterations in COX-2 gene expression were not related to COX-2 mRNA [30, 46]. How NO influences COX-2 gene expression is not yet known.

Physiological implications of NO-mediated COX activation

The activation of COX-1 by NO released from the constitutive form of NOS has important consequences in normal physiological conditions. This could indeed represent an important mechanism through which NO and PGs exert their beneficial cytoprotective effects in the cardiovascular system and in the central nervous systems.

The production of small amounts of NO and PGs from the constitutive enzymes regulate various physiological processes including the inhibition of platelet aggregation and white blood cell adhesion, regulation of blood vessel tone, cytoprotection in the kidney and intestinal mucosa. The main difference between the effects of NO and PGs in mediating these effects lies at the level of their respective intracellular transduction mechanisms. Thus, NO activates the soluble guanylate cyclase leading to increased cGMP and PG activate the adenylate cyclase leading to increase in cAMP. This raises the possibility that the increased platelet aggregation, vasoconstriction and elevation of systemic blood pressure induced by inhibition of endogenous NO production by non-selective NOS inhibitors could be due not only to removal of endogenous NO, but also to a concurrent reduction of antiplatelet and vasodilator COX products. Dual inhibition of NO and PG by non-selective NOS inhibitors may well explain the deleterious effects observed with these drugs in organs such as the kidneys and the gastrointestinal tract where both NO and PG are cytoprotective [20, 47].

An interesting effect of NO on COX-1 is perhaps in the regulation of neuropeptide release. Norepinephrine (NE) mediates the release of luteinizing hormone-releasing hormone (LHRH) from LHRH terminals and it is known that LHRH release from these terminals requires increased release of PGE_2 [48]. In an elegant study, Rettori and collegues demonstrated that the release LHRH following NE-stimulated hypothalamic slices was prevented by NOS inhibition and subsequent blockade of NE-mediated PGE_2 release [48]. These results have opened the possibility that through COX activation, NO may mediate exocytosis of secretory granules not only for LHRH, but also for other neuropeptides that are released by PGE_2. NO-driven COX-1 activation also seems to have a role in reproduction in that NO also modulates uterine motility [49] by activating COX-1 and releasing PGE_2. The potential interaction of NO and COX-1 and its implications in reproduction remains an exciting area for future investigation.

Pathological implications of NO-mediated COX activation

In vivo studies revealed that the regulation of COX by NO is a powerful mechanism that is used by NO to amplify the course of the inflammatory response. Indeed, we and others observed that iNOS and COX-2 are induced in a number of inflammatory models including rabbit hydronephrotic kidney [50], endotoxin-induced septic shock [51, 52] and carrageenan-induced pouch and paw inflammation [53–55]. The prolonged release of large amounts of NO and PG may subsequently lead to deleterious effects. Thus, inhibition of either NOS or COX activity is protective in several diseases. The interesting observation was that inhibition of NO by selective iNOS inhibitors is associated with profound inhibition of not only NO, but also of PG release; the anti-inflammatory potency of the iNOS inhibitors correlated with their respective ability to block both NO and PG (see the references cited). For instance, in an acute model of inflammation, namely carrageenan-induced paw edema in rats, inhibition of edema with L-NIL is associated with a dose-dependent inhibition of NO release and a clear inhibition of pro-inflammatory PG [54]. That the proinflammatory roles of NO have a PG component has also been demonstrated by showing that the injection of SNP elicits edema in the footpad of rats and the formation of edema is blocked by NSAID [56]. Therefore, the effects of endogenously released NO on COX-2 are mimicked by exogenous NO. Inhibition of NO in lungs taken from endotoxin-treated rats resulted in an inhibition of PGI_2 release [57]. In acute pancreatis, the increased production of PG was inhibited by NOS inhibitors indicative of the participation of NO in this process [58].

Furthermore, injection of carrageenan into the preformed air pouch of a rat induces an inflammatory response characterised by iNOS and COX-2 induction, white blood cell infiltration, edema and protein leakage into the pouch [53]. Selective inhibition of iNOS by L-NIL and AG inhibited not only NO, but also PG production [53]. All other parameters of inflammation were attenuated and histological examination of the pouch lining taken from animals treated with the iNOS inhibitor revealed a lack of inflammation [53]. In this scenario, we were able to demonstrate that in the presence of L-NIL, COX-2 was activated at least seven-fold by exogenous injection of NO-donors such as sodium nitroprusside or nitroglycerin; this activation resulted in a profound increase in PGE_2 release [53]. Similar results have been observed in the hydronephrotic rabbit model of inflammation [50]. Nonselective NOS inhibitors such as L-NMMA are also anti-inflammatory in these models and block both NO and PG. Nevertheless, when compared to a more selective iNOS inhibitor their antiinflammatory profile is weaker. This may stem from the fact that non-selective NOS inhibitors also block release of NO and PG from the constitutive enzymes which are known to play key cytoprotective roles. This would mask to some degree protective effects that would arise from their inhibitory effects on iNOS. This adds support to the notion that it is imperative to preserve cNOS and COX-1 activity in an inflammatory setting and this can be achieved by the use of glucocorticoids. The potent anti-inflammatory glucocorticoid dexamethasone is a good example of an agent able to inhibit the induction of both iNOS [2] and COX-2 [60]. Selective inhibition of iNOS or COX-2 is also antiinflammatory in a number of models. Besides its proinflammatory role, a feature of NO that is not shared by PG is its potent cytotoxic effect. Although there is some evidence that massive amounts of PGE_2 inhibit the formation of NO [60, 61] the relevance of these observations is questionable. We and others have found that *in vivo* inhibition of PG release by selective inhibition of COX-2 in inflammation has only minimal effects on the NO production, indicating that products of the COX pathway do not play a major role in the regulation of NOS activity. This could explain why in arthritis a NSAIDs such as indomethacin, by blocking PG but not NO production, alleviates the symptoms associated with the inflammatory insult, but does not modify the course of the disease [62]. Since selective iNOS inhibitors have the potential of reducing both NO and PG, it is then exciting to conceive that the utilization of these selective iNOS inhibitors may have the advantage of not only alleviating inflammatory symptoms through dual inhibition of NO and NO-driven COX-2 activation, but would also eliminate further cytotoxic damage of NO which may prove to be important disease modifying drugs in chronic inflammatory diseases such rheumatoid arthritis. Activation of COX pathway by NO was found to have a significant role in PG-mediated bone resoption in inflammatory bone disease processes [63, 64] and potential interactions between the two systems has been extended to osteoarthritis [65].

COX-2 activation by NO may also contribute to ischemic brain injury and possibly other brain diseases associated with inflammation. Thus, Nogawa et al. [66] demonstrated that cerebral ischemia in rats following middle cerebral artery occlusion leads to an induction of iNOS and COX-2. At 24 h after the infarct iNOS immunoreactivity was found in PMNs at close proximity to COX-2 positive cells at the periphery of the infarct. Blockade of iNOS by aminoguanidine reduced the levels of PGE_2 in the infarct where both iNOS and COX-2 were expressed and reduced the extent of the infarct. Role of iNOS on COX-2 expression was confirmed in iNOS knockout mice where less PGE_2 was found when compared to wild type controls [66].

Finally, NO from the neuronal form of the enzyme (expressed in the macula densa) has been shown to regulate renal COX-2 expression seen in volume depletion: this suggests an important interaction between these two pathways in the regulation of arteriolar tone and the rennin-angiotensin system by the macula densa [67].

NO-donors and cyclooxygenase activation: therapeutic implications

The fact that NO activates COX-1 enzyme has given a new dimension to the usefulness of exogenous NO therapy and has uncovered additional mechanisms by which NO-donors might exert their beneficial effects in the clinic. It is known that NO release from clinically useful NO-donors such as GTN or SIN-1 accounts for their vasodilatory and antithrombotic actions and that these properties are pertinent to the therapeutic effects of the NO-donors in conditions such as myocardial ischemia, thrombosis and atherosclerosis that are associated with a failing endogenous NO pathway [68]. For instance, since NO-donors do not require an intact endothelium in order to be effective [69] they can restore the desired vascular dilation and suppress platelet aggregation despite advanced atherosclerosis [70, 71]. The cardiovascular effects exerted by endogenously produced NO are often mediated in conjunction with prostacyclin (PGI_2) a potent vasodilator and platelet inhibitory COX metabolite released from the endothelium. NO released from the NO-donors activates COX-1 *in vitro* in endothelial cells as well as *in vivo* promoting the release of PGI_2 [72, 73]. Activation of COX is a cGMP-independent process.

Our work indicates that the vasodilator and antithrombotic effects of NO (and NO-donors) occur *via* two steps; (a) direct NO-stimulated soluble guanylate cyclase activation and cGMP elevation and (b) NO-mediated activation of cyclooxygenase in the endothelial cells leading to PGI_2 release and cAMP elevation [73]. During the progression of atherosclerosis or hypertension, defects at the level of the soluble guanylate cyclase have been observed. This may theoretically hamper the effectiveness of NO donors in restoring their vasodilator and antithrombotic (cGMP dependent) properties. However, since NO does not have to rely on the soluble guanylate cyclase to activate COX, NO-donors will still be able to provide adequate satisfactory vasodilation and antithrombotic effects (dual increase of NO and PGI_2 locally in the heart). Indeed, the beneficial protective effects of newly developed NO-donors, such as NCX4016, are associated with local delivery of NO and increased release of PGI_2 in the infarcted heart muscle [74].

Inhibition of PG by nitric oxide

A few investigators have reported an inhibitory effect of NO on both the expression and the activity COX in cells including mouse macrophage cell line J774.2, rat Kupffer cells and rat peritoneal macrophages [75–77]. In endotoxin-stimulated J774.2 macrophages sodium nitroprusside inhibits expression of COX-2 as well as its activity and the inhibition of endogenous NO by NOS inhibitor increased PGI_2 release and COX-2 expression [75]. Nevertheless, when these cells were treated first with a NOS inhibitor and then stimulated with a NO-donor, an increased release of PGI_2 was observed, indicative of the ability of NO to increase COX activity [75]. Most of the data collected has been performed in *in vitro* cells or tissue. Overall, the experimental data obtained so far on an inhibitory effect of NO on the COX pathway is controversial and insufficient. Thus the *in vivo* significance of a possible negative effect of NO on COX needs to be assessed in future studies.

Modulation of NO pathway by COX products

Products of the COX pathway may inhibit or increase the release of NO. Large amounts of PGI_2 inhibit LPS-stimulated iNOS induction in J774.2 macrophages or murine peritoneal macrophages [60, 61, 78, 79] perhaps by inhibiting NF-κB activation [80].

A role for PG as enhancers of NO production as been reported. In rat Kupffer cells stimulated with endotoxin, inhibition of endogenously produced PG by indomethacin resulted in a concommittant inhibition of NO release [81]. On the other hand, indomethacin did not inhibit NO release in mouse RAW 264.7 cells [1] nor in J774.2 macrophages [75].

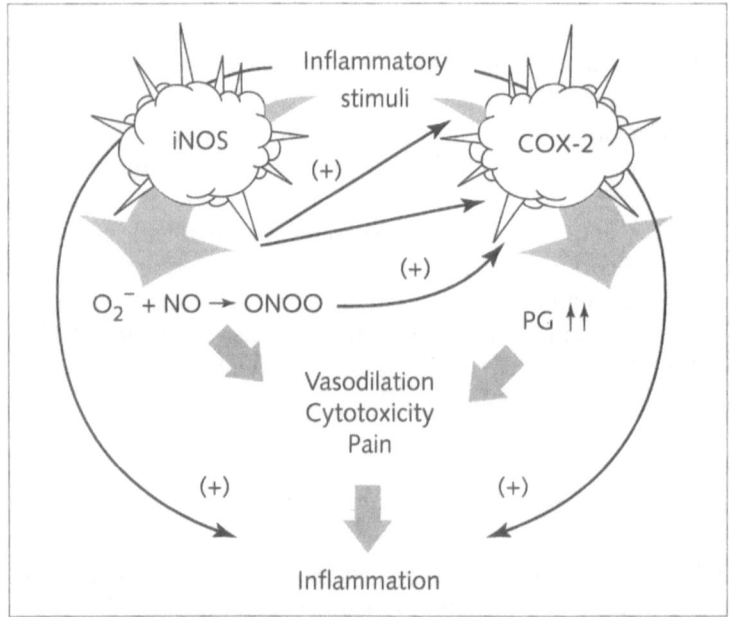

Figure 2
Nitric oxide and reactive oxygen species in inflammation. In those conditions where both the iNOS and COX-2 systems are induced, there is an NO-mediated increase in the production of pro-inflammatory PG resulting in an exacerbated inflammatory response. NO or its by-product, peroxynitrite (ONOO⁻) can increase PGs release by either activating or inducing the COX-2 enzyme. Thus, regulation of COX-2 by NO or peroxynitrite represent a powerful mechanism which amplifies the course of the inflammatory response.

The mechanism of action of the PG on the NOS pathway has been attributed in most instances to activation of adenylate cyclase system with subsequent increase in cyclic AMP (cAMP) levels [78, 79, 82]. For instance, in rat vascular smooth muscle, agents such as forskolin or ditutyrylcAMP increase iNOS mRNA as well as the formation of NO [83, 84].

Again, the experimental data obtained so far on the inhibitory/stimulatory effects of PG on the NOS pathways is controversial and insufficient. The *in vivo* significance of possible effects of PG on the NOS system both in physiology and pathology needs to be evaluated. We and others have found that *in vivo* inhibition of PG release by selective inhibition of COX-2 in inflammation has only minimal effects on the NO production indicating that products of the COX pathway do not play a major role in the regulation of NOS activity.

Conclusions

Compelling data has been generated over the last 9 years supporting the concept that NO plays a major role in the regulation of cyclooxygenase enzyme. NO can thus augment eicosanoid production by acting at several levels. NO activates COX-1 and COX-2 through mechanisms depicted in Figure 2. Furthermore, NO can induce COX-2 expression. Thus, in inflammatory conditions where both the iNOS and COX-2 systems are induced, there is an NO-mediated induction of COX-2 leading to increased formation of pro-inflammatory PG resulting in an exacerbated inflammatory response. Dual inhibition of NO and PGs accounts for the anti-inflammatory effects of nitric oxide synthase inhibitors. Data is also emerging to suggest that peroxynitrite, the product of the reaction between nitric oxide and superoxide, plays an important role in regulating the COX enzymes. At present, we cannot assess the relative contribution of $ONOO^-$ in the overall effects of NO. This area will be expanded as novel and selective inhibitors/catalysts for $ONOO^-$ become available.

The cyclooxygenase enzymes are clearly important "receptor" targets for the action of nitric oxide and other reactive oxygen species such as peroxynitrite: once activated or induced these represent important transduction mechanisms for their multifaceted actions.

The challenge in the future will be to understand the molecular mechanisms used by such species in modifying key steps of the cyclooxygenase pathway as this will undoubtedly elucidate important molecular targets for future pharmacological intervention.

References

1   Salvemini D, Misko TP, Masferrer JL, Seibert K, Currie MG, Needleman P (1993) Nitric oxide activates cyclooxygenase enzymes. *Proc Natl Acad Sci USA* 90: 7240–7244

2   Moncada S, Higgs EA (1995) Molecular mechanisms and therapeutic strategies related to nitric oxide. *FASEB J* 9: 1319–1330

3   Clancy RM, Abramson SB (1995) Nitric oxide: a novel mediator of inflammation. *Proc Soc Exp Biol Med* 23: 93–101

4   Kroncke K-D, Fehsel K, Kolb-Bachofen V (1995) Inducible nitric oxide synthase and its product nitric oxide, a small molecule with complex biological activities. *Biol Chem* 376: 327–343

5   Salvemini D, Jensen MP, Riley DP, Misko TP (1998) Therapeutic manipulations of peroxynitrite. *Drug News and Perspectives* 11: 204–214

6   Szabó C (1999) Nitric oxide, peroxynitrite and poly (ADP-ribose) synthetase: biochemistry and pathophysiological implications. In: GM Rubanyi (ed): *Pathophysiology and clinical applications of nitric oxide*. Harwood Academic Publishers, Newark, NJ, 69–98

7   Beckman JS, Crow JP (1993) Pathological implications of nitric oxide, superoxide and peroxynitrite formation. *Biochem Soc Trans* 21: 330–334

8   Salvemini D, Wang ZQ, Stern, MK, Currie, MG, Misko, TP (1998) Peroxynitrite decomposition catalysts: novel therapeutics for peroxynitrite-mediated pathology. *Proc Natl Acad Sci USA* 95: 2659–2663

9   Misko TP, Highkin MK, Veenhuizen AW, Manning PT, Stern MK, Currie MD, Salvemini D (1998) Characterization of the cytoprotective action of peroxynitrite decomposition catalysts. *J Biol Chem* 273: 15646–15653

10   Salvemini D, Riley DP, Lennon PJ, Wang ZQ, Currie MG, Macarthur H, Misko TP (1999) Protective effects of a superoxide dismutase mimetic and peroxynitrite decomposition catalysts in endotoxin-induced intestinal damage. *Br J Pharmacol* 127: 685–692

11   Beckman JS, Beckman TW, Chen J, Marshall PM, Freeman BA (1990) Apparent hydroxyl radical production by peroxynitrite: implications for endothelial injury from nitric oxide and superoxide. *Proc Natl Acad Sci USA* 87:1620–1624

12   Needleman P, Turk J, Jakschik BA, Morrison AR, Lefkowith JB (1986) Arachidonic acid. *Metabolism Annu Rev Biochem* 55: 69–102

13   Miyamoto T, Ogino N, Yamammoto S, Hayaishi O (1976) Purification of prostaglandin endoperoxide synthetase from bovine vesicular gland microsomes. *J Biol Chem* 251: 2629–2636

14   Van der Ouderaa F, Buyenhek M, Nugteren D, Van Dorp D (1977) Purification and characterisation of prostaglandin endoperoxide synthase from sheep vesicular glands. *Biochim Biophys Acta* 367: 315

15   DeWitt DL, Smith WL (1988) Primary structure of prostaglandin G/H synthase from sheep vesicular gland determined from the complementary DNA sequence *Proc Natl Acad Sci USA* 85: 1412–1416

16   Merlie JP, Fagan D, Mudd J, Needleman P (1988) Isolation and characterization of the complementary DNA for sheep seminal vesicle prostaglandin endoperoxide synthase (cyclooxygenase) *J Biol Chem* 263: 3550–3553

17   Bailey JM, Muza B, Hla T, Salata K (1985) Restoration of prostacyclin synthase in vascular smooth muscle cells after aspirin treatment: regulation by epidermal growth factor. *J Lipid Res* 26: 54–61

18   DeWitt DL (1991) Prostaglandin endoperoxide synthase: regulation of enzyme expression. *Biochim Biophys Acta* 1083: 121–134

19   Sano H, Hla T, Maier JAM, Crofford LJ, Case JP, Maciag T, Wilder RL (1992) *In vivo* cyclooxygenase expression in synovial tissues of patients with rheumatoid arthritis and osteoarthritis and rats with adjuvant and streptococcal cell wall arthritis. *J Clin Invest* 89: 97–10

20   Wu KK (1995) Inducible cyclooxygenase and nitric oxide synthase. *Adv Pharmacol* 33: 179–207

21   Seibert K, Zhang Y, Leahy K, Hauser S, Masferrer JL, Perkins W, Lee L, Isakson P

(1994) Pharmacological and biochemical demonstration of the role of cyclooxygenase 2 in inflammation and pain. *Proc Natl Acad Sci USA* 91: 12013–12017

22 Masferrer JL, Zweifel BS, Manning PT, Hauser SD, Leahy KM, Smith WG, Isakson PC, Seibert K (1994) Selective inhibition of inducible cyclooxygenase 2 *in vivo* is antiinflammatory and nonulcerogenic. *Proc Natl Acad Sci USA* 91: 3228–3232

23 Salvemini D, Masferrer JL (1996) Interactions of nitric oxide with cyclooxygenase: *in vitro*, ex vivo and *in vivo* studies. In: L Packer (ed): *Methods in enzymology*. Academic Press, Inc, San Diego, 269: 15–26

24 Salvemini D, MiskoTP, Masferrer J, Seibert K, Currie MG, Needleman P (1995) In: S Moncada, M Feelish, R Busse (eds): *Biology of nitric oxide, enzymology, biochemistry and immunology*. Portland Press, London, 4: 304–309

25 Corbett JA, Tilton RG, Chang K, Hasan KS, Ido Y, Wang JL, Sweetland MA, Lancaster JR Jr, Williamson JR, McDaniel ML (1992) Aminoguanidine, a novel inhibitor of nitric oxide formation, prevents diabetic vascular dysfunction. *Diabetes* 41: 552–556

26 Misko TP, Moore WM, Kasten TP, Nickols GA, Corbett JA, Tilton RG, McDaniel ML, Williamson JR, Currie MG (1993) Selective inhibition of the inducible nitric oxide synthase by aminoguanidine. *Eur J Pharmacol* 233: 119–125

27 Moore WM, Webber RK, Jerome GM, Tjoeng FS, Misko TP, Currie, MG (1994) L-N[6]-(1-Iminoethyl)lysine: A selective inhibitor of inducible nitric oxide synthase. *J Med Chem* 37: 3886–3888

28 Connor J, Manning PT, Settle SL, Moore WM, Jerome GM, Webber RK, Tjoeng FS, Currie MG (1995) Suppression of adjuvant-induced arthritis by selective inhibition of inducible nitric oxide synthase. *Eur J Pharmacol* 273: 15–24

29 Zingarelli B, Southan GJ, Gilad E, O'Connor M, Salzman AL, Szabo C (1997) The inhibitory effects of mercaptoalkylguanidines on cyclooxygenase activity. *Br J Pharmacol* 120: 357–366

30 Perkins DJ, Kniss DA (1999) Blockade of nitric oxide formation down-regulates cyclooxygenase-2 and decreases PGE_2 biosynthesis in macrophages. *J Leuk Biol* 65: 792–799

31 Corbett JA, Kwon G, Tur J, McDaniel ML (1993) IL1β induces the coexpression of both nitric oxide synthase and cyclooxygenase by islets of langerhans: activation of cyclooxygenase by nitric oxide. *Biochem* 32: 13767–13770

32 Inoue T, Fukuo K, Morimoto S, Koh E, Ogihara T (1993) Nitric oxide mediates interleukin-1-induced prostaglandin E_2 production by vascular smooth muscle cells. *Biochem Biophys Res Commun* 194: 420–424

33 Mollace V, Colasanti V, Rodino P, Lauro GM, Rotiroti D, Nistico G (1995) NMDA-dependent prostaglandin E_2 release by human cultured astroglial cells is driven by nitric oxide. *Biochem Biophys Res Commun* 215: 793–799

34 Misko TP, Trotter JL, Cross AH (1995) Mediation of inflammation by encephalitogenic cells: interferon gamma induction of nitric oxide and cyclooxygenase 2. *J Neuroimmunol* 61: 195–204

35 Watkins DN, Garlepp MJ, Thompson PJ (1997) Regulation of the inducible cyclo-oxy-

genase pathway in human culture airway epithelial (A549) cells by nitric oxide. *Br J Pharm* 121: 1482–1488

36 Von Knethen A, Brune, B (1997) Cyclooxygenase-2: an essential regulator of NO-mediated apoptosis. *FASEB J* 11: 887–895

37 Tsai AL, Wei C, Kulmacz RJ (1994) Interaction between nitric oxide and prostaglandin H synthase. *Arch Biochem Biophys* 313: 367–372

38 Egan RW, Paxton J, Kuehl FA, Jr (1976) Mechanism for irreversible self-deactivation of prostaglandin synthetase. *J Biol Chem* 251: 7329–7335

39 Gryglweski RJ, Palmer RMJ, Moncada S (1987) Superoxide anion is involved in the breakdown of endothelium-derived vascular relaxing factor. *Nature* 320: 454–456

40 Hajjar DP, Lander HM, Pearce FS, Upmacis RK, Pomerantz KB (1995) Nitric oxide enhances prostaglandin-H synthase activity by a heme-independent mechanism: evidence implicating nitrosothiols. *J Am Chem Soc* 117: 3340–3346

41 Landino LM, Crews BC, Timmons MD, Morrow JD, Marnett LJ (1996) Peroxynitrite, the coupling product of nitric oxide and superoxide, activates prostaglandin biosynthesis *Proc Natl Acad Sci USA* 93: 15069–15074

42 Upmacis RK, Deeb RS, Hajjar DP (1999) Regulation of prostaglandin H_2 synthase activity by nitrogen oxides. *Biochemistry* 38: 12505–12513

43 Markey CM, Alward A, Weller PE, Marnett LJ (1987) Quantitative studies of hydroperoxide reduction by prostaglandin H synthase Reducing substrate specificity and the relationship of peroxidase to cyclooxygenase activities. *J Biol Chem* 262, 6266–6279

44 Alvarez B, Ferrer-Sueta G, Freeman BA, Radi R (1999) Kinetics of peroxynitrite reaction with amino acids and human serum albumin. *J Biol Chem* 274: 842–848

45 Notoya K, Jovanovic DV, Reboul P, Martel-Pelletier J, Mineau F, Pelletier JP (2000) The induction of cell death in human osteoarthritis chondrocytes by nitric oxide is related to the production of prostaglandin E_2 *via* the induction of cyclooxygenase-2. *J Immunol* 165: 3402–3410

46 Tetsuka T, Daphna-Iken D, Miller BW, Guan Z, Baier LD, Morrison AR (1996) Nitric oxide amplifies interleukin1-induced cyclooxygenase-2 expression in rat mesangial cells. *J Clin Invest* 97: 2051–2056

47 Salvemini D, Marino MH (1998) Inducible nitric oxide synthase and inflammation. *Exp Opin Invest Drugs* 7: 65–75

48 Rettori V, Gimeno M, Lyson K, McCann SM (1992) Nitric oxide mediates norepinephrine-induced prostaglandin E_2 release from the hypothalamus. *Proc Natl Acad Sci USA* 89: 11543–11546

49 Franchi AM, Chaud M, Rettori V, Suburu A, McCann SM, Gimeno M (1994) Role of nitric oxide in eicosanoid synthesis and uterine motility in estrogen-treated rat uteri. *Proc Natl Acad Sci USA* 91: 539–543

50 Salvemini D, Seibert K, Masferrer JL, Misko TP, Currie MG, Needleman P (1994) Endogenous nitric oxide enhances prostaglandin production in a model of renal inflammation. *J Clin Invest* 93: 1940–1947

51 Salvemini D, Settle SL, Masferrer JL, Seibert K, Currie MG, Needleman P (1995) Reg-

ulation of prostaglandin production by nitric oxide; an *in vivo* analysis. *Br J Pharmacol* 114: 1171–1178

52 Swaisgood CM, Zu HX, Perkins DJ, Wu S, Garver C, Zimmerman PD, Iams JD, Kniss DA (1997) Coordinate expression of inducible nitric oxide synthase and cyclooxygenase-2 genes in uterine tissues of endotoxin-treated mice. *Am J Obstet Gynecol* 177: 1253–1262

53 Salvemini D, Manning PT, Zweifel BS, Seibert K, Connor J, Currie MG, Needleman P, Masferrer JL (1995) Dual inhibition of nitric oxide and prostaglandin production contributes to the antiinflammatory properties of nitric oxide synthase inhibitors. *J Clin Invest* 96: 301–308

54 Salvemini D, Wang ZQ, Wyatt PS, Bourdon DM, Marino MH, Manning PT, Currie MJ (1996) Nitric oxide: a key mediator in the early and late phase of carrageenan-induced rat paw inflammation. *Br J Pharmacol* 118: 829–838

55 Vane JR, Mitchell JA, Appleton I, Tomlinson A, Bishop-Bailey D, Croxtall J, Willoughby DA (1994) Inducible isoforms of cyclooxygenase and nitric-oxide synthase in inflammation. *Proc Natl Acad Sci USA* 91: 2046–2050

56 Sautebin L, Ialenti A, Ianaro A, Di Rosa M (1995) Modulation by nitric oxide of prostaglandin biosynthesis in the rat. *Br J Pharmacol* 114: 323–328

57 Sautebin L, Di Rosa M (1994) Nitric oxide modulates prostacyclin biosynthesis in the lung of endotoxin-treated rats. *Eur J Pharmacol* 262: 193–196

58 Closa D, Hotter G, Prats N, Bulbena O, Rosello-Catafau J, Fernandez-Cruz L, Gelpi E (1994) Prostanoid generation in early stages of acute pancreatis: a role for nitric oxide. *Inflammation* 18: 469–480

59 Masferrer JL, Seibert K (1994) Regulation of prostaglandin synthesis by glucocorticoids. *Receptor* 94: 25–30

60 Marotta P, Sautebin L, Di Rosa M (1992) Modulation of the induction of nitric oxide synthase by eicosanoids in the murine macrophage cell line J774. *Br J Pharmacol* 107: 640–641

61 Milano S, Arcoleo F, Dieli M, D'Agostino R, D'Agostino P, De Nucci G, Cillari, E (1995) Prostaglandin E$_2$ regulates inducible nitric oxide synthase in the murine macrophage cell line J774. *Prostaglandins* 49: 105–115

62 Flynn BL (1994) Rheumatoid arthritis and osteoarthritis: current and future therapies. *Am Pharm* NS 34: 31–42

63 Hughes FJ, Buttery LDK, Hukkanen MVJ, O'Donnell A, Maclouf J, Polak JM (1999) Cytokine-induced prostaglandin E$_2$ synthesis and cyclooxygenase-2 activity are regulated both by a nitric oxide-dependent and -independent mechanism in rat osteoblasts *in vitro*. *J Biol Chem* 274: 1776–1782

64 Kanematsu M, Ikeda K, Yamada Y (1997) Interaction between nitric oxide synthase and cyclooxygenase pathways in osteoblastic MC3T3-E1 cells. *J Bone Min Res* 12: 1789–1796

65 Needleman P, Manning PT (1999) Interactions between the inducible cyclooxygenase

(COX-2) and nitric oxide synthase (iNOS) pathways: implications for therapeutic intervention in osteoarthritis. *Osteoarthritis and Cartilage* 7: 367–370

66   Nogawa S, Forster C, Zhang F, Nagayama M, Ross ME, Iadecola C (1998) Interaction between inducible nitric oxide synthase and cyclooxygenase-2 after cerebral ischemia. *Proc Natl Acad Sci USA* 95:10966–10971

67   Cheng HF, Wang JL, Zhang MZ, McKanna JA, Harris RC (2000) Nitric oxide regulates renal cortical cyclooxygenase-2 expression. *Am J Physiol Renal Physiol* 279: F122–F1229

68   Anggard EE (1991) Endogenous nitrates-implications for treatment and prevention. *Eur Heart J* 12: 5–8

69   Luscher TF, Richard V,Yang Z (1990) Interaction between endothelium-derived nitric oxide and SIN-1 in human and porcine blood vessels. *J Cardiovasc Pharmacol* 14: 76–80

70   Parker JO (1987) Nitrate therapy in stable angina pectoris. *N Eng J Med* 31: 1635-1642

71   Stamler JS, Loscalzo J (1991) The antiplatelet effects of organic nitrates and related nitrous compounds *in vitro* and *in vivo* and their relevance to cardiovascular disorders. *J Am Coll Cardiol* 18: 1529–1536

72   Davidge ST, Baker PN, Mclaughlin MK, Roberts JM (1995) Nitric oxide produced by endothelial cells increases production of eicosanoids through activation of prostaglandin H synthase. *Circ Res* 77: 274–283

73   Salvemini D, Currie MG, Mollace V (1996) Nitric oxide-mediated cyclooxygenase activation A key event in the antiplatelet effects of nitrovasodilators *J Clin Invest* 97: 2562–2568

74   Yamamoto T, Kakar NR, Vina ER, Johnson PE, Bing RJ (2000) The effect of aspirin and two nitric oxide donors on the infarcted heart *in situ*. *Life Sci* 67: 839–846

75   Swierkosz TA, Mitchell JA, Warner TD, Botting RM, Vane R (1995) Co-induction of nitric oxide synthase and cyclooxygenase: interactions between nitric oxide and prostanoids. *Br J Pharmacol* 114: 1335–1342

76   Stadler J, Harbrecht BC, DiSilvio M, Curran RD, Jordan ML, Simmons RL, Billiar TR (1993) Endogenous nitric oxide inhibits the synthesis of cyclooxygenase products and interleukin-6 by rat Kuppfer cells. *J Leukocyte Biol* 53: 165–172

77   Habib A, Bernard C, Tedgui A, Maclouf J (1994) Evidence of cross-talks between inducible nitric oxide synthase and cyclooxygenase II in rat peritoneal macrophages. Abstracts of the 9th International Conference on Prostaglandins and Related Compounds, Florence (Italy), June 6–10: 57

78   Raddassi K, Petit JF, Lemaire G (1993) LPS-induced activation of primed murine peritoneal macrophages is modulated by prostaglandins and cyclic nucleotides. *Cell Immunol* 149: 50–64

79   Bulut V, Severn A, Liew FY (1993) Nitric oxide production by murine macrophages is inhibited by prolonged elevation of cyclic AMP. *Biochem Biophy Res Commun* 195: 1134–1138

80   D'Acquisto F, Sautebin L, Iuvone T, Di Rosa M, Carnuccio, R (1998) Prostaglandins

prevent inducible nitric oxide synthase protein expression by inhibiting nuclear factor-κB activation in J774 macrophages. *FEBS Letters* 440: 76–80

81 Gaillard T, Mulsch A, Klein H, Decker K (1992) Regulation by prostaglandin E_2 of cytokine-elicited nitric oxide synthesis in rat liver macrophages. *Biol Chem* 373: 897–902

82 Pang L, Hoult JRS (1997) Repression of inducible nitric oxide synthase and cyclooxygenase-2 by prostaglandin E_2 and other cyclic AMP stimulants in J774 macrophages. *Biochem Pharm* 53: 493–500

83 Ima T, Hirata, Y, Kanno K, Marumo F (1994) Induction of nitric oxide synthase by cyclic AMP in rat vascular smooth muscle cells. *J Clin Invest* 93: 543–549

84 Hirokawa K, O'Shaughnessy K, Moore K, Ramrakha P, Wilkins MR (1994) Induction of nitric oxide synthase in cultured vascular smooth muscle cells: the role of cyclic AMP. *Br J Pharmacol* 112: 396–402

Local and systemic inflammation: role of poly (ADP-ribose) synthetase activation by reactive nitrogen species

Jon Mabley[1], Lucas Liaudet[1,2], Francisco Garcia Soriano[1,2,3], László Virág[1], Prakash Jagtap[1], Anita Marton[1], Clara Batista Lorigados[3], Ferenc Gallyas[4], Éva Szabó[1], Galaleldin E. Abdelkarim[1], György Haskó[1,2], Garry J. Southan[1], Andrew L. Salzman[1] and Csaba Szabó[1,2]

[1]Inotek Corporation, Suite 419E, 100 Cummings Center, Beverly, MA 01915, USA; [2]Department of Surgery, New Jersey Medical School, UMDNJ, Newark, NJ 01703, USA; [3]Hospital das Clinicas FMUSP3, Saõ Paulo, SP, Brazil; [4]Department of Biochemistry, Pécs University Medical School, Pécs, Hungary

Poly (ADP)-ribosyltransferase (PARS): a nuclear enzyme with multiple functions

Poly (ADP)-ribosyltransferase (PARS), also known as poly(ADP-ribose) polymerase (PARP) is an abundant nuclear enzyme present throughout the phylogenetic spectrum [1]. The precise physiologic roles of PARS remain undefined: its traditional role as a DNA-repair enzyme has been questioned by recent studies [2]. PARS appears to play diverse roles, participating in DNA repair [3, 4], chromatin relaxation [5], cell differentiation [6], DNA replication [7], transcriptional regulation [8], control of cell cycle [9], p53 expression and apoptosis [10], and transformation [11]. In the last decade, the novel concept emerges that under various pathophysiological conditions, PARS plays a crucial role in the regulation and generation of the inflammatory response. Here, we summarize the evidence favoring this new role for PARS in various forms of local and systemic inflammation and propose therapeutic opportunities afforded by PARS inhibition.

Role of nitric oxide-derived reactive species, oxidative stress and peroxynitrite in stimulating PARS

Free radicals and oxidants are formed by parenchymal cells and infiltrating leukocytes, in various pathophysiological conditions of local and systemic inflammation. Nitrogen and oxygen centered free radicals and oxidants play key roles as effectors of tissue injury. In addition, oxidants are generated by the conversion of oxygen-centered free radicals to hydrogen peroxide and hydroxyl radical and by the inter-

Nitric Oxide and Inflammation, edited by Daniela Salvemini, Timothy R. Billiar and Yoram Vodovotz

action of superoxide anion and nitric oxide to form peroxynitrite. All of these species are formed during inflammation and play varied roles in the activation of PARS and the mediation of tissue damage.

Nitric oxide (NO) is synthesized from the guanidino group of L-arginine by a family of enzymes termed NO synthases (NOS). Three isoforms have been described and cloned: endothelial cell NOS (eNOS), brain NOS (bNOS), and an inducible macrophage type NOS (iNOS) [12]. Whereas eNOS is responsible for many physiological effects (e.g. maintaining basal vasodilator tone, inhibiting platelet and neutrophil adhesion and activation), many pathophysiological conditions are associated with the production of *large amounts* of NO, produced by the inducible isoform of NOS (iNOS), with consequent cytotoxic effects [13, 14]. The inducible isoform of NO synthase (iNOS), which generates NO for longer periods of time (several hours to days) and at rates several orders of magnitude greater than the constitutive isoforms [15], is not present in most tissues to any significant extent under resting conditions, but the enzyme is newly synthesized in response to infection and proinflammatory cytokines. Upregulation of NO synthesis has been associated with functional derangements in multiple cell types [12, 13].

The oxygen-centered free radical superoxide anion appears to play a major role in the pathogenesis of inflammatory injury [14–24]. Superoxide anion is generated by xanthine oxidase (XO) and NADPH oxidase from the partial reduction of molecular oxygen. Neutrophils and macrophages are known to produce superoxide free radicals and hydrogen peroxide, which normally are involved in the killing of ingested or invading microbes [25]. Under physiological conditions XO is ubiquitously present in the form of a dehydrogenase (XDH). In mammals, XDH is converted from the NAD-dependent dehydrogenase form to the oxygen-dependent oxidase form, either by reversible sulfhydryl oxidation or irreversible proteolytic modification [26]. XO then no longer uses NAD^+ as an electron acceptor, but transfers electrons onto oxygen, generating superoxide radical, peroxide, and hydroxyl radical as purines are degraded to uric acid [27, 28]. Inflammatory activation converts XDH to XO, mainly by oxidizing structurally important sulfhydryls. Inflammation also markedly upregulates the conversion of xanthine dehydrogenase [29].

XO levels increase during various types of inflammation (> 400-fold in bronchoalveolar fluid in pneumonitis), ischemia-reperfusion injury, and atherosclerosis [30, 31]. Plasma levels of XO, due to the spillover of tissue XO into the circulation, may be detected in adult respiratory distress syndrome, ischemia-reperfusion injury, arthritis, sepsis, hemorrhagic shock, and other inflammatory conditions [21–25]. Inflammatory-induced histamine release by mast cells and basophils lowers the Km values for XO substrates, thereby enhancing the activity of XO [23]. Oxygen radicals are involved in the microvascular and parenchymal cell injury associated with organ transplant rejection, circulatory shock, stroke, myocardial infarction, zymosan-induced systemic inflammation, intestinal ischemia, and auto-immune disease [14–25]. Superoxide is also readily catalyzed to form the oxidants hydrogen peroxide and hydroxyl radical, which mediate cellular injury to a greater extent than superoxide anion per se. In addition, superoxide readily reacts in a diffusion-limited manner with the nitrogen-centered free radical NO, producing peroxynitrite. Although all oxidants have been implicated in DNA strand breakage, and subsequent activation of PARS, the role of peroxynitrite has received particular attention in various inflammatory processes.

In vitro and *in vivo* data demonstrate that NO and superoxide anion are probably not the most relevant final effector species in a variety of forms of inflammatory injury [26–50]. Peroxynitrite, a potent oxidant anion formed from their interaction, appears rather to be the proximate cause of cytotoxicity and tissue injury. Peroxynitrite is formed in inflammatory conditions such as inflammatory bowel disease, as well as other inflammatory disorders, as evidenced by the formation of nitrotyrosine, a product of the reaction of peroxynitrite with tyrosine residues [31]. Peroxynitrite has been shown to have a wide variety of toxic actions, including damage to membranes, oxidation of intracellular proteins, and nitrosation of critical tyrosine residues. Both exogenous and endogenously generated peroxynitrite have also been shown to potently induce DNA strand breaks in a variety of cell types, including macrophages [26], vascular smooth muscle cells [30], pulmonary epithelial cells [32], and intestinal epithelial cells [33] (Fig. 1). In contrast to the potent effects of peroxynitrite on the production of DNA single strand breaks, its precursor NO has no such effects [30–33]. The existence of DNA single strand breaks has now been confirmed in experimental models of inflammation, and in the clinical setting. In colonic biopsies of patients with ulcerative colitis, for example, there are significantly increased levels of 8-hydroxyguanine, 2-hydroxyadenine, 8-hydroxyadenine and 2,6-diamino-5-formamido-pyrimidine [34, 35], providing indirect evidence of DNA injury.

DNA single strand breakage: the trigger of PARS activation in inflammation

Under basal conditions *in vivo*, PARS activity is relatively quiescent. Under conditions of redox stress, the N-terminal domain of PARS recognizes oxidant-induced DNA single strand breaks, resulting in a conformational change that activates its C-terminal catalytic domain [36]. Activated PARS cleaves the substrate NAD^+ into ADP-ribose and nicotinamide. During this process, PARS covalently attaches ADP-ribose to various proteins, including an auto-modification domain of PARS itself, and then extends the initial ADP-ribose group into a branched nucleic acid-like homopolymer, poly(ADP) ribose [36]. Simultaneously, poly-ADP ribose is degraded by various nuclear enzymes, including poly ADP-ribose glycohydrolase. The catalysis of poly ADP-ribose results in depletion of NAD, inhibition of glycolysis and mitochondrial respiration, and the ultimate reduction of intracellular high energy phosphates [26, 30, 33, 37, 48, 49]. The coincident activities of PARS and poly

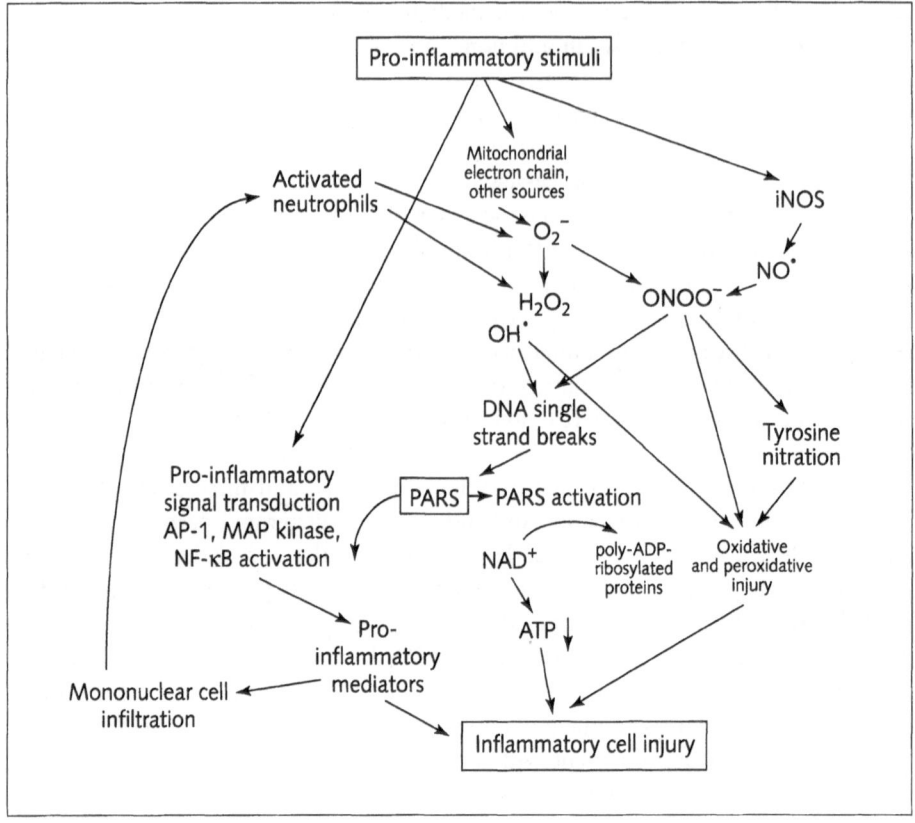

Figure 1
Proposed scheme of PARS-dependent and PARS-independent cytotoxic pathways involving nitric oxide (NO•), hydroxyl radical (OH•) and peroxynitrite (ONOO−) in local and systemic inflammation. Pro-inflammatory stimuli trigger the release of proinflammatory mediators, which, in turn, induce the expression of the inducible NO synthase (iNOS). NO, in turn, combines with superoxide to yield peroxynitrite. Hydroxyl radical (produced from superoxide via the iron-catalyzed Haber-Weiss reaction) and peroxynitrite or peroxynitrous acid induce the development of DNA single strand breakage, with consequent activation of PARS. Depletion of the cellular NAD+ leads to inhibition of cellular ATP-generating pathways leading to cellular dysfunction. NO alone does not induce DNA single strand breakage, but may combine with superoxide (produced from the mitochondrial chain or from other cellular sources) to yield peroxynitrite. Under conditions of low cellular L-arginine NOS may produce both superoxide and NO, which then can combine to form peroxynitrite. PARS activation, via a not yet characterized fashion, promotes the activation of NF-κB, AP-1, MAP kinases, and the expression of pro-inflammatory mediators, adhesion molecules, and of iNOS. PARS-independent, parallel pathways of cellular metabolic inhibition can be activated by NO, hydroxyl radical, superoxide and by peroxynitrite.

ADP-ribose glycohydrolase may be regarded functionally as an NADase. Loss of intracellular energetic stores has deleterious consequences on a broad range of cellular activities, that may be substantially delayed (hours) from the time of oxidant exposure.

This PARS-dependent loss of intracellular energetics and cellular function has been well demonstrated in studies of multiple cell types. It appears that the mechanism by which PARS activation leads to cell death is related to the triggering of cell necrosis (rather than apoptosis), which occurs because of the severe energetic crisis of the cell [47–49] (Fig. 1). In fact, pharmacological inhibition of PARS shifts the necrotic cell population into the normal, as well as the apoptotic population, as determined by flow cytometry studies in thymocytes exposed to peroxynitrite or hydrogen peroxide [47–49]. The shift of cell death from necrotic to apoptotic, in the absence of functional PARS, is considered beneficial, for necrotic cells (but not apoptotic cells) release their content into the extracellular space, thereby further triggering the inflammatory process. Recently, we investigated the role PARS in intestinal epithelial barrier function, an active process that is highly dependent upon cellular ATP concentration [50]. Exposure of human Caco-2BBe enterocyte cell monolayers to peroxynitrite rapidly induced DNA strand breaks and triggered an energy consuming pathway catalyzed by PARS [33]. The consequent reduction of cellular stores of ATP and NAD^+ was associated with the development of hyperpermeability of the epithelial monolayer to a fluorescent anionic tracer. Pharmacological inhibition of PARS activity had no effect on the development of peroxynitrite-induced DNA single strand breaks, but attenuated the decrease in intracellular stores of NAD and ATP and the functional loss of intestinal barrier function. Similar studies, in which peroxynitrite has been generated by the endogenous production of superoxide anion and nitric oxide, have implicated PARS activation as a major pathway of oxidant-induced cellular necrosis.

PARS as a regulator of pro-inflammatory signaling pathways

Initial studies of the role of PARS in experimental models of disease focused on its effects on intracellular energetics and resultant cellular dysfunction. In the last several years, however, a new series of *in vivo* investigations has revealed that inhibition of PARS activation, or its genetic deficiency, has unexpected actions in oxidant-driven diseases that are not associated with reperfusion injury. These effects, which are demonstrated in a broad range of inflammatory conditions, appear to be related to the effect of PARS on the expression, activation, and nuclear translocation of key pro-inflammatory genes and proteins. The absence of PARS or its pharmacologic inhibition has been shown to suppress the activation of MAP kinase [41], AP-1 complex [51], and NF-κB [52, 53]. Consequently, PARS inhibition interferes with the expression of pro-inflammatory genes, such as iNOS and ICAM-1, that are

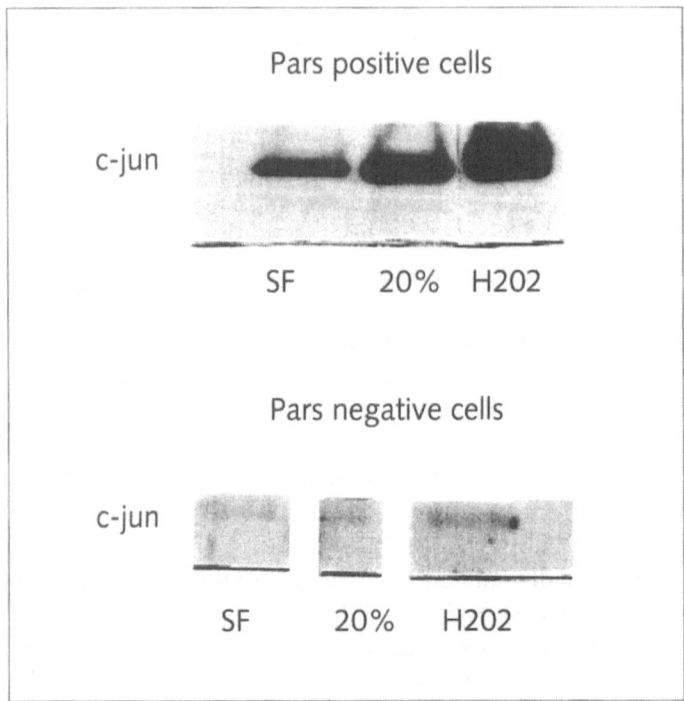

Figure 2
Fibroblasts lacking PARS do not induce c-jun in response to 20% serum stimulation or
100 µM hydrogen peroxide. SF = serum-free medium. Similar results were observed when
IL-1β was used to stimulate c-jun (not shown). Data shown are representative of n = 3
independent experiments.

dependent upon these signaling pathways [52–55]. These observations have been revealed in *in vitro* systems, examining a broad range of cell types, and in various experimental models of inflammation [52–61].

In an experimental model of enterocolitis, PARS knock-out mice have marked suppression of inflammatory-induced upregulation of ICAM-1 expression [54]. PARS inhibition also blocks ICAM-1 expression in cultured endothelial cells stimulated *in vitro* by a combination of pro-inflammatory cytokines [54]. PARS inhibition suppresses the expression of the chemokine MIP-1α in immunostimulated macrophages and fibroblasts *in vitro* (Fig. 2). We have also observed that PARS inhibition attenuates IL-1β mediated induction of C3 in cultured intestinal enterocytes (unpublished observations). Since C3 is an early component of the complement pathway that generates the potent chemotaxin C5a, PARS inhibition may reduce neutrophil recruitment into inflammatory foci. Experimental evidence indeed

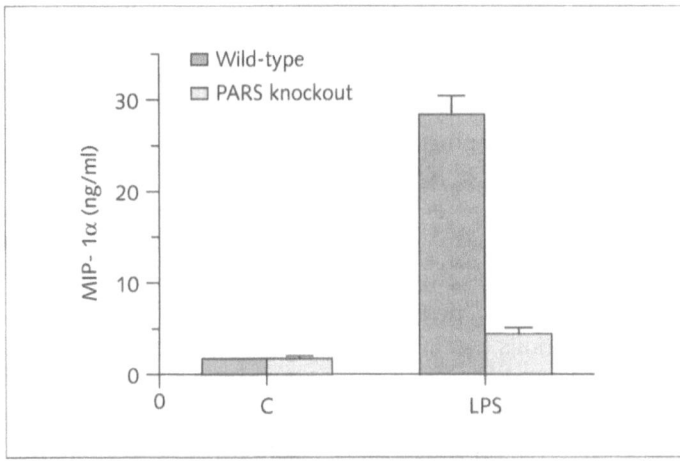

Figure 3

Effect of PARS negative phenotype on the production of MIP-1α in response to stimulation by LPS (10 ng/ml) in RAW macrophages. The production of MIP-1α increased from 1.5 ± 0.1 ng/ml to 28.1 ± 2.2 ng/ml in response to LPS. PARS negative phenotype decreased MIP-1α release induced by LPS. There was a significant suppression of LPS-induced MIP-1α production in the absence of functional PARS (p < 0.01; n = 8).

demonstrates that PARS inhibition suppresses neutrophil infiltration in experimental models of endotoxicosis, carrageenan-induced pleurisy, and splanchnic ischemia-reperfusion injury [39, 40, 54, 55].

The regulation by PARS of gene expression may involve the poly-ADP ribosylation of transcription factors or by the repair of DNA strand breaks which interfere with transcription. PARS may also alter the activation of pro-inflammatory pathways *via* its influence on the expression of AP-1, a heterodimer composed of *c-fos* and *jun* factors. High levels of transcriptional activation of human ICAM-1, C3, and *c-fos* require AP-1 binding to 5' flanking regulatory regions [51]. In cultured cells PARS inhibition blocks oxidant-induced *c-fos* mRNA expression and AP-1 activation (Fig. 3) [8]. Since the *c-fos* promoter contains an AP-1 consensus site, *c-fos* activation could trigger a positive-feedback cycle of gene expression. Superoxide anion has also been reported to induce the post-translational poly ADP-ribosylation of *c-fos* [51].

PARS inhibition attenuates LPS and gamma interferon induced iNOS expression in fibroblasts [58], pancreatic beta islet cells [59] and macrophages [60]. Similar anti-inflammatory effects have been noted *in vitro* in murine macrophages and *in vivo* in rats. PARS inhibition has been shown, for example, to suppress endotoxin-induced expression of TNFα, IL-6 and iNOS [41, 53] and to elevate the expression of the anti-inflammatory cytokine IL-10 [41]. These effects are associated with the suppression of LPS-mediated induction of NF-κB activation [53] and of MAP kinase activity [41]. Since MAP kinase plays a major role in the pleiotropic transduction of intracellular inflammatory cascades, the anti-inflammatory effects of PARS inhibition may be accounted for at this level of gene regulation. One may also expect that PARS-dependent regulation of NF-κB activation has a pleiotropic effect on the expression of pro-inflammatory genes, given the broad role that NF-κB plays in the transcriptional activation of cytokine and chemokine genes. A microchip analysis study recently completed has investigated the changes in the expression of 15,000 genes in wild-type and PARS deficient fibroblasts. The study has demonstrated that under baseline conditions (i.e. in the absence of specific pro-inflammatory stimuli), there is a significant alteration in the expression of a whole host of genes [62]. It is expected that even more significant differences will be found in immunostimulated cells. However, systematic survey experiments comparing gene expression in immunostimulated wild-type and PARS deficient cells using the microchip method, have, to our knowledge, not yet been performed.

Role of PARS activation in local inflammatory responses

The effect of PARS inhibition, or PARS deficiency, on the expression of pro-inflammatory genes and signaling pathways *in vitro* led us to explore the potential role of PARS activation on *in vivo* inflammation. These studies have included a broad range of models, ranging from carrageenan-induced paw edema, colitis, arthritis, and endotoxic shock. Pharmacologic studies, using diverse inhibitors, have consistently supported data from murine gene deletion models, providing strong support for the role of PARS in the inflammatory process. Our data clearly demonstrate that PARS activation is a critical regulatory step in these experimental models of inflammatory injury.

To confirm that PARS plays a relevant role in intestinal inflammatory injury and dysfunction, we evaluated the biological effect of *in vivo* pharmacological inhibition of PARS activity in a rat model of trinitrobenzenesulfonic acid (TNBS)-induced colitis, a classic model of hapten-induced autoimmune inflammatory bowel disease. Treatment with the PARS inhibitor 3-AB reduced tissue injury, as evaluated by the improvement in histology and body weight, reduction in colonic myeloperoxidase activity and prostaglandin levels, and preserved ATP concentration. The cecum, colon and rectum showed evidence on gross examination of mucosal congestion, erosion, and hemorrhagic ulcerations 4 days after intracolonic administration of TNBS. The histopathological features included transmural necrosis and edema and a diffuse leukocytic cellular infiltrate in the submucosa. Inhibition of PARS activation by intraperitoneal administration of 3-AB decreased the extent and severity of the colonic damage. The inflammation of the intestinal tract was also accompanied by a significant loss in body weight in comparison to control rats. PARS inhibition significantly reduced the loss in body weight, which correlated well with the amelioration of colonic injury. Treatment with 3-AB reduced leukocytic infiltration and the elevation of 6-keto-PGF$_{1\alpha}$ levels, indicative of activation of the inflammatory response by cyclooxygenase. Treatment with 3-AB also reduced the extent of ATP depletion in colonic tissue [54].

In a subsequent study, PARS$^{-/-}$ mice and their littermate wild-type controls were subjected to colitis by intraluminal administration of TNBS/ethanol, a procedure that induces colonic epithelial injury with ulceration in mice. PARS$^{+/+}$ mice appeared markedly more sensitive to the injurious effects of TNBS: all developed bloody diarrhea, 50% died within 4 days, and 78% within 7 days after TNBS administration. In contrast, PARS$^{-/-}$ mice appeared healthy, with a very mild diarrhea; only 20% died within 7 days. Weight loss was more pronounced in wild-type than in PARS$^{-/-}$ mice. 4 days after TNBS treatment there were multiple sites of grossly visible colonic mucosal congestion, erosion, and hemorrhagic ulcerations in wild-type animals, whereas the colon of most of the TNBS-treated PARS$^{-/-}$ mice was indistinguishable from those of mice treated with 50% ethanol only. At the histologic level, TNBS-treated wild-type mice evidenced mucosal erosions, edema, large stretches of denuded epithelia, and a diffuse leukocyte infiltration in the submucosa. The histological features of TNBS-treated PARS$^{-/-}$ mice were typical of normal or healing mucosa with an intact epithelium [54]. Colonic injury in PARS$^{+/+}$ animals was also associated with increased neutrophil infiltration into the inflamed tissue [54]. The level of myeloperoxidase activity, a marker of neutrophil infiltration, paralleled the increase of tissue malondialdehyde, an indicator of lipid peroxidation. A positive staining for nitrotyrosine, a marker of nitrosative injury, was present throughout the inflamed colon in PARS$^{+/+}$ animals [54]. TNBS-treated PARS$^{-/-}$ mice had substantially less infiltration of neutrophils and formation of malondialdehyde and nitrotyrosine [64].

The diminished neutrophil infiltration in the PARS$^{+/+}$ animals implicated PARS in the regulation of pro-inflammatory signaling pathways. In support of this concept, TNBS-treated wild-type mice showed immunoreactivity for the neutrophil adhesion molecule ICAM-1 in the endothelium in the submucosal vasculature [54]. In contrast, TNBS-treated PARS$^{-/-}$ mice did not reveal upregulated expression of ICAM-1, which was constitutively expressed in the endothelium along the vascular wall [54]. Thus, PARS activation appears to mediate neutrophil recruitment *via* its effect on the expression of adhesion molecules.

In addition to the TNBS models described above, pharmacological inhibition of PARS also exerts protective effects in dextran sulfate induced colitis (unpublished data), and in the spontaneous autoimmune colitis that develops in animals deficient in interleukin-10 [61]. IL-10 gene-deficient mice demonstrated significant alterations in colonic cellular energy status in conjunction with increased permeability, proinflammatory cytokine release, and nitrosative stress. After 14 days of treatment with the PARS inhibitor 3-aminobenzamide, IL-10 gene-deficient mice demonstrated normalized colonic permeability; reduced tumor necrosis factor-alpha and interferon-gamma secretion, inducible nitric oxide synthase expression, and nitrotyrosine levels; and significantly attenuated inflammation. Time-course studies demonstrated that 3-aminobenzamide rapidly altered cellular metabolic activity and decreased cellular lactate levels. This was associated with normalization of colonic permeability and followed by a downregulation of proinflammatory cytokine release [61]. Thus, taken together, the data obtained in multiple models of colitis demonstrate that inhibition of PARP activity results in a marked improvement of colonic inflammatory disease and a normalization of cellular metabolic function and intestinal permeability.

Free radicals and oxidants have also been implicated in the pathophysiology of auto-immune arthritis [68–71]. Upregulated expression of iNOS and production of toxic quantities of NO have been measured ex vivo in chondrocytes obtained from experimental animals and clinical biopsies [72–76]. In addition, plasma levels of nitrite/nitrate (the breakdown products of NO) and plasma and synovial levels of nitrotyrosine are increased in clinical disease [77]. Experimental studies in a murine model of collagen-induced arthritis have also demonstrated increased nitrotyrosine formation [78]. Given the existence of redox stress in experimental and clinical arthritis, we hypothesized that PARS activation could represent a final common effector mechanism of injury.

Similar to the findings in enterocolitis, there are now direct experimental data demonstrating that PARS activation plays a role in the pathophysiology of joint inflammation. Blockade of PARS activity with the weak inhibitor nicotinamide, or with nicotinic acid amide, reduced the onset of the disease in a murine model of arthritis [58, 63–72]. In experimental systems, PARS inhibitors have been shown to prevent both the incidence of joint inflammation as well as the progression of established collagen induced arthritis [58, 70–72]. Furthermore, treatment with the PARS inhibitor 5-iodo-6-amino-1,2-benzopyrone produced substantial protection in a murine model of collagen-induced arthritis and reduced the incidence and severity of joint disease [58]. Vehicle-treated arthritic animals, in contrast, revealed signs of severe suppurative arthritis, with massive infiltration of neutrophils, macrophages and lymphocytes. PARS inhibition markedly reduced the extent of neutrophil infiltration into the larger joints, and decreased necrosis and hyperplasia of the synovium [58]. Similarly, inhibition of PARS with a novel, potent, phenantridinone derivative PARS inhibitor designated as PJ34 [73] exerts marked protective effects in a murine model of collagen induced arthritis (Fig. 4). Taken together, these data provide strong support for the concept that PARS activation mediates the leukocytic trafficking and end-organ damage in models of inflammatory joint disease.

Additional local inflammatory diseases, or disease conditions with strong local inflammatory components, where PARS may play a pathogenetic role include aller-

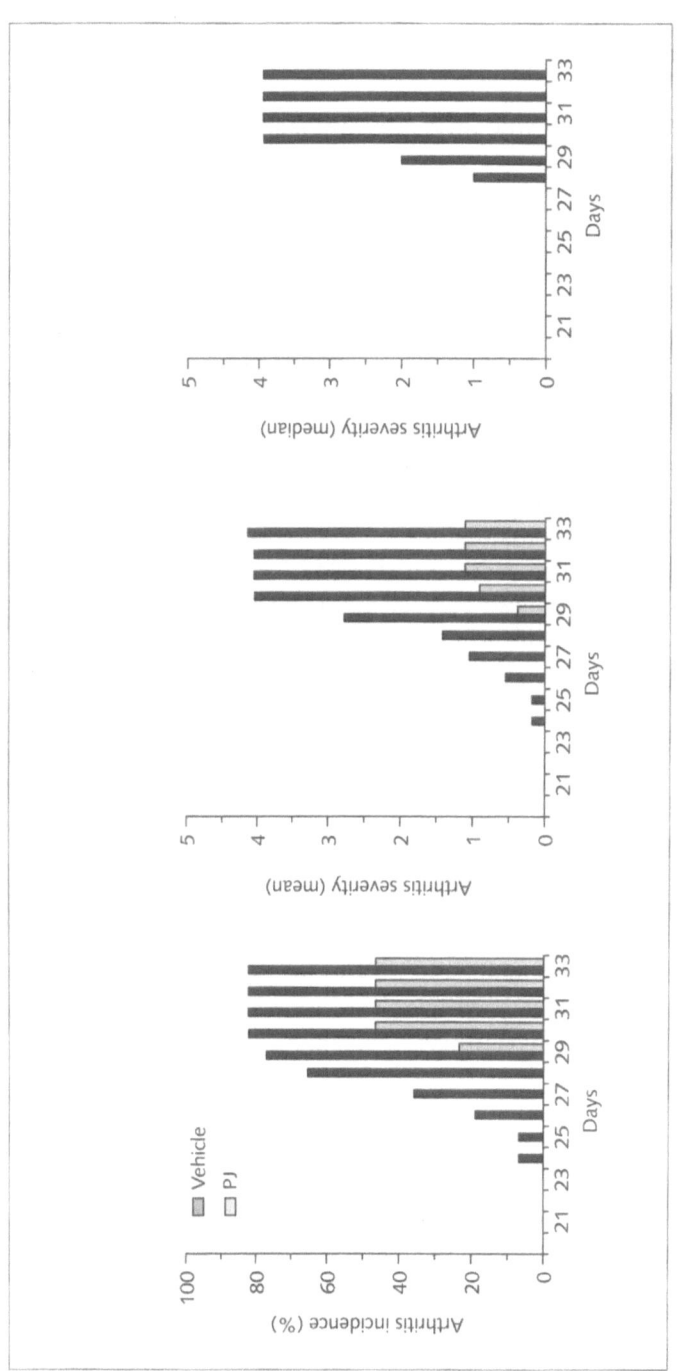

Figure 4

Anti-arthritic effect of the phenantridinone PARS inhibitor PJ34. The PARS inhibitor compound (or appropriate vehicle in the control group) was administered at 10 mg/kg oral gavage, twice a day, starting simultaneously with the second injection of collagen on Day 21 on arthritis development in a mouse model of collagen-induced arthritis in male DBA/1J mice. Arthritis was induced as previously described [58]. Mice were evaluated daily for arthritis by using a macroscopic scoring system (0–4 scale). Arthritic index for each mouse was calculated by adding the four scores of individual paws. n = 16 animals per group. PJ34 provided a significant protection against the development of arthritis in this model.

gic encephalomyelitis [74], uveitis [75] and the primary process of autoimmune islet destruction associated with diabetes mellitus [76].

Role of PARS activation in systemic inflammatory responses

Circulatory shock, a systemic inflammatory condition, is associated with a reduced responsiveness of arteries and veins to exogenous or endogenous vasoconstrictor agents (vascular hyporeactivity), myocardial dysfunction and disrupted intracellular energetic processes, culminating in multiple organ failure and death. Some of these alterations have previously been suggested to be related to NO overproduction, due to the activation of the endothelial isoform of NO in the early stage and expression of a distinct inducible isoform of NOS in the later stage or the disease [77–82]. Shock is associated with pro-inflammatory cytokine production, and subsequent stimulation of oxygen-centered free radical and peroxynitrite production [77–82]. Many of the features of systemic inflammation and shock, including the vascular failure, the hemodynamic decompensation, the gut failure and the neutrophil infiltration and multiple organ dysfunction are related to PARS activation, as it has been demonstrated in shock models induced by bacterial lipopolysaccharide, zymosan, hemorrhage and resuscitation and splanchnic occlusion and reperfusion [30, 38, 39, 41–43, 53, 56, 57]. The vascular contractile failure associated with circulatory shock is well known to be closely related to overproduction of NO within the blood vessels.

The evidence that PARP is involved in the peroxynitrite-induced vascular hyporeactivity in shock is multiple. First, in studies in anesthetized rats, inhibition of PARP with 3-aminobenzamide and nicotinamide were able to reduce the suppression of the vascular contractility of the thoracic aorta in ex vivo experiments [30, 42]. These findings are similar to the *in vitro* results with authentic peroxynitrite, which also causes a vascular hyporeactivity in thoracic aortic rings, and which is also reduced by pharmacological inhibition of PARS [43, 83]. Second, the vascular hyporeactivity associated with hemorrhagic shock is attenuated in animals deficient of functional PARS [56]. Peroxynitrite production has also been suggested to contribute to endothelial injury in shock states. In isolated perfused hearts, infusion of authentic peroxynitrite results in an impairment of the endothelium-dependent relaxations [84]. Data, demonstrating protective effects of 3-aminobenzamide against the development of endothelial dysfunction in vascular rings obtained from rats with endotoxic shock [43] suggest that DNA strand breakage and PARS activation occur in endothelial cells during shock and that the subsequent energetic failure reduces the ability of the cells to generate NO in response to acetylcholine-induced activation of the muscarinic receptors on the endothelial membrane. This effect may be related to a PARS-dependent consumption of cellular NADPH, an obligatory co-factor for endothelial NOS [73].

Similar findings were reported in pulmonary vessels challenged with endotoxin [85]. Indeed, several lines of *in vitro* data demonstrate DNA injury, PARS activation and consequent cytotoxicity in endothelial cells exposed to hydroxyl radical generators [86–88], or in response to peroxynitrite [43]. The PARS pathway has also been implicated in the pathophysiology of the cellular energetic failure associated with endotoxin shock by demonstration of increased DNA strand breakage, decreased intracellular NAD^+ and ATP levels and mitochondrial respiration in peritoneal macrophages obtained from rats subjected to endotoxin shock [89]. This cellular energetic failure was reduced by pretreatment of the animals with the PARS inhibitors 3-aminobenzamide or nicotinamide [89]. There is an overall reduction in pro-inflammatory mediator production, neutrophil infiltration, and the degree of organ injury in PARS deficient animals or in animals pretreated with various PARS inhibitors in diverse models of systemic inflammation and shock [30, 38–43, 56, 57]. Importantly, the intestinal leakage, which is considered by many investigators as an important trigger of multiple organ failure, is markedly reduced in PARS deficient animals subjected to endotoxic shock, hemorrhagic shock or splanchnic occlusion shock [56, 57, 90]. In the guts of the animals subjected to shock, there is a marked activation of PARS, as demonstrated by poly(ADP-ribose) immunostaining (Fig. 5), which is absent in the PARS deficient mice, which also show a markedly improved gut morphology [56, 57, 90]. Also, in a model of sepsis induced by live *E. coli* sponge implantation in pigs, pharmacological inhibition of PARS provides marked hemodynamic improvements and massive survival benefit (Marton, Szabo, Goldfarb, unpublished observations). It is likely that the improved hemodynamic status due to improved vascular function, and possibly, the improved cellular energetic status in some organs, results in an overall survival benefit in this condition.

Summary and implications: role of PARS in local and systemic inflammation

The following working hypothesis summarizes our current understanding on the role of PARS activation in the development of inflammatory injury (Fig. 1). Pro-inflammatory cytokines stimulate free radical formation by stimulating xanthine oxidase activity and *de novo* iNOS expression and by recruiting activated neutrophils which express NADPH oxidase. As a consequence, the oxidants peroxynitrite, hydrogen peroxide, and hydroxyl radical are formed from the interaction of superoxide and NO and by iron-catalyzed oxidation of superoxide. Oxidant stress induces AP-1 formation and generates DNA single-strand breaks. DNA strand breaks then activate PARS, which in turn potentiates NF-κB activation and AP-1 expression, resulting in greater expression of the AP-1 and NF-κB dependent genes, such as iNOS, ICAM-1, MIP-1α, TNFα, and C3. Generation of C5a (derived from C3), in combination with increased endothelial expression of ICAM-1, recruits more activated leukocytes to inflammatory foci, producing greater oxidant stress.

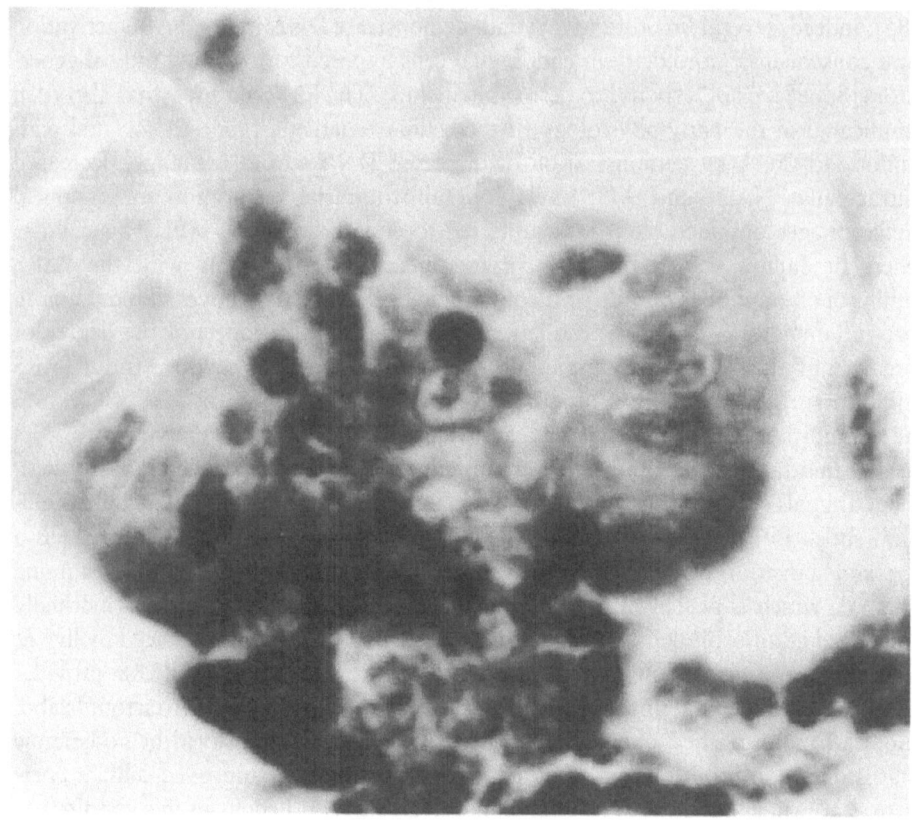

Figure 5

*Immunohistochemical detection of poly(ADP-ribose) in the gut of mice subjected to hemor-
rhagic shock and resuscitation Guts were removed from wild-type mice after hemorrhagic
shock and resuscitation and tissue sections were stained for poly(ADP-ribose). Poly(ADP-
ribose) has been detected in the epithelial cells with strongest immuno-positivity at the tip
of the villi. Several stromal cells also displayed poly(ADP-ribose) positivity.*

The cycle is thus renewed as the increase in oxidant stress triggers more DNA strand
breakage. The proposed cycle of inflammatory activation will be augmented in systems where PARS-dependent MAP kinase activation and NF-κB translocation contribute importantly to free radical and oxidant formation and granulocyte recruitment. According to this proposed model, which still requires validation but is supported by multiple lines of evidence, PARS occupies a critical position in a
positive-feedback loop of inflammatory injury. NAD depletion induced by PARS

activation is likely to accelerate this positive-feedback cycle by preventing the ener-gy-dependent reduction of oxidized glutathione, the chief intracellular anti-oxidant and most abundant thiol in eukaryotic cells. NAD is the precursor for NADP, a cofactor that plays a critical role in bioreductive synthetic pathways and the main-tenance of reduced glutathione pools [91]. Depletion of reduced glutathione, as a consequence of intracellular energetic failure or overwhelming oxidant exposure [84], leaves further oxidant stress unopposed, resulting in greater DNA strand breakage.

PARS occupies a critical position in a self-amplifying cycle of oxidant-driven damage. It is appropriate then to ask whether PARS inhibition is a candidate for clinical treatment of inflammation. A variety of PARS inhibitors are in pre-clinical development, many with potency that greatly exceeds the prototypic agents used in experimental proof-of-concept studies of inflammation. PARS inhibitors may be particularly useful in the treatment of acute inflammatory disorders, such as circu-latory shock, where issues of potential toxicity related to chronic administration are unimportant. Although the exact physiologic role of PARS is still unclear, and remains a matter of dispute, it is logical to suppose it plays an important role since it is one of the most abundant proteins in the nucleus. PARS has been implicated in many physiologic housekeeping functions, such as gene repair, transcription, and cell cycling. Until such time as its true physiologic functions are more precisely defined, there should exist a considerable caution in the long-term administration of PARS inhibitors to man. Chronic *in vitro* administration of high doses of the PARS inhibitor nicotinamide, for example, has been shown in experimental models to reduce β-islet cell function [92]. Since nicotinamide is a weak PARS inhibitor, and has additional pharmacological activities beyond PARS inhibition, these data do not directly imply that chronic inhibition of the enzyme is problematic. PARS inhibition has also been associated with an increase in sister chromatid exchange [93], a con-cerning finding that raises the risk of malignant transformation. PARS activation clearly leads to cell death and some have argued that its physiologic role is to elim-inate genetically damaged cells, thereby reducing oncogenic potential. Indeed, PARS inhibition has been shown to facilitate the rapid ligation of DNA excision-repair patches [94] and to suppress malignant transformation in cells with DNA damage induced by irradiation and chemical carcinogens [95]. Whether chronic PARS inhi-bition predisposes to malignant transformation is open to question. The PARS defi-cient mice have not been reported to present increased frequency of spontaneous of induced malignancies, although, to our knowledge, this issue has not yet been sys-tematically investigated. A clear distinction must also be made between chronic PARS inhibition, *versus* chronic PARS deficiency: the latter condition will also affect cellular processes due to the absence of protein-protein interactions that PARS is known to participate in. Nevertheless, these issues must be adequately addressed prior to considering the development of PARS inhibitors to treat chronic inflamma-tory conditions.

Acknowledgements

This work was supported by the following grants from the National Institutes of Health: R01GM60915, R01GM60699 and R29GM 54773.

References

1 Lautier D, Lageux J, Thibodeau J, Ménard L, Poirier GG (1993) Molecular and biochemical features of poly (ADP-ribose) metabolism. *Mol Cell Biochem* 122: 171–193

2 Wang ZQ, Auer B, Sting L, Berghammer H, Haidacher D, Schweiger M, Wagner EF (1995) Mice lacking ADPRT and poly (ADP-ribosylation) develop normally but are susceptible to skin disease. *Genes and Development* 9: 510–552

2 Durkacz BW, Omidiji O, Gray DA, Shall S (1980) (ADP-ribose)n participates in DNA excision repair. *Nature* 283: 593–596

3 Satoh MS, Lindahl T (1992) Role of poly(ADP-ribose) formation in DNA repair. *Nature* 356: 356–358

4 Poirier, GG, de Murcia G, Jongstra-Bilen J, Niedergang C, Mandel P (1982) Poly(ADP-ribosyl)ation of polynuclesomes causes relaxation of chromatin structure. *Proc Natl Acad Sci USA* 79: 3423–3427

6 Ohashi Y, Ueda K, Hayaisha O, Ikai K, Niwa O (1984) Induction of murine teratocarcinoma cell differentiation by suppression of poly(ADP-ribose) synthesis. *Proc Natl Acad Sci USA* 81: 7132–7136

7 Simbulan-Rosenthal CM, Rosenthal DS, Hilz H, Hickey R, Malkas L, Applegren N, Wu Y, Bers G, Smulson ME (1996) The expression of poly(ADP-ribose) polymerase during differentiation-linked DNA replication reveals that it is a component of the multiprotein DNA replication complex. *Biochem* 35: 11622–11633

8 Amstad PA, Krupitza G, Cerutti PA (1992) Mechanism of c-fos induction by active oxygen. *Cancer Res* 52: 3952–3960

9 Berger NA, Kaichi AS, Steward PG, Klevecz RR, Forrest GL, Gross SD (1978) Synthesis of poly(adenosine diphosphate ribose) in synchronized Chinese hamster cells. *Experimental Cell Research* 117: 127–135

10 Whitacre CM, Hashimoto H, Tsia ML, Chatterjee S, Berger SJ, Berger NA (1995) Involvement of NAD-poly(ADP-ribose) metabolism in p53 regulation and its consequences. *Cancer Res* 55: 3697–3701

11 Kun E, Kirsten E, Milo GE, Kurian P, Kumari HL (1983) Cell cycle-dependent intervention by benzamide of carcinogen-induced neoplastic transformation and *in vitro* poly(ADP-ribosyl)ation of nuclear proteins in human fibroblasts. *Proc Natl Acad Sci USA* 80: 7219–7223

12 Nathan C (1992) Nitric oxide as a secretory product of mammalian cells. *FASEB J* 6: 3051–3064

13 Southan GJ, Szabó C (1995) Selective pharmacological inhibition of distinct nitric oxide synthase isoforms. *Biochem Pharmacol* 51: 383–394

14   Oda T, Akaike T, Hamamoto T, Suzuki F, Hirano T, Maeda H (1989) Oxygen radicals in influenza-induced pathogenesis and treatment with pyran polymer-conjugated SOD. *Science* 244: 974–976

15   Tan S, Yokoyama Y, Dickens E, Cash TG, Freeman BA, Parks DA (1993) Xanthine oxidase activity in the circulation of rats following hemorrhagic shock. *Free Radic Biol Med* 15: 407–414

16   McCord JM (1985) Oxygen-derived free radicals in postischemic tissue injury. *New Engl J Med* 312: 159–163

17   Miesel R, Zuber M, Sanocka D, Graetz R, Kroeger H (1994) Effects of allopurinol on *in vivo* suppression of arthritis in mice and *ex vivo* modulation of phagocytic production of oxygen radicals in whole human blood. *Inflammation* 18: 597–612

18   Engerson TD, McKelvey TG, Rhyne DB, Boggio EB, Snyder SJ, Jones HP (1987) The conversion of xanthine dehydrogenase to oxidase in ischaemic rat tissue. *J Clin Invest* 79: 1564–1570

19   Akaike T, Ando M, Tatsuya O, Doi T, Ijiri S, Araki S, Maeda H (1990) Dependence on O_2 generation by xanthine oxidase of pathogenesis of influenza virus infection in mice. *J Clin Invest* 85: 739–745

20   Mohacsi A, Kozlovszky B, Kiss I, Seres I, Fulop T Jr (1996) Neutrophils obtained from obliterative atherosclerotic patients exhibit enhanced resting respiratory burst and increased degranulation in response to various stimuli. *Biochim Biophys Acta* 1316: 210–216

21   Grum CM, Ragsdale RA, Ketai LH, Simon RH (1987) Plasma hypoxanthine and exercise. *Am Rev Resp Dis* 136: 98–101

22   Friedl HP, Smith DJ, Till GO, Thomson PD, Louis DS, Ward PA (1990) Ischemia-reperfusion in humans. Appearance of xanthine oxidase activity. *Am J Path* 136: 491–495

23   Friedl HP, Till GO, Trentz O, Ward PA (1989) Role of histamine, complement and xanthine oxidase in thermal injury of the skin. *Am J Path* 135: 203–217

24   Parks DA, Bulkley GB, Granger DN (1983) Role of oxygen free radicals in shock, ischemia, and organ preservation. *Surgery* 94: 428–432

25   Demling R, LaLonde C, Youn YK, Daryani R, Campbell C, Knox J (1992) Lung oxidant changes after zymosan peritonitis: relationship between physiologic and biochemical changes. *Am Rev Respir Dis* 146: 1272–1278

26   Szabó C, Zingarelli B, O'Connor M, Salzman AL (1996) DNA strand breakage, activation of poly-ADP ribosyl synthetase, and cellular energy depletion are involved in the cytotoxicity in macrophages and smooth muscle cells exposed to peroxynitrite. *Proc Natl Acad Sci USA* 93: 1753–1758

27   Szabó C, Salzman AL (1995) Endogenous peroxynitrite is involved in the inhibition of cellular respiration in immunostimulated J774.2 macrophages. *Biochem Biophys Res Comm* 209: 739–743

28   Szabó A, Hake P, Salzman AL, Szabó C (1998) Inhibition of poly (ADP-ribose) synthetase exerts protective effects in a porcine model of hemorrhagic shock. *Shock* 10: 347–353

29 Szabó C, Salzman AL, Ischiropoulos H (1995) Peroxynitrite-mediated oxidation of dihydrorhodamine 123 occurs in early stages of endotoxic and hemorrhagtic shock and ischemia-reperfusion injury. *FEBS Lett* 372: 229–232

30 Szabó C, Zingarelli B, Salzman AL (1996) Role of poly-ADP ribosyltransferase activation in the vascular contractile and energetic failure elicited by exogenous and endogenous nitric oxide and peroxynitite. *Circ Res* 78: 1051–1063

31 Singer II, Kawka DW, Scott S, Weidner JR, Mumford RA, Riehl TE, Stenson WF (1996) Expression of inducible nitric oxide synthase and nitrotyrosine in colonic epithelium in inflammatory bowel disease. *Gastroenterol* 111: 871–885

32 Szabó C, Saunders C, O'Connor M, Salzman AL (1996) Peroxynitrite causes energy depletion and increases permeability *via* activation of poly-ADP ribosyl synthetase in pulmonary epithelial cells. *Am J Resp Mol Biol* 60: 105–109

33 Kennedy MS, Denenberg A, Szabó C, Salzman AL (1998) Poly (ADP-ribose) synthetase (PARS) mediates increased permeability induced by peroxynitrite in Caco-2BBe cells. *Gastroenterol* 114: 510–518

34 Cochrane CG (1996) Damage to DNA by reactive oxygen and nitrogen species: role in inflammatory diosease and progression to cancer. *Biochem J* 313: 17–29

35 Lih-Brody L, Powell SR, Collier KP, Reddy GM, Cerchia R, Kahn E, Weissman GS, Katz S, Floyd RA, McKinley MJ (1996) Increased oxidative stress and decreased antioxidant defenses in mucosa of inflammatory bowel disease. *Dig Dis Sci* 41: 2078–2086

36 Ueda K, Hayaishi O (1985) ADP-ribosylation. *Ann Rev Biochem* 54: 73–100

37 Zhang J, Dawson VL, Dawson TM, Snyder SH (1994) Nitric oxide activation of poly (ADP-ribose) synthetase in neurotoxicity. *Science* 263: 687–689

38 Cuzzocrea S, Zingarelli B, Constantino G, Szabó A, Salzman AL, Caputi AP, Szabó C (1997) Beneficial effects of 3-aminobenzamide, an inhibitor of poly (ADP-ribose) synthetase in a rat model of splanchnic artery occlusion and reperfusion. *Br J Pharm* 121: 1065–1074

39 Szabó C, Lim LH, Cuzzocrea S, Getting SJ, Zingarelli B, Flower RJ, Salzman AL, Perretti M (1997) Inhibition of poly (ADP-ribose) synthetase attenuates neutrophil recruitment and exerts antiinflammatory effects. *J Exp Med* 186: 1041–1049

40 Cuzzocrea S, Zingarelli B, Gilad E, Hake P, Salzman AL, Szabó C (1998) Protective effects of 3-aminobenzamide, an inhibitor of poly (ADP-ribose) synthase in a carrageenan-induced model of local inflammation. *Eur J Pharm* 342: 67–76

41 Szabó C, Wong H, Bauer PI, Kirsten E, O'Connor M, Zingarelli B, Mendeleyev J, Hasko G, Vizi ES, Salzman AL Kun E (1997) Regulation of components of the inflammatory response by 5-iodo-6-amino-1,2-benzopyrone, an inhibitor of poly (ADP-ribose) synthetase and pleiotropic modifier of cellular signal pathways. *Int J Oncol* 10: 1093–1104

42 Zingarelli B, Salzman AL, Szabó C (1996) Protective effects of nicotinamide against nitric oxide mediated vascular failure in endotoxic shock: potential involvement of poly ADP ribosyl synthetase. *Shock* 5: 258–264

43 Szabó C, Cuzzocrea S, Zingarelli B, O'Connor M, Salzman AL (1997) Endothelial dys-

function in endotoxic shock: importance of the activation of poly (ADP ribose) synthetase (PARS) by peroxynitrite. *J Clin Invest* 100: 723–735

44 Zingarelli B, Cuzzocrea S, Zsengeller Z, Salzman AL, Szabó C (1997) Beneficial effect of inhibition of poly-ADP ribose synthetase activity in myocardial ischemia-reperfusion injury. *Cardiovasc Res* 36: 205–215

45 Gilad E, Zingarelli B, Salzman AL, Szabó C (1997) Protection by inhibition of poly (ADP-ribose) synthetase against oxidant injury in cardiac myoblasts *in vitro. J Mol Cell Cardiol* 29: 2585–2597

46 Cuzzocrea S, Zingarelli B, O'Connor M, Salzman AL, Caputi AP, Szabó C (1997) Role of peroxynitrite and activation of poly (ADP-ribose) synthetase in the vascular failure induced by zymosan-activated plasma. *Br J Pharm* 122: 493–503

47 Virag L, Scott GS, Cuzzocrea S, Marmer D, Salzman AL, Szabo C (1998) Peroxynitrite-induced thymocyte apoptosis: the role of caspases and poly (ADP-ribose) synthetase (PARS) activation. *Immunology* 94: 345–355

48 Virag L, Salzman AL, Szabo C (1998) Poly(ADP-ribose) synthetase activation mediates mitochondrial injury during oxidant-induced cell death. *J Immunol* 161: 3753–3759

49 Ha HC, Snyder SH (1999) Poly(ADP-ribose) polymerase is a mediator of necrotic cell death by ATP depletion. *Proc Natl Acad Sci USA* 96: 13978–13982

50 Unno N, Menconi MJ, Salzman AL, Smith M, Hagan S, Ye GE, Ezzel RM, Fink MP (1996) Hypermeability and ATP depletion induced by chronic hypoxia or glycolytic inhibition in Caco-2BBe monolayers. *Am J Phys* 270: G1010–G1021

51 Roebuck KA, Rahman A, Lakshminarayanan V, Janakidevi K, Malik AB (1995) H_2O_2 and tumor necrosis factor-alpha activate intercellular adhesion molecule 1 (ICAM-1) gene transcription through distinct cis-regulatory elements within the ICAM-1 promoter. *J Biol Chem* 270: 18996–18974

52 Le Page C, Sanceau J, Drapier JC, Wietzerbin J (1998) Inhibitors of ADP-ribosylation impair inducible nitric oxide synthase gene transcription through inhibition of NF kappa B activation. *Biochem Biophys Res Comm* 243: 451–457

53 Oliver FJ, Menissier-de Murcia J, Nacci C, Decker P, Andriantsitohaina R, Muller S, De la Rubia G, Stoclet JC, De Murcia G (1999) Resistance to endotoxic shock as a consequence of defective NF-kappaB activation in poly (ADP-ribose) polymerase-1 deficient mice. *EMBO J* 18, 4446–4454

54 Zingarelli B, Szabo C, Salzman AL (1999) Blockade of Poly(ADP-ribose) synthetase inhibits neutrophil recruitment, oxidant generation, and mucosal injury in murine colitis. *Gastroenterology* 116: 335–45

55 Zingarelli B, Salzman AL, Szabo C (1998) Genetic disruption of poly (ADP-ribose) synthetase inhibits the expression of P-selectin and intercellular adhesion molecule-1 in myocardial ischemia/reperfusion injury. *Circ Res* 83: 85–94

56 Liaudet L, Soriano FG, Szabo E, Virag L, Mabley JG, Salzman AL, Szabo C (2000) Protection against hemorrhagic shock in mice genetically deficient in poly(ADP-ribose)polymerase. *Proc Natl Acad Sci USA* 97: 10203–10208

57 Liaudet L, Szabo A, Soriano FG, Zingarelli B, Szabo C, Salzman AL (2000) Poly (ADP-

ribose) synthetase mediates intestinal mucosal barrier dysfunction after mesenteric ischemia. *Shock* 14: 134–41

58 Szabó C, Virág L, Cuzzocrea S, Scott GJ, Hake P, O'Connor M, Zingarelli B, Salzman AL, Kun E (1998) Protection against peroxynitrite-induced fibroblast injury and arthritis development by inhibition of poly (ADP-ribose) synthetase. *Proc Natl Acad Sci USA* 95: 3867–3872

59 Akabane A, Kato I, Takasawa S, Unno M, Yonekura H, Yoshimoto T, Okamaoto H (1995) Nicotinamide inhibits IRF-1 mRNA induction and prevents IL-1 beta-induced nitric oxide synthase expression in pancreatic beta cells. *Biochem Biophys Res Comm* 215: 524–530

60 Le Page C, Pellat-Deceunynck C, Drapier JC, Wietzerbin J (1997) Effects of inhibitors of ADP-ribosylation on macrophage activation. *Adv Exp Med Biol* 419: 203–207

61 Jijon HB, Churchill T, Malfair D, Wessler A, Jewell LD, Parsons HG, Madsen KL (2000) Inhibition of poly(ADP-ribose) polymerase attenuates inflammation in a model of chronic colitis. *Am J Physiol* 279: G641–G651

62 Simbulan-Rosenthal CM, Ly DH, Rosenthal DS, Konopka G, Luo R, Wang ZQ, Schultz PG, Smulson ME (2000) Misregulation of gene expression in primary fibroblasts lacking poly(ADP-ribose) polymerase. *Proc Natl Acad Sci USA* 97: 11274–11279

63 Oyanagui Y (1994) Nitric oxide and superoxide radical are involved in both initiation and development of adjuvant arthritis in rats. *Life Sci* 54: PL285–PL259

64 Santos L, Tipping PG (1994) Attenuation of adjuvant arthritis in rats by treatment with oxygen radical scavengers. *Immunol Cell Biol* 72: 406–414

65 Kaur H, Halliwell B (1994) Evidence for nitric oxide-mediated oxidative damage in chronic inflammation. Nitrotyrosine in serum and synovial fluid from rheumatoid patients. *FEBS Lett* 350: 9–12

66 Hauselmann HJ, Opplinger L, Michel BA, Stefanovic-Racic M, Evans CH (1994) Nitric oxide and proteoglycan synthesis by human articular chondrocytes in alginate culture. *FEBS Lett* 352: 361–364

67 Sakurai H, Kohsaka H, Liu MF, Higashiyama H, Hirata Y, Kanno K, Saito I, Miyaska N (1995) Nitric oxide production and inducible nitric oxide synthase expression in inflammatory arthritides. *J Clin Invest* 96: 2357–2363

68 Murrell GA, Jang D, Williams RJ (1995) Nitric oxide activates metalloprotease enzymes in articular cartilage. *Biochem Biophys Res Comm* 206: 15–21

69 Farrell AJ, Blake DR, Palmer RM, Moncada S (1992) Increased concentrations of nitrite in synovial fluid and serum samples suggest increased nitric oxide synthesis in rheumatic diseases. *Ann Rheumat Dis* 51: 1219–1222

70 Miesel R, Kurpis M, Kroger H (1998) Modulation of inflammatory arthritis by inhibition of poly(ADP ribose) polymerase. *Inflammation* 19: 379–387

71 Ehrlich W, Huser H, Kroger H (1998) Inhibition of the induction of collagenase by interleukin-1 beta in cultured rabbit synovial fibroblasts after treatment with the poly(ADP-ribose)-polymerase inhibitor 3 aminobenzamide. *Rheumatol Int* 15: 171–172

72 Kroger KD, Miesel R, Dietrich A, Ohde M, Rajnavolgyi E, Ockenfels H (1998) Syner-

gistic effects of thalidomide and poly (ADP-ribose) polymerase inhibition on type II collagen-induced arthritis in mice. *Inflammation* 20: 203–215

73   Garcia Soriano F, Virag L, Jagtap P, Szabo E, Mabley JG, Liaudet L, Marton A, Hoyt DG, Murthy KG, Salzman AL et al (2001) Diabetic endothelial dysfunction: the role of poly (ADP-ribose) polymerase activation. *Nature Med* 7: 108–113

74   Scott GS, Hake P, Salzman AL, Szabó C (1998) Suppression of experimental allergic encephalomyelitis by administration of 5-iodo-6-amino-1,2,benzopyrone, a novel inhibitor of poly(ADP-ribose) synthetase. *Crit Care Med* 26 (Suppl): A36

75   Prendergast RA, Szabó C (1999) The role of poly (ADP-ribose) synthase in endotoxin-induced uveitis in the rat. ARVO Annual Meeting. *Inv Opht Vis Sci* 40: S570

76   Pieper AA, Verma A, Zhang J, Snyder SH (1999) Poly (ADP-ribose) polymerase, nitric oxide and cell death. *Trends Pharmacol Sci* 20: 171–181

77   Szabó C (1995) Alterations in nitric oxide production in various forms of circulatory shock. *New Horizons* 3: 2–32

78   Kilbourn RG, Szabó C, Traber D (1997) Beneficial versus detrimental effects of nitric oxide synthase inhibitors in circulatory shock: lessons learned from experimental and clinical studies. *Shock* 7: 235–246

79   Szabó C, Salzman AL, Ischiropoulos H (1995) Endotoxin triggers the expression of an inducible isoform of NO synthase and the formation of peroxynitrite in the rat aorta *in vivo*. *FEBS Lett* 363: 235–238

80   Szabó C, Day BJ, Salzman AL (1996) Evaluation of the relative contribution of nitric oxide and peroxynitrite to the suppression of mitochondrial respiration in immunostimulated macrophages, using a novel mesoporphyrin superoxide dismutase analog and peroxynitrite scavenger. *FEBS Lett* 381: 82–86

81   Wizemann T, Gardner C, Laskin J, Quinones S, Durham S, Goller N, Ohnishi T Laskin D (1994) Production of nitric oxide and peroxynitrite in the lung during acute endotoxemia. *J Leukoc Biol* 56: 759–768

82   Rees DD (1995) Role of nitric oxide in the vascular dysfunction of septic shock. *Biochem Soc Transact* 23: 1025–1029

83   Chabot F, Mitchell JA, Quinlan GJ, Evans TW (1997) Characterization of the vasodilator properties of peroxynitrite on rat pulmonary artery: role of poly (adenosine 5'-diphosphoribose) synthase. *Br J Pharmacol* 121: 485–490

84   Villa LM, Salas E, Darley-Usmar M, Radomski ME, Moncada S (1994) Peroxynitrite induces both vasodilatation and impaired vascular relaxation in the isolated perfused rat heart. *Proc Natl Acad Sci USA* 91: 12383–12387

85   Pulido EJ, Shames BD, Selzman CH, Barton HA, Banerjee A, Bensard DD, McIntyre RC (1999) Inhibition of poly (ADP-ribose) synthetase attenuates endotoxin-induced dysfunction of pulmonary vasorelaxation. *Am J Physiol* 277: L769–L776

86   Spragg RG (1991) DNA strand break formation following exposure of bovine pulmonary artery and aortic endothelial cells to reactive oxygen products. *Am J Respir Cell Mol Biol* 4: 4–10

87   Thies RL, Autor AP (1991) Reactive oxygen injury to cultured pulmonary artery

endothelial cells: mediation by polyADP-ribose polymerase activation causing NAD depletion and altered energy balance. *Arch Biochem Biophys* 286: 353–363

88   Junod AF, Jornot L, Petersen H (1991) Differential effects of hyperoxia and hydrogen peroxide on DNA damage, polyadenosine diphosphate-ribose polymerase activity, and nicotinamide adenine dinucleotide and adenosine triphosphate contents in cultured endothelial cells and fibroblasts. *J Cell Physiol* 140: 177–185

89   Zingarelli B, O'Connor M, Wong H, Salzman AL, Szabó C (1996) Peroxynitrite-mediated DNA strand breakage activates poly-ADP ribosyl synthetase and causes cellular energy depletion in macrophages stimulated with bacterial lipopolysaccharide. *J Immunol* 156: 350–358

90   Szabó A, Salzman AL, Szabó C (1998) Inhibition of poly (ADP-ribose) synthetase ameliorates endotoxin-induced intestinal and pulmonary leakage. *Life Sci* 63: 2133–2139

91   Schoenberg MH, Beger HG (1990) Oxygen radicals in intestinal ischemia and reperfusion. *Chem Biol Inter* 76: 141–161

92   Reddy S, Salari-Lak N, Sandler S (1995) Long-term effects of nicotinamide-induced inhibition of poly(adenosine diphosphate-ribose) polymerase activity in rat pancreatic islets exposed to interleukin-1 beta. *Endocrinology* 136: 1907–1912

93   Oikawa A, Tohda H, Kanai M, Miwa M, Sugimura T (1980) Inhibitors of poly(adenosine diphosphate ribose) polymerase induce sister chromatid exchanges. *Biochem Biophys Res Comm* 97: 1311–1316

94   Cleaver JE, Park SD (1986) Enhanced ligation of repair sites under conditions of inhibition of poly(ADP-ribose) synthesis by 3-aminobenzamide. *Mutation Res* 173: 287–290

95   Borek C, Morgan WF, Ong A, Cleaver JE (1984) Inhibition of malignant transformation *in vitro* by inhibitors of poly(ADP-ribose) synthesis. *Proc Natl Acad Sci USA* 81: 243–247

Nitric oxide regulation of leukocyte adhesion molecule expression

Martin Spiecker[1] and James K. Liao[1]

[1]Medizinische Klinik II, St. Josef Hospital, Ruhr-Universität Bochum, Gudrunstrasse 56, 44791 Bochum, Germany; [2]James K. Liao, Department of Medicine, Brigham & Women's Hospital and Harvard Medical School, 221 Longwood Avenue, Boston, MA 02115, USA

Introduction

The vascular endothelium serves as an important autocrine/paracrine organ that regulates vascular wall contractile state and cellular composition [1, 2]. The endothelium interacts with both cellular and hormonal mediators from the blood and the vascular wall. These interactions are of crucial importance in inflammatory reactions. One of the initial events in vascular inflammation is endothelial activation [3, 4]. Upon activation, endothelial cells express surface adhesion molecules such as intercellular adhesion molecule-1 (ICAM-1), E-selectin, and vascular cell adhesion molecule 1 (VCAM-1) [5].

Leukocyte endothelial interaction is a multi-step process starting with rolling of leukocytes along the vessel wall, activation of leukocyte ligands (triggering), tight adhesion, and finally the transmigration [6, 7]. Different endothelial adhesion molecules and their leukocyte counter-receptors allow a differential regulation of endothelial-leukocyte interaction. According to structural homologies, adhesion molecules and their counter-receptors are classified in at least three families: the immunoglobulin superfamiliy, the integrin family, and the selectin family.

Adhesion molecules and integrins

Both ICAM-1 and VCAM-1 belong to the immunoglobulin superfamily. Common feature of these glycoproteins is an immunoglobulin like domain and a short carboxyterminal protruding into the cytoplasm. ICAM-1 has five immunoglobulin like domains, each VCAM-1 molecule six to seven. ICAM-1 is expressed on endothelial cells, certain epithelial cells, fibroblasts, tissue macrophages, dendritic cells in lymph nodes, and on certain lymphoblasts [8]. ICAM-1 is constitutively expressed at low levels on endothelial cells. Upon stimulation with tumor necrosis factor α (TNFα) or interleukin 1 (IL-1), ICAM-1 cell surface expression is increased by transcriptional induction. In contrast, VCAM-1 is not detectable on unstimulated, cultured endothelial cells. Bacterial lipopolysaccharide (LPS) , IL-1, TNFα, and IL-4 induce endothelial VCAM-1 expression, maximal activity is reached by 6 to 12 h [9]. The counterreceptor for VCAM-1 is VLA-4, a member of the integrin family. VLA-4 is expressed on lymphcytes, monocytes, basophils and eosinophils [10–12]. VCAM-1 binds to these cells *via* VLA-4. Expression of VCAM-1 has been described in acute and chronic inflammatory reactions [13]. Both ICAM-1 and VCAM-1, mediate the tight adhesion of leukocytes to the endothelium, a process which is one important requirement for transmigration. Interaction of endothelial ICAM-1 and VCAM-1 with leukocytes is dependent on the expression of the immunoglobulin superfamily members and the functional activity of their counterreceptors, the integrins.

Integrins are heterodimeric transmembrane proteins composed of noncovalently associated α- and β-subunits [14, 15]. The ligand for VCAM-1, VLA-4, belongs to the group of β_1-integrins [16]. The ligands for ICAM-1 belong to β_2-integrins [17]. LFA-1 is expressed on all leukocytes, Mac-1 is expressed only on monocytes and myeloic cells. Although integrins are constitutively expressed, they need to be functionally activated by triggers such as chemokines. For example, Mac-1 is activated by platelet activating factor (PAF), and IL-8, VLA-4 and LFA-1 are activated by macrophage inflammatory protein 1β (MIP-1β), monocyte chemoattractant protein (MCP-1), and RANTES [18–22].

Selectins are a family of transmembraneous adhesion molecules. Members of this family are P-selectin, L-selectin, and E-selectin. E-selectin is expressed on activated endothelial cells. Interaction with its ligands on neutrophils results in rolling of these leukocytes [23]. Additionally, this interaction triggers the activation of the ICAM-1 ligand Mac-1 [24]. Like ICAM-1 and VCAM-1, E-selectin is essentially regulated by the transcription factor NF-κB [25].

Adhesion molecules and vascular inflammation

One of the proximal event in atherogenesis and vascular inflammation is the activation of endothelial cells. The activated endothelium expresses monocyte chemotactic protein (MCP)-1, macrophage-colony stimulating factor (M-CSF or CSF-1), and cell-surface adhesion molecules such as intercellular and vascular cell adhesion molecules (ICAM-1 and VCAM-1) and E-selectin which facilitate the recruitment and attachment of circulating leukocytes to the vessel [4, 26–28]. Indeed, monocyte adhesion to the vessel wall and its subsequent differentiation into macrophages is crucial for the development of macrophage-derived foam cells in atherosclerotic plaques [27, 29–31].

Another condition associated with vascular inflammation is reperfusion following myocardial ischemia. The leukocytes involved are predominantly neutrophils. Expression of ICAM-1 and functional activation of its ligand Mac-1 play a major role in this pathophysiolgic condition [32]. The rolling of leukocytes along the vascular endothelium appears to be mediated by the interaction of P-selectin on endothelial cells and PSGL-1 on leukocytes [33]. Attachment of leukocytes and their subsequent migration in the vessel wall requires endothelial expression of these adhesion molecules. Factors that modulate endothelial cell adhesion molecule expression, therefore, may be important in regulating vascular inflammation and atherosclerosis. One such endogenous modulator is nitric oxide (NO).

Vascular effects of NO

NO has numerous effects on the vessel wall including vasodilatation [34-36], inhibition of platelet aggregation [37], inhibition of MCP-1 and M-CSF production [38, 39], changes in vascular permeability [40], inhibition of smooth muscle cell proliferation [41], and inhibition of leukocyte-endothelium interaction [42–45]. As a consequence of these effects, NO is cytoprotective in experimental models of atherosclerosis [46], thrombosis [47], intima hyperplasia following endothelial injury [48, 49], and ischemia/reperfusion injury [40, 50].

Indeed, *in vivo* studies have shown that inhibition of endogenous NO production by N-nitro-L-arginine methlyester (L-NAME) promotes leukocyte adhesion to the endothelium during ischemia/reperfusion injury in splanchnic vessels [42, 44]. Similarly, decreased endogenous NO-production increases neutrophil adhesion in coronary vessels [32]. Administration of NO donors or an increase in endogenous NO induced by its precursor, L-arginine, decreases neutrophil adhesion in the coronary vasculature [50, 51].

Endothelial dysfunction is a pathophysiologic condition associated with decreased synthesis, release, and/or activity of NO [1]. Endothelial dysfunction is an important feature of atherosclerosis and acute coronary syndromes. Indeed, atherosclerotic risk factors, chronic infections, environmental factors, and genetic factors can all lead to endothelial dysfunction [52]. One important example is hypercholesterolemia, where NO production is reduced [53, 54]. Endothelial dysfunction in hypercholesterolemia results in expression of endothelial adhesion molecules and increased leukocyte attachment [4, 26, 55]. Treatment with NO donors or L-arginine reverses this increase in leukocyte adhesion [43, 56, 57]. Taken together, these studies support the belief that NO possess anti-inflammatory properties.

NO and adhesion molecules

Although many effects of NO are mediated by activation of soluble guanylyl cyclase, the ability of NO to attenuate leukocyte attachment to the endothelial surface appears to be cGMP independent [58–60]. For example, several structurally unrelated NO donors, but not cGMP analogues, inhibit cytokine-induced surface expression of VCAM-1, VCAM-1 mRNA, and VCAM-1 promotor activity [58, 59]. The NO donor S-nitrosoglutathione (GSNO) inhibits VCAM-1 expression in a concentration-dependent manner with a maximum 75% inhibition achieved with 200 µM of GSNO [61]. Similar effects with several structurally unrelated NO donors suggest a NO-specific effect. Inhibition of VCAM-1 expression by NO is not due to cytotoxicity since measurements of cell viability, protein synthesis, and constitutive expression of endothelial cell surface antigens (MHC-1, E1/1) were not affected by 200 µM of GSNO [58]. Interestingly, GSNO is not only an exogenous NO donor, but also an endogenous storage form of NO [62]. In the presence of physiologic glutathione concentrations, GSNO is a reaction product of NO derived from eNOS [63, 64].

To confirm the effects of NO donors, a co-culture system is useful to assess the effects of endogenously derived NO. In this system, murine macrophage-like cells, RAW264.7, were grown on culture inserts above human endothelial cell monolayers within the same culture medium [61]. Using this separate co-culture setting, no basal VCAM-1 expression is detected. Stimulation with LPS induces endothelial VCAM-1. In combination with the species specific murine IFNγ, iNOS expression and NO production can be induced in RAW264.7, but not in endothelial cells. Co-stimulation with LPS and murine IFNγ strongly inhibits endothelial VCAM-1 expression compared to LPS stimulation alone. Whereas LPS alone is unable to stimulate NO-production, co-stimulation with murine IFNγ significantly increases NO-production by RAW264.7 cells. Pre-incubation of the co-culture system with the NO synthase inhibitor LNMA abolishes the NO-production induced by LPS and murine IFNγ. A strong VCAM-1 expression under this experimental conditions suggests a causal role of macrophage-like cell derived NO as an inhibitor of endothelial VCAM-1 expression.

Activation of NF-κB and transcriptional induction of adhesion molecules

The genes that encode a number of cellular adhesion molecules and cytokines implicated in atherogenesis share specific DNA binding motifs in their promoters which interact with the transcription factor, NF-κB (Tab. 1). NF-κB was originally described as a heterodimeric cytosolic protein in B cells, which upon activation, translocates into the nucleus where it binds to specific decameric sequences in the IgG κ light chain enhancer [65–67]. Subsequent studies have shown that this nuclear binding protein can also activate viral enhancer elements [68, 69]. Members of the mammalian NF-κB family possess *Rel* homology domains which are necessary for dimerization, nuclear translocation, and DNA binding [70, 71]. The *Rel*-related proteins were initially used to describe factors which determine the relative spatial orientation during differentiation of the *Drosophila* body (i.e. dorsal vs. ventral) [72].

Table 1 - NF-κB responsive genes

Cellular adhesion molecules	Intercellular adhesion molecule-1 (ICAM-1)
	Vascular cell adhesion molecule-1 (VCAM-1)
	Endothelial leukocyte adhesion molecule-1 (ELAM-1 or E-Selectin)
Inflammatory cytokines	Interleukin (IL)-2, -6, and -8
	Tumor necrosis factor (TNF) α and β
	Macrophage-colony stimulating factor (M-CSF or CSF-1)
	Granulocyte colony stimulating factor (G-CSF)
	Granulocyte/Macrophage-colony stimulating factor (GM-CSF)
	Interferon-β
	Tissue factor
	Macrophage chemotactic protein-1 (MCP-1)
Immunologic mediators	Immunoglobulin (IgG) κ light chain
	T cell receptor α and β chain
	Major histocompatability complex (MHC) class I
	Major histocompatability complex (MHC) class II invariant chain (Ii)
	$β_2$-microglobulin
	Type II inducible nitric oxide synthase (iNOS)
Viral enhancers	Human immunodeficiency virus-1 (HIV-1)
	Cytomegalovirus (CMV)
	Adenovirus
	Simian virus 40 (SV40)
Transcription factors	IκBα
	c-Rel
	NF-κB p105
	c-myc
	Interferon regulatory factor-1 (IRF-1)

The NF-κB family can be further divided into two groups based upon their structure and function. The first group consists of RelA, c-Rel, and RelB, which contain transcriptional activation domains necessary for gene induction [73]. The second group consists of p100 and p105, which on proteolytic processing give rise to p50 (NF-κB1) and p52 (NF-κB2), respectively [74, 75]. The activation of NF-κB is mediated by NF-κB inducing kinase (NIK) which is a member of the mitogen-activated protein kinase kinase kinase family (MAP3K) [76]. NIK activates the IκB kinase (IKK) which directly activates NF-κB by phosphorylating IκBs [77].

The IKK is a complex comprising at least three IKK subunits, IKK-α (CHUK), IKK-β, and IKK-γ [78–82]. Both IKK-α and IKK-β phosphorylate specific serine residues of IκBα at position 32 and 36, which targets IκBα for ubiquitination and rapid degradation by the 26S proteasome [83] . Upon degradation of its cytoplasmic inhibitor protein, NF-κB translocates to the nucleus and transactivates enhancer elements of proinflammatory genes such as ICAM-1, VCAM-1, and E-selectin [84]. An additional requirement for NF-κB activation is phosphorylation of the RelA subunit by protein kinase A [85, 86]. Since adhesion molecules are predominantly regulated at the level of gene transcription, the activation of NF-κB activity is a key regulatory step in the induction of endothelial cell adhesion molecule expression.

As mentioned, NF-κB is bound to its own inhibitor in the cytoplasm and degradation of IκB proteins are required for NF-κB translocation to the nucleus. The best characterized IκB molecule is IκBα, which is present in all mammalian cells [87]. IκBα is a 36 kDa protein which binds to the Rel homology domain of NF-κB subunits. The nuclear localization sequence (NLS) of Rel proteins is masked by IκBα [88]. Upon phoshorylation of IκBα on serine residues 32 and 36, the polypeptide, ubiquitin, is attached to lysine residues of IκBα. For IκBβ, specific phosphorylation sites are serine residues 19 and 23 [77, 82]. Ubiquitination of IκB triggers its recognition for rapid degradation by a high molecular ATP-dependent protease, the 26S proteasome [89–91]. Several cell permeable protease inhibitors such as peptide aldehydes (i.e. MG132) inhibit NF-κB activation by inhibiting the 26S proteasome, which is necessary for IκB protein degradation [92]. The activation of NF-κB also results in the induction of IκBα since the IκBα promoter contains several κB-binding motifs [93]. Thus, the ability of NF-κB to induce its own inhibitor suggests an autoregulatory feedback mechanism for terminating its own activation.

Inhibition of NF-κB activation by NO

NO is produced by three different NO synthases depending upon tissue distribution and stimulation (Tab. 2). Vascular endothelial cells produce NO constitutively and can express the inducible isoform of NO synthase in response to cytokine stimulation [94–96]. Thus, the net activation of NF-κB in vascular wall cells during inflammation probably depends on a complex balance between stimulatory and inhibitory factors. The finding that inhibition of endogenous endothelial NO production by L-NMA could activate NF-κB, induce VCAM-1 expression, and stimulate endothelial-leukocyte adhesion suggests that constitutively-produced NO may play an important physiologic role in tonically inhibiting endothelial cell activation under basal conditions [58]. This inhibitory effect of NO is also supported by the finding *in vivo* that inhibition of endogenous NO production by L-NAME promotes

Table 2 - NO synthases

Isoforms	Cell types	Basal NO levels	Stimulated NO levels
Type I (nNOS)	Neurons, skeletal muscle, ? smooth muscle	Low	Transient, low
Type II (iNOS)	Macrophages, myocytes, smooth muscle, hepatocytes	None	Sustained, high
Type III (eNOS)	Endothelial cells, platelets	Low	Transient, high

endothelial-leukocyte interactions through the expression of NF-κB-dependent adhesion molecules [97].

The activation of NF-κB is required for the transcriptional induction of many pro-inflammatory mediators, such as cytokines, growth factors, and endothelial cell adhesion molecules [5, 39]. Consequently, NO is able to inhibit other NF-κB-dependent genes such as IL-8, MCP-1, and MCS-F [38, 39, 58]. Although two other endothelial adhesion molecules, E-selectin and ICAM-1, are transcriptionally regulated by NF-κB, their expressions are less affected by NO compared to that of VCAM-1. This is due, in part, to the complex interaction of transcription factors and other regulatory elements which are required to transactivate these genes [84].

Although under static conditions, cultured endothelial cells do not produce sufficient NO to inhibit cytokine-induced activation of NF-κB, higher levels of NO may be produced by endothelial cells *in vivo* in response to fluid shear stress which is known to stimulate endothelial cell Type III NO synthase (eNOS) gene transcription [98, 99]. As eNOS expression increases with shear stress, regions of normal laminar flow may have sufficient NO production to suppress NF-κB activation. However, regions of distrubed flow, lacking the stimulus to augment NO production, may lose this potentially protective action of NO. This phenomenon could help explain why the regions of physiologic shear stress tend to be less susceptible to the development of nascent atherosclerotic lesions than regions of disturbed flow (i.e. near branch points or flow dividers) which have increased predilection to develop these lesions [100].

In addition to NO produced by eNOS, endothelial cells may encounter higher levels of NO generated by inducible Type II NO synthase (iNOS) at sites of vascular inflammation [101–103]. Exposure of rodent macrophages and human vascular smooth muscle cells to cytokines leads to the induction of iNOS which produces substantially higher levels of NO compared to that of eNOS [104]. Furthermore, compared to *in vitro* studies, higher NO concentrations could be achieved locally since endothelial cells are in close proximity to cells expressing iNOS *in vivo*. Thus, the amount of NO produced by iNOS can be approximated with NO donors which have been shown to inhibit NF-κB activation [58]. Indeed, in the separated co-culture system with endothelial cells and RAW264.7 cells, LPS induced nuclear translocation of endothelial RelA is inhibited by iNO produced by RAW264.7 cells [105].

Mechanistic differences between NO and antioxidants on NF-κB activation

Our initial data had suggested that NO inhibited IκBα degradation as an essential mechanism for NO's inhibitory effect on NF-κB activation [106]. However, a more detailed analysis using shorter stimulation intervals indicated that stabilization of latent IκBα is probably not responsible for inhibition of NF-κB activity [61]. This is in contrast to antioxidants such as N-acetylcysteine (NAC) and pyrrolidine dithiocarbamate (PDTC) which prevent IκBα phosphorylation and degradation [60]. These findings were confirmed by analysis of IKK activity. Endothelial IKK (IKK-1 and -2) directly phoshorylates IκBα at serine residues 32 and 36 within 10 min following TNFα stimulation. Pre-incubation with NAC completely prevented IKK activity, whereas the NO donor, GSNO, had no effect on IKK activity [60]. These results suggest that NO inhibits NF-κB activation by mechanisms which are distinct from NAC and PDTC.

Enhanced nuclear translocation of IκB by NO

Higher protein levels of IκBα may result in a different subcellular distribution of the protein. Whereas under physiological conditions IκBα is exclusively localized in the cytoplasm, when synthesized in excess, IκBα can translocate into the nucleus and terminate NF-κB-induced gene transcription [107–109]. It is somewhat surprising though that IκBα can enter the nucleus since the carboxy terminus of IκBα contains multiple ankyrin repeat motifs which may inhibit its entry into the cell nucleus [110]. Nevertheless, the nuclear translocation of IκBα has been documented by several investigators and appears to constitute an effective mechanism which can rapidly terminate NF-κB-mediated transactivation of pro-inflammatory genes.

It is not known for certain, however, whether enhanced nuclear translocation of IκBα results from an active IκBα nuclear transporter or the result of passive diffusion of increased amounts of newly-synthesized IκBα. For example, nuclear translocation of IκBα occurs following stimulation with TNFα which also induces IκBα synthesis indirectly *via* activation of NF-κB [93, 111, 112]. Thus, the process

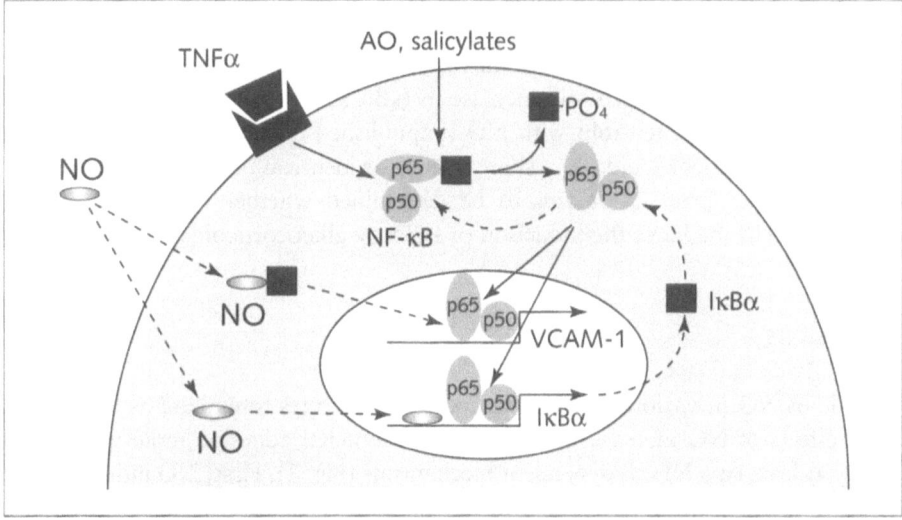

Figure 1
Mechanisms by which NO inhibits NF-κB activation. NO enhances the nuclear translocation of IκB-α and induces IκB-α gene transcription. IκB-α functions as an autoregulatory inhibitor of NF-κB activation. AO: antioxidants; VCAM-1: vascular cell adhesion molecule-1.

of nuclear translocation of IκBα may not be restricted to the actions of NO, but rather, occurs through a more general mechanism for terminating NF-κB transactivation.

Induction of IκBα gene transcription by NO

Transfection studies using the IκBα promoter linked to the chloramphenicol acetyltransferase reporter gene suggests that the induction of IκBα by NO occurs at the transcriptional level [60]. Previous analyses of the human, porcine, and murine IκBα promoters have revealed multiple functional κB sites necessary for transcriptional induction by NF-κB [111, 113–115]. All of these sites are located within −350 bp of the transcriptional start site and provide for an inducible autoregulatory pathway for terminating the activation of NF-κB. However, NO's effects on IκBα gene transcription is probably not mediated by NF-κB since NO inhibits NF-κB, and alone does not induce VCAM-1 gene transcription. Further analyses of the upstream IκBα promoter will be necessary to determine which DNA binding domain(s) constitute the NO-responsive cis-regulatory element(s) in the IκBα promoter.

The induction of IκBα gene transcription also occurs following treatment with corticosteroids in Jurkat or T cells [116, 117]. However, we have observed that the induction of IκBα by glucocorticoids in vascular endothelial cells is modest at best, producing only about a two-fold increase in IκBα steady-state mRNA levels compared to greater than ten-fold with NO (unpublished observations). It is possible that NO and glucocorticoids may share similar or identical pathways for transactivating the IκBα gene. It remains to be determined whether NO production in endothelial cells mediates the induction of IκBα by glucocorticoids.

Conclusions

The role of NO in various biological processes continues to expand as knowledge of the effects of NO increases. NO inhibits endothelial adhesion molecule expression by at least two NF-κB dependent mechanisms (Fig. 1). First, NO induces IκBα, the newly synthesized inhibitor binds to cytoplasmic NF-κB resulting in prevention of further NF-κB translocation to the nucleus. The induction of IκBα by NO is independent of cytokine stimulation and occurs also in unstimulated endothelial cells. Second, NO causes nuclear accumulation of IκBα which may be able to terminate signaling of already activated NF-κB. This would also explain the time delay observed for NF-κB inhibition. Whether IκBα translocates into the nucleus by active or passive mechanisms, remains to be established. No doubt, continued exploration of NO's effects will yield further insight into its role in vascular biology.

References

1   Gimbrone MA Jr (1995) Vascular endothelium: an integrator of pathophysiologic stimuli in atherosclerosis. *Am J Cardiol* 75: 67B–70B

2   Vane JR, Anggard EE, Botting RM (1990) Regulatory functions of the vascular endothelium. *N Engl J Med* 323: 27–36

3   Pober JS, Collins T, Gimbrone MA, Jr., Cotran RS, Gitlin JD, Fiers W, Clayberger C, Krensky AM, Burakoff SJ, Reiss CS (1983) Lymphocytes recognize human vascular endothelial and dermal fibroblast Ia antigens induced by recombinant immune interferon. *Nature* 305: 726–729

4   Cybulsky MI, Gimbrone MA Jr (1991) Endothelial expression of a mononuclear leukocyte adhesion molecule during atherogenesis. *Science* 251: 788–791

5   Collins T (1993) Endothelial nuclear factor-kappa B and the initiation of the atherosclerotic lesion. *Lab Invest* 68: 499–508

6   Butcher EC (1991) Leukocyte-endothelial cell recognition: three (or more) steps to specificity and diversity. *Cell* 67: 1033–1036

7   Mackay CR, Imhof BA (1993) Cell adhesion in the immune system. *Immunol Today* 14: 99–102

8   Dustin ML, Rothlein R, Bhan AK, Dinarello CA, Springer TA (1986) Induction by IL-1 and interferon-gamma: tissue distribution, biochemistry, and function of a natural adherence molecule (ICAM-1). *J Immunol* 137: 245–254

9   Rice GE, Munro JM, Bevilacqua MP (1990) Inducible cell adhesion molecule 110 (INCAM-110) is an endothelial receptor for lymphocytes. A CD11/CD18-independent adhesion mechanism. *J Exp Med* 171: 1369–1374

10   Osborn L, Hession C, Tizard R, Vassallo C, Luhowskyj S, Chi-Rosso G, Lobb R (1989) Direct expression cloning of vascular cell adhesion molecule 1, a cytokine-induced endothelial protein that binds to lymphocytes. *Cell* 59: 1203–1211

11   Dobrina A, Menegazzi R, Carlos TM, Nardon E, Cramer R, Zacchi T, Harlan JM, Patriarca P (1991) Mechanisms of eosinophil adherence to cultured vascular endothelial cells. Eosinophils bind to the cytokine-induced ligand vascular cell adhesion molecule-1 *via* the very late activation antigen-4 integrin receptor. *J Clin Invest* 88: 20–26

12   Carlos TM, Schwartz BR, Kovach NL, Yee E, Rosa M, Osborn L, Chi-Rosso G, Newman B, Lobb R, Rosso M, et al (1990) Vascular cell adhesion molecule-1 mediates lymphocyte adherence to cytokine-activated cultured human endothelial cells. *Blood* 76: 965–970

13   Rice GE, Munro JM, Corless C, Bevilacqua MP (1991) Vascular and nonvascular expression of INCAM-110. A target for mononuclear leukocyte adhesion in normal and inflamed human tissues. *Am J Pathol* 138: 385–393

14   Hynes RO (1987) Integrins: a family of cell surface receptors. *Cell* 48: 549–554

15   Plow EF, Ginsberg MH (1989) Cellular adhesion: GPIIb-IIIa as a prototypic adhesion receptor. *Prog Hemost Thromb* 9: 117–156

16   Maxfield SR, Moulder K, Koning F, Elbe A, Stingl G, Coligan JE, Shevach EM, Yokoyama WM (1989) Murine T cells express a cell surface receptor for multiple extracellular matrix proteins. Identification and characterization with monoclonal antibodies. *J Exp Med* 169: 2173–2190

17   Sanchez-Madrid F, Nagy JA, Robbins E, Simon P, Springer TA (1983) A human leukocyte differentiation antigen family with distinct alpha-subunits and a common beta-subunit: the lymphocyte function-associated antigen (LFA-1), the C3bi complement receptor (OKM1/Mac-1), and the p150,95 molecule. *J Exp Med* 158: 1785–1803

18   Weber C, Alon R, Moser B, Springer TA (1996) Sequential regulation of alpha 4 beta 1 and alpha 5 beta 1 integrin avidity by CC chemokines in monocytes: implications for transendothelial chemotaxis. *J Cell Biol* 134: 1063–1073

19   Szabo MC, Butcher EC, McIntyre BW, Schall TJ, Bacon KB (1997) RANTES stimulation of T lymphocyte adhesion and activation: role for LFA-1 and ICAM-3. *Eur J Immunol* 27: 1061–1068

20   Schall TJ (1991) Biology of the RANTES/SIS cytokine family. *Cytokine* 3: 165–183

21   Zimmerman GA, Prescott SM, McIntyre TM (1992) Endothelial cell interactions with granulocytes: tethering and signaling molecules. *Immunol Today* 13: 93–100

22   Huber AR, Kunkel SL, Todd RFD, Weiss SJ (1991) Regulation of transendothelial neutrophil migration by endogenous interleukin-8 [published errata appear in *Science* 1991 Nov 1; 254 (5032): 631 and 1991 Dec 6; 254 (5037): 1435]. *Science* 254: 99–102

23   Lawrence MB, Springer TA (1991) Leukocytes roll on a selectin at physiologic flow rates: distinction from and prerequisite for adhesion through integrins. *Cell* 65: 859–873

24   Lo SK, Lee S, Ramos RA, Lobb R, Rosa M, Chi-Rosso G, Wright SD (1991) Endothelial-leukocyte adhesion molecule 1 stimulates the adhesive activity of leukocyte integrin CR3 (CD11b/CD18, Mac-1, alpha m beta 2) on human neutrophils. *J Exp Med* 173: 1493–1500

25   Whitley MZ, Thanos D, Read MA, Maniatis T, Collins T (1994) A striking similarity in the organization of the E-selectin and beta interferon gene promoters. *Mol Cell Biol* 14: 6464–6475

26   Li H, Cybulsky MI, Gimbrone MA Jr, Libby P (1993) An atherogenic diet rapidly induces VCAM-1, a cytokine-regulatable mononuclear leukocyte adhesion molecule, in rabbit aortic endothelium. *Arterioscler Thromb* 13: 197–204

27   Libby P, Sukhova G, Lee RT, Liao JK (1997) Molecular biology of atherosclerosis. *Int J Cardiol* 62 (Suppl 2): S23–S29

28   Davies MJ, Gordon JL, Gearing AJ, Pigott R, Woolf N, Katz D, Kyriakopoulos A (1993) The expression of the adhesion molecules ICAM-1, VCAM-1, PECAM, and E-selectin in human atherosclerosis. *J Pathol* 171: 223–229

29   Berliner JA, Navab M, Fogelman AM, Frank JS, Demer LL, Edwards PA, Watson AD, Lusis AJ (1995) Atherosclerosis: basic mechanisms. Oxidation, inflammation, and genetics. *Circulation* 91: 2488–2496

30   Ross R, Harker L (1976) Hyperlipidemia and atherosclerosis. *Science* 193: 1094–1100

31   Dong ZM, Chapman SM, Brown AA, Frenette PS, Hynes RO, Wagner DD (1998) The combined role of P- and E-selectins in atherosclerosis. *J Clin Invest* 102: 145–152

32   Ma XL, Weyrich AS, Lefer DJ, Lefer AM (1993) Diminished basal nitric oxide release after myocardial ischemia and reperfusion promotes neutrophil adherence to coronary endothelium. *Circ Res* 72: 403–412

33   Hafezi-Moghadam A, Ley K (1999) Relevance of L-selectin shedding for leukocyte rolling *in vivo*. *J Exp Med* 189: 939–948

34   Darius H, Ahland B, Rucker W, Klaus W, Peskar BA, Schror K (1984) The effects of molsidomine and its metabolite SIN-1 on coronary vessel tone, platelet aggregation, and eicosanoid formation *in vitro* – inhibition of 12-HPETE biosynthesis. *J Cardiovasc Pharmacol* 6: 115–121

35   Rees DD, Palmer RM, Moncada S (1989) Role of endothelium-derived nitric oxide in the regulation of blood pressure. *Proc Natl Acad Sci USA* 86: 3375–3378

36   Vallance P, Collier J, Moncada S (1989) Effects of endothelium-derived nitric oxide on peripheral arteriolar tone in man. *Lancet* 2: 997–1000

37   Radomski MW, Palmer RM, Moncada S (1987) The anti-aggregating properties of vascular endothelium: interactions between prostacyclin and nitric oxide. *Br J Pharmacol* 92: 639–646

38   Zeiher AM, Fisslthaler B, Schray-Utz B, Busse R (1995) Nitric oxide modulates the expression of monocyte chemoattractant protein 1 in cultured human endothelial cells. *Circ Res* 76: 980–986

39   Peng HB, Rajavashisth TB, Libby P, Liao JK (1995) Nitric oxide inhibits macrophage-colony stimulating factor gene transcription in vascular endothelial cells. *J Biol Chem* 270: 17050–17055

40   Kurose I, Kubes P, Wolf R, Anderson DC, Paulson J, Miyasaka M, Granger DN (1993) Inhibition of nitric oxide production. Mechanisms of vascular albumin leakage. *Circ Res* 73: 164–171

41   Garg UC, Hassid A (1989) Nitric oxide-generating vasodilators and 8-bromo-cyclic guanosine monophosphate inhibit mitogenesis and proliferation of cultured rat vascular smooth muscle cells. *J Clin Invest* 83: 1774–1777

42   Gauthier TW, Davenpeck KL, Lefer AM (1994) Nitric oxide attenuates leukocyte-endothelial interaction *via* P-selectin in splanchnic ischemia-reperfusion. *Am J Physiol* 267: G562–568

43   Gauthier TW, Scalia R, Murohara T, Guo JP, Lefer AM (1995) Nitric oxide protects against leukocyte-endothelium interactions in the early stages of hypercholesterolemia. *Arterioscler Thromb Vasc Biol* 15: 1652–1659

44   Kubes P, Suzuki M, Granger DN (1991) Nitric oxide: an endogenous modulator of leukocyte adhesion. *Proc Natl Acad Sci USA* 88: 4651–4655

45   Niu XF, Smith CW, Kubes P (1994) Intracellular oxidative stress induced by nitric oxide synthesis inhibition increases endothelial cell adhesion to neutrophils. *Circ Res* 74: 1133–1140

46   Cooke JP, Singer AH, Tsao P, Zera P, Rowan RA, Billingham ME (1992) Antiatherogenic effects of L-arginine in the hypercholesterolemic rabbit. *J Clin Invest* 90: 1168–1172

47   Groves PH, Lewis MJ, Cheadle HA, Penny WJ (1993) SIN-1 reduces platelet adhesion and platelet thrombus formation in a porcine model of balloon angioplasty. *Circulation* 87: 590–597

48   Guo JP, Panday MM, Consigny PM, Lefer AM (1995) Mechanisms of vascular preservation by a novel NO donor following rat carotid artery intimal injury. *Am J Physiol* 269: H1122–1131

49   von der Leyen HE, Gibbons GH, Morishita R, Lewis NP, Zhang L, Nakajima M, Kaneda Y, Cooke JP, Dzau VJ (1995) Gene therapy inhibiting neointimal vascular lesion: *in vivo* transfer of endothelial cell nitric oxide synthase gene. *Proc Natl Acad Sci USA* 92: 1137–1141

50   Siegfried MR, Carey C, Ma XL, Lefer AM (1992) Beneficial effects of SPM-5185, a cysteine-containing NO donor in myocardial ischemia-reperfusion. *Am J Physiol* 263: H771–777

51   Weyrich AS, Ma XL, Lefer AM (1992) The role of L-arginine in ameliorating reperfusion injury after myocardial ischemia in the cat. *Circulation* 86: 279–288

52   Liao JK (1998) Endothelium and acute coronary syndromes. Clin Chem 44: 1799–1808

53   Creager MA, Cooke JP, Mendelsohn ME, Gallagher SJ, Coleman SM, Loscalzo J, Dzau VJ (1990) Impaired vasodilation of forearm resistance vessels in hypercholesterolemic humans. *J Clin Invest* 86: 228–234

54   Zeiher AM, Drexler H, Saurbier B, Just H (1993) Endothelium-mediated coronary blood flow modulation in humans. Effects of age, atherosclerosis, hypercholesterolemia, and hypertension. *J Clin Invest* 92: 652–662

55   Lefer AM, Ma XL (1993) Decreased basal nitric oxide release in hypercholesterolemia increases neutrophil adherence to rabbit coronary artery endothelium. *Arterioscler Thromb* 13: 771–776

56   Hamon M, Vallet B, Bauters C, Wernert N, McFadden EP, Lablanche JM, Dupuis B, Bertrand ME (1994) Long-term oral administration of L-arginine reduces intimal thickening and enhances neoendothelium-dependent acetylcholine-induced relaxation after arterial injury. *Circulation* 90: 1357–1362

57   Tsao PS, McEvoy LM, Drexler H, Butcher EC, Cooke JP (1994) Enhanced endothelial adhesiveness in hypercholesterolemia is attenuated by L-arginine. *Circulation* 89: 2176–2182

58   De Caterina R, Libby P, Peng HB, Thannickal VJ, Rajavashisth TB, Gimbrone MA Jr, Shin WS, Liao JK (1995) Nitric oxide decreases cytokine-induced endothelial activation. Nitric oxide selectively reduces endothelial expression of adhesion molecules and proinflammatory cytokines. *J Clin Invest* 96: 60–68

59   Khan BV, Harrison DG, Olbrych MT, Alexander RW, Medford RM (1996) Nitric oxide regulates vascular cell adhesion molecule 1 gene expression and redox-sensitive transcriptional events in human vascular endothelial cells. *Proc Natl Acad Sci USA* 93: 9114–9119

60   Spiecker M, Darius H, Kaboth K, Hubner F, Liao JK (1998) Differential regulation of endothelial cell adhesion molecule expression by nitric oxide donors and antioxidants. *J Leukoc Biol* 63: 732–739

61   Spiecker M, Peng HB, Liao JK (1997) Inhibition of endothelial vascular cell adhesion molecule-1 expression by nitric oxide involves the induction and nuclear translocation of IκBα. *J Biol Chem* 272: 30969–30974

62   Stamler JS, Singel DJ, Loscalzo J (1992) Biochemistry of nitric oxide and its redox-activated forms. *Science* 258: 1898–1902

63   Hogg N, Singh RJ, Kalyanaraman B (1996) The role of glutathione in the transport and catabolism of nitric oxide. *FEBS Lett* 382: 223–228

64   Mayer B, Pfeiffer S, Schrammel A, Koesling D, Schmidt K, Brunner F (1998) A new pathway of nitric oxide/cyclic GMP signaling involving S-nitrosoglutathione. *J Biol Chem* 273: 3264–3270

65   Wirth T, Baltimore D (1988) Nuclear factor NF-κB can interact functionally with its cognate binding site to provide lymphoid-specific promoter function. *Embo J* 7: 3109–3113

66   Sen R, Baltimore D (1986) Multiple nuclear factors interact with the immunoglobulin enhancer sequences. *Cell* 46: 705–716

67 Sen R, Baltimore D (1986) Inducibility of kappa immunoglobulin enhancer-binding protein N-κB by a posttranslational mechanism. *Cell* 47: 921–928

68 Speir E, Shibutani T, Yu ZX, Ferrans V, Epstein SE (1996) Role of reactive oxygen intermediates in cytomegalovirus gene expression and in the response of human smooth muscle cells to viral infection. *Circ Res* 79: 1143–1152

69 Perkins ND, Edwards NL, Duckett CS, Agranoff AB, Schmid RM, Nabel GJ (1993) A cooperative interaction between NF-κB and Sp1 is required for HIV-1 enhancer activation. *Embo J* 12: 3551–3558

70 Thanos D, Maniatis T (1995) NF-κB: a lesson in family values. *Cell* 80: 529–532

71 Baeuerle PA, Baltimore D (1996) NF-κB: ten years after. *Cell* 87: 13–20

72 Lemaitre B, Nicolas E, Michaut L, Reichhart JM, Hoffmann JA (1996) The dorsoventral regulatory gene cassette spatzle/Toll/cactus controls the potent antifungal response in *Drosophila* adults. *Cell* 86: 973–983

73 Ballard DW, Dixon EP, Peffer NJ, Bogerd H, Doerre S, Stein B, Greene WC (1992) The 65-kDa subunit of human NF-κB functions as a potent transcriptional activator and a target for v-Rel-mediated repression. *Proc Natl Acad Sci USA* 89: 1875–1879

74 Rice NR, MacKichan ML, Israel A (1992) The precursor of NF-κB p50 has IκB-like functions. *Cell* 71: 243–253

75 Scheinman RI, Beg AA, Baldwin AS Jr (1993) NF-κB p100 (Lyt-10) is a component of H2TF1 and can function as an IκB-like molecule. *Mol Cell Biol* 13: 6089–6101

76 Malinin NL, Boldin MP, Kovalenko AV, Wallach D (1997) MAP3K-related kinase involved in NF-κB induction by TNF, CD95 and IL-1. *Nature* 385: 540–544

77 Regnier CH, Song HY, Gao X, Goeddel DV, Cao Z, Rothe M (1997) Identification and characterization of an IκB kinase. *Cell* 90: 373–383

78 Woronicz JD, Gao X, Cao Z, Rothe M, Goeddel DV (1997) IκB kinase-β: NF-κB activation and complex formation with IκB kinase-α and NIK. *Science* 278: 866–869

79 Zandi E, Rothwarf DM, Delhase M, Hayakawa M, Karin M (1997) The IκB kinase complex (IKK) contains two kinase subunits, IKKα and IKKβ, necessary for IκB phosphorylation and NF-κB activation. *Cell* 91: 243–252

80 Rothwarf DM, Zandi E, Natoli G, Karin M (1998) IKK-γ is an essential regulatory subunit of the IκB kinase complex. *Nature* 395: 297–300

81 DiDonato JA, Hayakawa M, Rothwarf DM, Zandi E, Karin M (1997) A cytokine-responsive IκB kinase that activates the transcription factor NF-κB. *Nature* 388: 548–554

82 Mercurio F, Zhu H, Murray BW, Shevchenko A, Bennett BL, Li J, Young DB, Barbosa M, Mann M, Manning A, et al (1997) IKK-1 and IKK-2: cytokine-activated IκB kinases essential for NF-κB activation. *Science* 278: 860–866

83 Brown K, Gerstberger S, Carlson L, Franzoso G, Siebenlist U (1995) Control of IκBα proteolysis by site-specific, signal-induced phosphorylation. *Science* 267: 1485–1488

84 Collins T, Read MA, Neish AS, Whitley MZ, Thanos D, Maniatis T (1995) Transcriptional regulation of endothelial cell adhesion molecules: NF-κB and cytokine-inducible enhancers. *FASEB J* 9: 899–909

85   Naumann M, Scheidereit C (1994) Activation of NF-κB *in vivo* is regulated by multiple phosphorylations. *EMBO J* 13: 4597–4607

86   Zhong H, SuYang H, Erdjument-Bromage H, Tempst P, Ghosh S (1997) The transcriptional activity of NF-κB is regulated by the IκB-associated PKAc subunit through a cyclic AMP-independent mechanism. *Cell* 89: 413–424

87   Haskill S, Beg AA, Tompkins SM, Morris JS, Yurochko AD, Sampson-Johannes A, Mondal K, Ralph P, Baldwin AS Jr (1991) Characterization of an immediate-early gene induced in adherent monocytes that encodes IκB-like activity. *Cell* 65: 1281–1289

88   Beg AA, Ruben SM, Scheinman RI, Haskill S, Rosen CA, Baldwin AS Jr (1992) IκB interacts with the nuclear localization sequences of the subunits of NF-κB: a mechanism for cytoplasmic retention. *Genes Dev* 6: 1899–1913

89   Palombella VJ, Rando OJ, Goldberg AL, Maniatis T (1994) The ubiquitin-proteasome pathway is required for processing the NF-κB1 precursor protein and the activation of NF-κB. *Cell* 78: 773–785

90   Chen Z, Hagler J, Palombella VJ, Melandri F, Scherer D, Ballard D, Maniatis T (1995) Signal-induced site-specific phosphorylation targets IκBα to the ubiquitin-proteasome pathway. *Genes Dev* 9: 1586–1597

91   DiDonato J, Mercurio F, Rosette C, Wu-Li J, Suyang H, Ghosh S, Karin M (1996) Mapping of the inducible IκB phosphorylation sites that signal its ubiquitination and degradation. *Mol Cell Biol* 16: 1295–1304

92   Traenckner EB, Wilk S, Baeuerle PA (1994) A proteasome inhibitor prevents activation of NF-kappa B and stabilizes a newly phosphorylated form of IκB-α that is still bound to NF-κB. *Embo J* 13: 5433–5441

93   Sun SC, Ganchi PA, Ballard DW, Greene WC (1993) NF-κB controls expression of inhibitor IκBα: evidence for an inducible autoregulatory pathway. *Science* 259: 1912–1915

94   Gross SS, Jaffe EA, Levi R, Kilbourn RG (1991) Cytokine-activated endothelial cells express an isotype of nitric oxide synthase which is tetrahydrobiopterin-dependent, calmodulin-independent and inhibited by arginine analogs with a rank-order of potency characteristic of activated macrophages. *Biochem Biophys Res Commun* 178: 823–829

95   Janssens SP, Simouchi A, Quertermous T, Bloch DB, Bloch KD (1992) Cloning and expression of a cDNA encoding human endothelium-derived relating factor/nitric oxide synthase. *J Biol Chem* 267: 22694

96   Lamas S, Marsden PA, Li GK, Tempst P, Michel T (1992) Endothelial nitric oxide synthase: molecular cloning and characterization of a distinct constitutive enzyme isoform. *Proc Natl Acad Sci USA* 89: 6348–6352

97   Tsao PS, Buitrago R, Chan JR, Cooke JP (1996) Fluid flow inhibits endothelial adhesiveness. Nitric oxide and transcriptional regulation of VCAM-1. *Circulation* 94: 1682–1689

98   Nadaud S, Philippe M, Arnal JF, Michel JB, Soubrier F (1996) Sustained increase in aor-

tic endothelial nitric oxide synthase expression *in vivo* in a model of chronic high blood flow. *Circ Res* 79: 857–863

99 Uematsu M, Ohara Y, Navas JP, Nishida K, Murphy TJ, Alexander RW, Nerem RM, Harrison DG (1995) Regulation of endothelial cell nitric oxide synthase mRNA expression by shear stress. *Am J Physiol* 269: C1371–1378

100 Golledge J, Turner RJ, Harley SL, Springall DR, Powell JT (1997) Circumferential deformation and shear stress induce differential responses in saphenous vein endothelium exposed to arterial flow. *J Clin Invest* 99: 2719–2726

101 Xie QW, Cho HJ, Calaycay J, Mumford RA, Swiderek KM, Lee TD, Ding A, Troso T, Nathan C (1992) Cloning and characterization of inducible nitric oxide synthase from mouse macrophages. *Science* 256: 225–228

102 Lyons CR, Orloff GJ, Cunningham JM (1992) Molecular cloning and functional expression of an inducible nitric oxide synthase from a murine macrophage cell line. *J Biol Chem* 267: 6370–6374

103 Lowenstein CJ, Glatt CS, Bredt DS, Snyder SH (1992) Cloned and expressed macrophage nitric oxide synthase contrasts with the brain enzyme. *Proc Natl Acad Sci USA* 89: 6711–6715

104 Dinerman JL, Lowenstein CJ, Snyder SH (1993) Molecular mechanisms of nitric oxide regulation. Potential relevance to cardiovascular disease. *Circ Res* 73: 217–222

105 Peng HB, Spiecker M, Liao JK (1998) Inducible nitric oxide: an autoregulatory feedback inhibitor of vascular inflammation. *J Immunol* 161: 1970–1976

106 Peng HB, Libby P, Liao JK (1995) Induction and stabilization of IκBα by nitric oxide mediates inhibition of NF-κB. *J Biol Chem* 270: 14214–14219

107 Zabel U, Henkel T, Silva MS, Baeuerle PA (1993) Nuclear uptake control of NF-κB by MAD-3, an IκB protein present in the nucleus. *Embo J* 12: 201–211

108 Arenzana-Seisdedos F, Thompson J, Rodriguez MS, Bachelerie F, Thomas D, Hay RT (1995) Inducible nuclear expression of newly synthesized IκBα negatively regulates DNA-binding and transcriptional activities of NF-κB. *Mol Cell Biol* 15: 2689–2696

109 Read MA, Neish AS, Gerritsen ME, Collins T (1996) Postinduction transcriptional repression of E-selectin and vascular cell adhesion molecule-1. *J Immunol* 157: 3472–3479

110 Beg AA, Baldwin AS Jr (1993) The IκB proteins: multifunctional regulators of Rel/NF-κB transcription factors. *Genes Dev* 7: 2064–2070

111 Chiao PJ, Miyamoto S, Verma IM (1994) Autoregulation of IκBα activity. *Proc Natl Acad Sci USA* 91: 28–32

112 Read MA, Whitley MZ, Williams AJ, Collins T (1994) NF-κB and IκBα: an inducible regulatory system in endothelial activation. *J Exp Med* 179: 503–512

113 de Martin R, Vanhove B, Cheng Q, Hofer E, Csizmadia V, Winkler H, Bach FH (1993) Cytokine-inducible expression in endothelial cells of an IκBα-like gene is regulated by NF-κB. *EMBO J* 12: 2773–2779

114 Ito CY, Kazantsev AG, Baldwin AS Jr (1994) Three NF-kappa B sites in the I kappa B-

alpha promoter are required for induction of gene expression by TNFα. *Nucleic Acids Res* 22: 3787–3792

115 Le Bail O, Schmidt-Ullrich R, Israel A (1993) Promoter analysis of the gene encoding the IκBα/MAD3 inhibitor of NF-κB: positive regulation by members of the rel/NF-κB family. *EMBO J* 12: 5043–5049

116 Scheinman RI, Cogswell PC, Lofquist AK, Baldwin AS Jr (1995) Role of transcriptional activation of IκBα in mediation of immunosuppression by glucocorticoids. *Science* 270: 283–286

117 Auphan N, DiDonato JA, Rosette C, Helmberg A, Karin M (1995) Immunosuppression by glucocorticoids: inhibition of NF-κB activity through induction of IκB synthesis. *Science* 270: 286–290

Nitric oxide and leukocyte recruitment

Graciela Andonegui and Paul Kubes

Immunology Research Group, University of Calgary, Health Sciences Center, 3330 Hospital Dr. N.W., Calgary, Alberta, T2N 4N1, Canada

Introduction

Leukocyte recruitment into sites of inflammation requires the activation of vascular endothelium by inflammatory mediators leading to a cascade of events. These include leukocyte rolling followed by leukocyte adhesion, and ultimately migration out of the circulation and into the inflammatory site. Although much attention has been attributed to the pro-adhesive mechanisms involved in leukocyte recruitment, the potential down-regulating or inhibitory factors that reduce leukocyte recruitment have not been studied in great detail. The purpose of this overview is to highlight some of the evidence that nitric oxide (NO) produced by the lining of blood vessels acts as an endogenous inhibitor of neutrophil adhesion to vascular endothelium.

In 1991, it was first proposed [1] that inhibition of nictric oxide synthase (NOS) in the microvasculature would lead to an increase in leukocyte recruitment. In that and subsequent studies it was demonstrated that an L-arginine analogue, L-NAME, increased PMN adherence to postcapillary venules as assessed by intravital microscopy and that this effect could be prevented by pretreatment with L-arginine the substrate for NO. Moreover, the L-NAME-induced adhesion could be reversed with either a cGMP analog [2] or a NO donor [3]. These data suggested that endogenous NO modulates PMN-endothelial cell interactions, but to date the mechanism of action has not been elucidated. A number of potential factors have been excluded. For example, a very real concern was that the NO inhibitor was functioning simply as a vasoconstrictor reducing blood flow and thereby decreasing the hydrodynamic shear rates that would normally push leukocytes along the length of venules. This would of course increase the propensity of the leukocytes to adhere. In an experiment where shear forces were reduced mechanically to mimic the shear forces with NO inhibition, the leukocyte adhesion that was induced by the former procedure was minor compared to the adhesion induced by NO synthesis inhibition [1]. Clearly, reduced blood flow could not account for the increased cell recruitment.

In addition, L-NAME was not directly activating the leukocytes either *in vivo* or *in vitro*. Direct exposure of leukocytes to L-NAME did not induce an increase in neutrophil adhesion to endothelium or various other substrata [4, 5]. Consistent with these data was the observation that addition of L-NAME did not increase the β_2-integrin expression on the surface of neutrophils [1]. This integrin is normally responsible for essentially all adhesion of neutrophils to various substrata. However, the adhesion was certainly dependent upon the β_2-integrin *in vivo* as an antibody directed against this molecule prevented the neutrophils from adhering to post-capillary venules [1]. Clearly, a factor or factors were missing in the *in vitro* leukocyte-endothelial cell experiments. In a separate series of experiments, Gaboury and colleagues [6] demonstrated the application of L-NAME to a tissue caused mast cell degranulation and subsequent neutrophil adhesion perhaps *via* pro-inflammatory phospholipids including PAF and LTB_4 [7]. Indeed, preventing mast cell stabilization prevented L-NAME-induced neutrophil adhesion. This was consistent with a series of *in vitro* experiments that demonstrated that L-NAME could activate mast cells to release pro-inflammatory mediators and that these mediators could induce very significant leukocyte adhesion *in vitro* [4]. Again, the dominant pro-inflammatory molecule in these acute experiments was PAF. It should be noted that in a series of experiments by Kitamura and colleagues using mast cell-deficient rats, leukocyte adhesion could still be induced with L-NAME [8]. Whether this suggests that the mast cell stabilizing drugs were affecting more than mast cells or whether the mast cell-deficient rats were compensating in some manner remains unclear.

In addition to leukocyte adhesion, Lefer and his colleagues [9] demonstrated that inhibition of nitric oxide synthesis induced rapid leukocyte recruitment. The selectin responsible for rolling (P-selectin) was rapidly expressed on the surface of post-capillary venules and the increase in rolling was inhibited with a P-selectin antibody. The increase in rolling appeared to be dependent upon oxidative stress as SOD also reduced the rolling. The latter observation is consistent with an increase in oxidant production following NO synthesis inhibition both *in vivo* and *in vitro* in mast cells and endothelium [4, 10].

The increase in rolling and adhesion following NO synthesis inhibition resulted in significant leukocyte migration into the extravascular space [1]. Scalia et al. [11] reported that the L-NAME–induced transendothelial migration of leukocytes was inhibited *in vivo* with an antibody directed against PECAM-1. Although the expression of PECAM-1 on the rat mesenteric endothelium was not affected by the superfusion with L-NAME, this is not surprising as this molecule is constitutively expressed in very abundant quantities.

Although much of the aforementioned work was completed in the rat mesenteric microvasculature, the observations have been reproduced in rabbit, cat, mouse and in lung, liver, muscle, heart and brain [2, 10, 12, 13]. Therefore, the concept that NO is an endogenous inhibitor of leukocyte adhesion may span many species and many organ systems. Whether NO synthesis inhibition also induces rapid leukocyte adhesion in humans is still debatable as the work has only been done *in vitro*. The suppressive action of NO on the adhesion process is not limited to neutrophils.

Hokari et al. [14], found that endogenous NO is an important modulator of lymphocyte migration in Peyer's patches and in nonlymphoid regions of the intestine. L-NAME significantly increased rolling and adherence of lymphocytes in postcapillary venules of Peyer's patches and submucosal venules. Anti-α_4-integrin and anti-P-selectin antibodies attenuated the L-NAME-induced lymphocyte-endothelial cell interaction. In addition, Bath et al. [15] reported that NO inhibits monocyte adhesion to endothelium *in vitro*, without altering expression of CD11b/CD18. Work by DeCaterina and colleagues [16] reported that NO donors (SNP, SIN-1 and GSNO) inhibit monocyte adhesion to IL-1α-stimulated-human saphenous vein endothelial cells. This inhibition was unaffected by cGMP analogues suggesting an alternative pathway of leukocyte recruitment.

Is inhaled NO also anti-adhesive?

Although both Neonatal and Adult Intensive Care Units are using NO inhalation with increasing frequency, it remains unclear whether inhaled NO is of any real benefit. It is used mainly because it reduces pulmonary hypertension which may thereby improve oxygenation of peripheral tissues [17–19]. Other effects have not been considered in the clinical setting, however there is a growing body of evidence that inhaled NO may affect neutrophil recruitment into the pulmonary vasculature. Inhaled NO has been shown to prevent hemodialysis-induced neutrophil accumulation into lungs [20], LPS-induced neutrophil accumulation into lungs [21], I/R-induced neutrophil infiltration and capillary leak in lungs [22], IL-1-induced neutrophil infiltration into the pulmonary vasculature [23] and neutrophil infiltration into lung allografts [24]. How this is occurring is not clear, but *in vitro* studies suggest that NO prevents the reduction in neutrophil deformability following activation *via* inhibition of F-actin assembly [25]. This is important with respect to the pulmonary circulation as neutrophils are thought to physically trap rather than adhere *via* adhesion molecules within the lung. Improved deformability could improve trafficking of neutrophils through the lung.

Inhaled NO is thought to have effects strictly within the lung. However, inhaled NO may also impact upon neutrophils as they circulate through the pulmonary vasculature to provide peripheral anti-adhesive effects. Indeed, there is evidence that NO may also directly affect neutrophil adhesive capacity. Four days of inhaled NO reduced CD18 upregulation on the surface of neutrophils [26]. However, the authors acknowledged that cytokine levels were also reduced in these patients relative to untreated patients. Reduced cytokine levels may have reduced the pro-inflammatory milieu, thereby reducing the pro-adhesive state of neutrophils. Although a direct assessment of inhaled NO on adhesion has not been performed, some studies suggest that inhaled NO may affect other components of neutrophil function including a reduction in superoxide production [21, 27]. In addition, numerous reports do suggest that inhaled NO may impact on platelet adhesive mechanisms in the peripheral microvasculature. For example, inhaled NO decreased platelet aggregation in patients with ARDS (1–100 ppm) [28], increased bleeding time in rabbits (30 ppm and 300 ppm) [29], swine (5–80 ppm) [30] and reduced the development of coronary reocclusion after thrombolysis in dogs [31].

All of the aforementioned studies assumed that the cells were affected during their movement through the pulmonary circulation. This seems reasonable in light of the prevailing view that inhaled NO is rapidly inactivated in the lung capillaries by reaction with oxyhemogloblin [19]. Indeed, neither systemic blood pressure, cerebral blood flow [32] nor myocardial blood flow [31] were affected by NO inhalation (20–80 ppm). However, all of these studies have been done in replete (normal) microvascular beds. Although we also saw no noticeable effects of inhaled NO in a distal unperturbed microcirculation, when NO was locally depleted from a vascular bed, inhaled NO in a rapid and effective manner reversed the responses to NO inhibition [33]. In fact the arteriolar vasoconstriction and leukocyte adhesion observed with L-NAME was completely prevented with inhaled NO. The work was further extended in a model of inflammation (ischemia/reperfusion) where endothelial NO is depressed and poor perfusion, elevated leukocyte adhesion and microvascular dysfunction are hallmark features [33]. Inhaled NO again reduced each of these effects not only supporting the view that inhaled NO can reach the distal vasculature, but for the first time demonstrating that it could reach the distal vasculature to functionally impact upon the inflamed microcirculation and improve perfusion, dampen adhesion and reduce vascular protein leak. Further work has revealed that the effects of inhaled NO are restricted to the microcirculation and not the extravascular compartment [34] and appears to have a major impact on oxidative stress situations [35]. Finally, in studies where blood was drawn from animals breathing NO and perfused over adhesion molecules, neutrophil adhesion was unimpaired, suggesting that perhaps NO was impacting upon the endothelium not upon the neutrophil [33].

These data would therefore suggest that NO must be carried in blood from lungs to peripheral tissues [33]. Although NO reacts very quickly with heme groups thereby allowing for rapid clearance of NO from blood, NO also undergoes nitrosylation with protein bound thiol groups under physiologic conditions producing stable S-nitroso-proteins [36]. These nitrosothiols may represent a stabilized form of NO in biological tissues. Indeed, Keaney et al. [37] have reported that S-nitroso-albumin possesses EDRF-like properties including vasodilation and inhibition of platelet aggregation. Although the responses were seven-fold less potent as a bolus than nitroprusside, it is very important that they lasted almost 10 min *versus* 19 s for nitroprusside. These data suggest that protein thiols can serve as an NO-adduct preserving bioactivity and increasing the half-life of NO in biological systems. An issue not considered is that these low levels of NO (inhaled NO) for prolonged periods may be more effective than large levels of NO (nitroprusside) for very short periods.

Additionally, Stamler's group reported that hemoglobin can be nitrosylated in the lung and the NO group may be released within peripheral vascular beds [38]. If this is the case, then continuous delivery of NO to blood in the form of inhaled NO could conceivably produce these and other NO-adducts and thereby continuously deliver small amounts of NO to peripheral tissues over long periods of time to function as potent anti-adhesive therapeutics.

NO and neutrophil adhesion induces vascular dysfunction

Inhibition of nitric oxide synthesis induces a rapid increase in microvascular permeability in the intestine that was partly neutrophil-dependent and partly neutrophil -independent [3]. Kurose et al. [2], extended this work by examining single vessels in the rat mesentery and reported that exposure of rat mesenteric venules to L-NAME elicited a rapid increase in albumin accumulation in the interstitial space that persisted for a prolonged duration. The initial phase of albumin leakage preceded the L-NAME-induced leukocyte adherence and emigration, whereas the magnitude of the albumin leakage observed in the late phase of L-NAME exposure was highly correlated with the number of adherent and emigrated leukocytes in the same segment of venule. L-NAME induced-albumin leakage was attenuated by MAbs directed against β_2-integrins, P-selectin as well as the platelet activating factor antagonist, WEB2086 [2]. Phalloidin, which promotes endothelial junctional integrity, inhibited both the early and late phases of albumin leakage [2]. The increase in albumin leakage is not consistent in all laboratories as some investigators have observed that inhibition of NO can decrease permeability [39]. There appears to be no direct explanation for these results at this time.

Nitric oxide reduces adhesion in ischemia-reperfusion (I/R)

The hallmark features of ischemia/reperfusion (I/R) include a reduction in NO release, increased oxidant production, increased neutrophil adhesion and a reduction in the physiological functions of the endothelium. Much evidence is available that in this acute condition, NO may interfere with the activation of the vascular endothelium and thereby attenuate the neutrophil-endothelial cell interactions that elicit the inflammatory component of reperfusion injury. The interrelationships between NO and cell adhesion molecules and the relevance of these relationships to ischemia-reperfusion were carefully studied by numerous investigators. Davenpeck and coworkers [40] using intravital microscopy of the rat mesenteric microvasculature found that ischemia-reperfusion of the mesenteric circulation resulted in a rapid increase in leukocyte rolling and adherence to the venular endothelium within the first 30 min following reperfusion. Moreover, immunohistochemistry of the intestinal microcirculation indicated a marked upregulation of P-selectin expression on the venular endothelial surface 30 min post reperfusion. These results clearly indicate that at a time when NO levels were known to be critically reduced, P-selectin was markedly upregulated at the endothelial site of enhanced leukocyte adherence, possibly due to increased superoxide and hydrogen peroxide levels. Gauthier et al. [40] also showed in the same model of ischemia-reperfusion of the rat mesenteric circulation, that the infusion of a NO donor, SNAP, markedly decreased post-reperfusion rolling and adherence of leukocyte on the venular endothelium. Moreover, infusion of SNAP concomitantly prevented P-selectin expression on the surface of the venular endothelium. In fact, SNAP infusion ameliorated the signs of circulatory shock that occur in mesenteric ischemia-reperfusion. It is quite interesting how closely the effects of I/R mimic the effects of L-NAME (described early) and lend credence to the view that a decrease in NO is a contributing and perhaps initiating factor of ischemia/reperfusion dysfunction.

Again the findings were not re65stricted to the mesentery as Liu et al. [41] showed that L-NAME administration significantly exacerbated hepatic ischemia-reperfusion injury reflected by an increase in plasma ALT activity in the I/R + L-NAME rats compared with that in I/R group. The mechanism of enhancement of hepatic ischemia-reperfusion injury by L-NAME was probably caused by the increase in generation of superoxide and neutrophil accumulation in the liver. Hepatic P-selectin and ICAM-1 mRNA expressions were increased after ischemia-reperfusion and further augmented by L-NAME, suggesting that some endogenous NO must still be produced during I/R and may dampen the expression of these adhesion molecules [42].

It is intriguing that in this disease state, but not other conditions, NO donors were as effective as a β_2-integrin-specific antibody in attenuating reperfusion-induced leukocyte adhesion [43]. Because neutrophils are important mediators of the postischemic tissue injury, the attenuation of neutrophil adhesion in this study may provide a physiological basis for the protective effect of NO donors in I/R injury. As already mentioned, inhaled NO was as effective as NO donors in inhibiting I/R-induced leukocyte recruitment without the complicating effects of hypotension.

Inducible NOS functions as an anti-adhesive molecule

Although to date many investigators consider NO produced from iNOS as strictly a pro-inflammatory molecule, the cytotoxic potential of iNOS is not a consistent finding. For example, iNOS-deficient mice have been reported to have less frequency of LPS-induced cardiovascular collapse [44, 45], but the same group [46] and other groups [47] have reported as much LPS-induced liver damage as their wild type counterparts and no improved survival or even enhanced mortality in iNOS-deficient mice. Zingarelli and colleagues [48] have observed that in a model of IBD (TNBS-colitis) more wild-type than iNOS deficient mice die, but in our own laboratory in a model of non-lethal TNBS-induced colitis the initial injury and leukocyte recruitment is worse in the iNOS deficient mice, but by 1 week the disease parameters are approximately the same [49]. Fenyk-Melody et al. [50] have reported a more than four-fold increase in incidence and severity of experimental autoimmune encephalomyelitis (EAE) in iNOS-deficient mice relative to their wild-type littermates, whereas in another autoimmune model, iNOS-deficient, MRL-lpr/lpr mice have less vasculitis associated with the glomerulonephritis that is a hallmark of this autoimmune disease [51]. In a model of hemorrhagic shock, Billiar's group reported a protective effect in iNOS-deficient mice [52], but in a skin injury model, the iNOS-deficient mice had a delayed healing response [53], highlighting the fact that in two different models from the same laboratory two opposing results are seen. Clearly, the role of iNOS is completely unpredictable from the aforementioned studies and appears to be dependent upon the type of pathology or perhaps the identity of the afflicted organ. It should also be noted that the presence of iNOS is not always involved in the inflammatory response or alternatively, the iNOS effects are sufficiently subtle that its inhibition is not manifested by increased or decreased inflammation. For example, iNOS was not a contributing factor to antigen-induced autoimmune myocarditis [54], lyme arthritis [64], bacterial septic arthritis [55] or colitis in IL10-deficient mice [56] despite increased iNOS production in each of these models.

Clearly the model may dictate whether iNOS is beneficial or detrimental. One possible explanation may be differing cellular sources of iNOS with different functions. Perhaps NO may be detrimental when produced in the presence of superoxide to produce more potent oxidants, but simultaneously in the same organism NO produced from a different source may reduce leukocyte adhesion. Indeed, endotoxemic iNOS-deficient animals were reported to have increased levels of leukocyte infiltration into tissues than their endotoxemic wild type littermates despite reduced hypotensive complications, suggesting that iNOS may function as a "turn off signal" or "feedback mechanism" for the activated immune system [44]. *In vitro* work revealed that leukocytes from septic iNOS -deficient mice interacted more avidly with E-selectin in a flow chamber than did leukocytes from wild-type septic mice suggesting the effects were on leukocytes. It remains to be established whether the source of iNOS was the leukocyte or whether the source was from some other cell impacting upon the leukocytes.

Nitric oxide attenuates adhesion molecule expression in endothelial cells

There is increasing evidence that NO may attenuate adhesion molecule expression on endothelial cells. Indeed, both ICAM-1 and VCAM-1synthesis by human and rodent endothelial cells is reduced with NO donors [16, 57, 58]. In addition, endogenously produced NO may downregulate the expression of VCAM-1 both from constitutive [59] and iNOS sources [60]. For example, DeCaterina and colleagues [16] reported that three structurally unrelated NO donors inhibit IL-1 stimulated VCAM-1 expression by 35–55% on human saphenous vein endothelial cells. This inhibition was unaffected by cGMP analogues, and was quantitatively similar after stimulation by either IL-1α, IL-1β, IL-4, TNFα, or LPS. NO also decreased the endothelial expression of other leukocyte adhesion molecules E-selectin and to a lesser extent, ICAM-1 and secretable cytokines (IL-6 and IL-8). Inhibition of endogenous NO production by L-NMA also induced the expression of VCAM-1, but did not augment cytokine-induced VCAM-1 expression. Nuclear run-on assays, transfection studies using various VCAM-1 promoter reporter gene constructs, and electrophorectic mobility shift assays indicated that NO represses VCAM-1 gene transcription, in part, by inhibiting NF-κB [16]. Similar results were observed by Shin et al. in smooth muscle cells, where NO repressed IFNγ-induced VCAM-1 gene transcription, in part, through inhibition of NF-κB [65].

Work by Spiecker et al. [61] showed that NO donors inhibited the expression of VCAM-1, ICAM-1 and E-selectin induced by TNFα in cultured human vascular endothelial cells. NO donors inhibited NF-κB primarily through the induction of IκBα. The inhibitory effects of these NO donors were not mediated by cGMP-dependent mechanisms because the cGMP analog, 8-bromo-cGMP, did not appreciably affect TNFα-induced adhesion molecule expression. Treatment with NO donors, however, did not inhibit IκBα phosphorylation or proteasome degradation in response to stimulation with TNFα, even at submaximal concentrations. These results, therefore, provide a potential novel mechanism whereby NO could downregulate the expression of NF-κB-dependent pro-inflammatory genes such as cellular adhesion molecules through modulating the expression of IκBα. It remains to be determined how NO induces IκBα gene transcription.

Yao et al. [62] demonstrated that exposure of rat mesangial cells to numerous structurally unrelated NO donors resulted in dose-dependent inhibition of mesangial cell adhesion and spreading on various extracellular matrix substrata, being more pronounced on collagen type I than on collagen type IV, laminin or fibronectin. The inhibitory effects were reversed by hemoglobin and enhanced by superoxide dismutase. Besides, a lipophilic analog of cGMP, 8-bromo-cGMP mimicked the ability of NO to inhibit mesangial cell adhesion, spreading, pp125[FAK] tyrosine phosphorylation, as well as to disturb α-actin organization. The inhibitory NO effect on mesangial cell adhesion was markedly reduced by pretreatment of these cells with ODQ, an inhibitor of the soluble guanylate cyclase. Thus, exogenous NO interferes with the establishment and maintenance of mesangial cells adhesion to extracellular components. This inhibitory NO effect is mediated predominantly by cGMP-signaling highlighting that adhesion in different cells is sensitive to NO *via* different mechanisms.

Khan et al. [58] showed that in human umbilical vein endothelial cells and human dermal microvascular endothelial cells, the NO donor diethylamine-NO (DETA-NO, 100 μM) reduced VCAM-1 gene expression induced by the cytokine tumor necrosis factor α (TNFα) at the cell surface level by 65% and intracellular adhesion molecule 1 (ICAM-1) gene expression by 35% without affecting E-selectin gene expression. Moreover, DETA-NO suppressed TNFα-induced mRNA accumulation of VCAM-1 and TNFα-mediated transcriptional activation of the human VCAM-1 promoter. Conversely, treatment with L-NMMA, an inhibitor of NO synthesis, augmented cytokine induction of VCAM-1 and ICAM-1 mRNA accumulation. Gel mobility shift analysis revealed that DETA-NO inhibited TNFα activation of DNA binding protein activity to the VCAM-1 NF-κB like binding sites. Interestingly, using thin-layer chromatography, DETA-NO suppressed formation of 13-hydroperoxydodecanoeic acid (linoleyl hydroperoxide), a peroxy-fatty acid that may serve as an intracellular signal for NF-κB activation. This suggests that DETA-NO modifies the reactivity of oxygen intermediates in the vascular endothelium. Through this mechanism, NO may modulate gene transcription. The precise pathway by which this occurs remains undefined, but is mimicked by other antioxidants, suggesting that NO may function through a redox-sensitive mechanism.

In a recent study *in vivo* using iNOS-deficient mice, Kawachi and colleagues [63] examined VCAM-1 expression following TNF. They observed some enhanced expression of VCAM-1 in iNOS deficient mice, predominantly in the gastrointestinal organs, and only at one, but not another, concentration – suggesting some impact of iNOS on regulation of adhesion molecule expression, albeit to a lesser degree than what has been reported *in vitro*.

In conclusion, there is a growing body of evidence that nitric oxide may function as an anti-adhesive molecule in inflammatory settings. However, it is clear that this does not always result in a predominantly beneficial phenotype as often the inflammation is lessened by NO inhibition. Clearly, depending on how important the leukocyte recruitment is to the inflammatory disease may dictate how beneficial NO synthesis inhibition or delivery will be. As our understanding of NO biology grows, we are beginning to appreciate that non-specific inhibition of NO and even inhibition of a single NO synthase may not be sufficiently selective to obtain satisfying anti-inflammatory results. We may ultimately have to accept that the only effective way of therapeutically targeting NO may be *via* inhibition of NO or delivery of NO to a specific cell at a specific time, a proposition that presently is very daunting.

Acknowledgment
Supported by a grant from the Heart and Stroke Foundation of Canada. Dr. P. Kubes is a Medical Research Council (MRC) scientist and Alberta Heritage Foundation for Medical Research (AHFMR) senior scholar. Dr. Andonegui is an Alberta Heritage Foundation for Medical Research (AHFMR) fellow.

References

1   Kubes P, Suzuki M, Granger DN (1991) Nitric oxide: An endogenous modulator of leukocyte adhesion. *Proc Natl Acad Sci USA* 88: 4651–4655

2   Kurose I, Kubes P, Wolf R, Anderson DC, Paulson J, Miyasaka M, Granger DN (1993) Inhibition of nitric oxide production: Mechanisms of vascular albumin leakage. *Circ Res* 73: 164–171

3   Kubes P, Granger DN (1992) Nitric oxide modulates microvascular permeability. *Am J Physiol* 262: H611–H615

4   Niu X-F, Ibbotson G, Kubes P (1996) A balance between nitric oxide and oxidants regulates mast cell-dependent neutrophil-endothelial cell interactions. *Circ Res* 79: 992–999

5   Niu X-F, Smith CW, Kubes P (1994) Intracellular oxidative stress induced by nitric oxide synthesis inhibition increases endothelial cell adhesion to neutrophils. *Circ Res* 74: 1133–1140

6   Kubes P, Kanwar S, Niu X-F, Gaboury J (1993) Nitric oxide synthesis inhibition induces leukocyte adhesion *via* superoxide and mast cells. *FASEB J* 7: 1293–1299

7   Arndt H, Russell JM, Kurose I, Kubes P, Granger DN (1993) Mediators of leukocyte adhesion in rat mesenteric venules elicited by inhibition of nitric oxide synthesis. *Gastroenterology* 105: 675–680

8   Kosaka H, Seiyama A, Terada N, Yoneyama H, Hirota S, Kitamura Y (1997) Absence of mast cell involvement in leukocyte adhesion and emigration induced by inhibition of nitric oxide synthase. *Lab Invest* 77: 575–80

9   Davenpeck KL, Gauthier TW, Lefer AM (1994) Inhibition of endothelial-derived nitric oxide promotes P-selectin expression and actions in the rat microcirculation. *Gastroenterology* 107: 1050–1058

10   Suematsu M, Tamatani T, Delano FA, Miyasaka M, Forrest M, Suzuki H, Schmid-Schönbein GW (1994) Microvascular oxidative stress preceding leukocyte activation elicited by *in vivo* nitric oxide suppression. *Am J Physiol* 266: H2410–H2415

11   Scalia R, Lefer AM (1998) *In vivo* regulation of PECAM-1 activity during acute endothelial dysfunction in the rat mesenteric microvasculature. *J Leukoc Biol* 64: 163–169

12   May GR, Crook P, Moore PK, Page CP (1991) The role of nitric oxide as an endogenous regulator of platelet and neutrophil activation within the pulmonary circulation of the rabbit. *Br J Pharmacol* 102: 759–763

13   Ma X-L, Weyrich AS, Lefer DJ, Lefer AM (1993) Diminished basal nitric oxide release after myocardial ischemia and reperfusion promotes neutrophil adherence to coronary endothelium. *Circ Res* 72: 403–412

14   Hokari R, Miura S, Fujimori H, Tsuzuki Y, Shigematsu T, Higuchi H, Kimura H, Kurose I, Serizawa H, Suematsu M, Yagita H, Granger DN, Ishii H (1998) Nitric oxide modulates T-lymphocyte migration in Peyer's patches and villous submucosa of rat small intestine. *Gastroenterology* 115: 618–627

15 Bath PMW, Hasall DG, Gladwin A-M, Palmer RMJ, Martin JF (1991) Nitric oxide and prostacyclin. Divergence of inhibitory effects on monocyte chemotaxis and adhesion to endothelium *in vitro*. *Arteriosclerosis Thromb* 11: 254–260

16 De Caterina R, Libby P, Peng HB, Thannickal VJ, Rajavashisth TB, Gimbrone MA Jr, Shin WS, Liao JK (1995) Nitric oxide decreases cytokine-induced endothelial activation. Nitric oxide selectively reduces endothelial expression of adhesion molecules and proinflammatory cytokines. *J Clin Invest* 96: 60–68

17 Kinsella JP, Neish SR, Ivy DD, Shaffer E, Abman SH (1993) Clinical responses to prolonged treatment of persistent pulmonary hypertension of the newborn with low doses of inhaled nitric oxide. *J Pediatrics* 123: 103–108

18 Abman SH, Kinsella JP, Schaffer MS, Wilkening RB (1993) Inhaled nitric oxide in the management of a premature newborn with severe respiratory distress and pulmonary hypertension. *Am Acad Pediatrics* 606–609

19 Edwards AD (1995) The pharmacology of inhaled nitric oxide. *Arch Dis Child Fetal Neon Ed* 72: F127–130

20 Malmros C, Blomquist S, Dahm P, Martensson L, Thorne J (1996) Nitric oxide inhalation decreases pulmonary platelet and neutrophil sequestration during extracorporeal circulation in the pig. *Crit Care Med* 24: 845–849

21 Bloomfield GL, Sweeney LB, Fisher BJ, Blocher CR, Sholley MM, Sugerman JH, Fowler AA III (1997) Delayed administration of inhaled nitric oxide preserves alveolar-capillary membrane integrity in porcine gram-negative sepsis. *Arch Surg* 132: 65–75

22 Barbotin-Larrieu F, Mazmanian M, Baudet B, Detruit D, Chapelier A, Libert JM, Dartevelle P, Herve P (1996) Prevention of ischemia-reperfusion lung injury by inhaled nitric oxide in neonatal piglets. *J Appl Physiol* 80: 782–788

23 Guidot DM, Hybertson BM, Kitlowski RP, Repine JE (1996) Inhaled NO prevents IL-1-induced neutrophil accumulation and associated acute edema in isolated rat lungs. *Am J Physiol* 2: L225–229

24 Fujino S, Nagahiro I, Triantafillou AN, Boasquevisque CH, Yano M, Cooper JD, Patterson GA (1997) Inhaled nitric oxide at the time of harvest improves early lung allograft function. *Ann Thorac Surg* 63: 1383–1389

25 Sato Y, Walley KR, Klut ME, English D, D'yachkova Y, Hogg JC, van Eeden SF (1999) Nitric oxide reduces the sequestration of polymorphonuclear leukocytes in lung by changing deformability and CD18 expression. *Am J Respir Crit Care Med* 159: 1469–1476

26 Chollet-Martin S, Gatecel C, Kermarrec N, Gougerot-Pocidalo M-A, Payen DM (1996) Alveolar neutrophil functions and cytokine levels in patients with the adult respiratory distress syndrome during nitric oxide inhalation. *Am J Respir Crit Care Med* 153: 985–990

27 Gessler P, Nebe T, Birle A, Mueller W, Kachel W (1996) A new side effect of inhaled nitric oxide in neonates and infants with pulmonary hypertension: functional impairment of the neutrophil respiratory burst. *Intensive Care Med* 22: 252–258

28 Samama CM, Diaby M, Fellahi JL, Mdhafar A, Eyraud D, Arock M, Guillosson JJ,

Coriat P, Rouby JJ (1995) Inhibition of platelet aggregation by inhaled nitric oxide in patients with acute respiratory distress syndrome. *Anesthesiol* 83: 56–65

29   Hogman M, Frostell C, Arnberg H, Sandhagen B, Hedenstierna G (1994) Prolonged bleeding time during nitric oxide inhalation in the rabbit. *Acta Physiol Scand* 151: 125–129

30   Gries A, Bottiger BW, Dorsam J, Bauer H, Weimann J, Bode C, Martin E, Motsch J (1997) Inhaled nitric oxide inhibits platelet aggregation after pulmonary embolism in pigs. *Anesthesiol* 86: 387–393

31   Adrie C, Bloch KD, Moreno PR, Hurford WE, Guerrero JL, Holt R, Zapol WM, Gold HK, Semigran MJ (1996) Inhaled nitric oxide increases coronary artery patency after thrombolysis. *Circulation* 94: 1919–1926

32   Rosenberg AA, Kinsella JP, Abman SH (1995) Cerebral hemodynamics and distribution of left ventricular output during inhalation of nitric oxide. *Crit Care Med* 23: 1391–1397

33   Fox-Robichaud A, Payne D, Hasan SU, Ostrovsky L, Fairhead T, Reinhardt P, Kubes P (1998) Inhaled NO as a viable antiadhesive therapy for ischemia/reperfusion injury of distal microvascular beds. *J Clin Invest* 101: 2497–2505

34   Fox-Robichaud A, Payne D, Kubes P (199) Inhaled NO reaches distal vasculatures to inhibit endothelium – but not leukocyte-dependent cell adhesion. *Am J Physiol* 277: L1224–L1231

35   Kubes P, Payne D, Grisham MB, Jourd-Heuil D, Fox-Robichaud A (1999) Inhaled NO impacts vascular but not extravascular compartments in postischemic peripheral organs. *Am J Physiol* 277: H676–H682

36   Stamler JS, Simon DI, Osborne JA, Mullins ME, Jaraki O, Singel DJ, Loscalzo J (1992) S-nitrosylation of proteins by nitric oxide: synthesis and characterization of novel biologically active compounds. *Proc Natl Acad Sci USA* 89: 444–448

37   Keaney JF Jr, Simon DI, Stamler JS, Jaraki O, Scharfstein J, Vita JA, Loscalzo J (1993) NO forms an adduct with serum albumin that has endothelium-derived relaxing factor-like properties. *J Clin Invest* 91: 1582–1589

38   Jia L, Bonaventura C, Bonaventura J, Stamler JS (1996) S-nitrosohaemoglobin: a dynamic activity of blood involved in vascular control. *Nature* 380: 221–226

39   Rumbaut RE, McKay MK, Huxley VH (1995) Capillary hydraulic conductivity is decreased by nitric oxide synthase inhibition. *Am J Physiol* 268: H1856–H1861

40   Gauthier TW, Davenpeck KL, Lefer AM (1994) Nitric oxide attenuates leukocyte-endothelial interaction *via* P-selectin in splanchnic ischemia-reperfusion. *Am J Physiol* 267: G562–G568

41   Liu P, Yin K, Nagele R, Wong PY (1998) Inhibition of nitric oxide synthase attenuates peroxynitrite generation, but augments neutrophil accumulation in hepatic ischemia-reperfusion in rats. *J Pharmacol Exp Ther* 284: 1139–1146

42   Liu P, Xu B, Hock CE, Nagele R, Sun FF, Wong PY (1998) NO modulates P-selectin and ICAM-1 mRNA expression and hemodynamic alterations in hepatic I/R. *Am J Physiol* 275: H2191–H2198

43 Kubes P, Kurose I, Granger DN (1994) NO donors prevent integrin-induced leukocyte adhesion, but not P-selectin-dependent rolling in postischemic venules. *Am J Physiol* 267: H931–H937

44 Hickey MJ, Sharkey KA, Sihota EG, Reinhardt PH, MacMicking JD, Nathan C, Kubes P (1997) Inducible nitric oxide synthase-deficient mice have enhanced leukocyte-endothelium interactions in endotoxemia. *FASEB J* 11: 955–964

45 Wei XQ, Charles IG, Smith A, Ure J, Feng GJ, Huang FP, Xu D, Muller W, Moncada S, Liew FY (1995) Altered immune responses in mice lacking inducible nitric oxide synthase. *Nature* 375: 408–411

46 Nicholson SC, Grobmyer SR, Shiloh MU, Brause JE, Potter S, MacMicking JD, Dinauer MC, Nathan CF (1999) Lethality of endotoxin in mice genetically deficient in the respiratory burst oxidase, inducible nitric oxide synthase, or both. *Shock* 11: 253-258

47 Laubach VE, Shesely EG, Smithies O, Sherman PA (1995) Mice lacking inducible nitric oxide synthase are not resistant to lipopolysaccharide-induced death. *Proc Natl Acad Sci USA* 92: 10688–10692

48 Zingarelli B, Szabo C, Salzman AL (1999) Reduced oxidative and nitrosative damage in murine experimental colitis in the absence of inducible nitric oxide synthase. *GUT* 45: 199–209

49 McCafferty D-M, Miampamba M, Sihota E, Sharkey KA, Kubes P (1999) Role of inducible nitric oxide synthase in trinitrobenzene sulphonic acid-induced colitis in mice. *Gut* 45: 864–873

50 Fenyk-Melody JE, Garrison AE, Brunnert SR, Weidner JR, Shen, F Shelton BA, Mudgett JS (1998) Experimental autoimmune encephalomyelitis is exacerbated in mice lacking the *NOS2* gene. *J Immunol* 160: 2940–2946

51 Gilkeson GS, Mudgett JS, Seldin MF, Ruiz P, Alexander AA, Misukonis MA, Pisetsky DS, Weinberg JB (1997) Clinical and serologic manifestations of autoimmune disease in MRL-1pr/1pr mice lacking nitric oxide synthase type 2. *J Exp Med* 186: 365–373

52 Hierholzer C, Harbrecht B, Menezes JM, Kane J, MacMicking J, Nathan CF, Peitzman AB, Billiar TR, Tweardy DJ (1998) Essential role of induced nitric oxide in the initiation of the inflammatory response after hemorrhagic shock. *J Exp Med* 187: 917–28

53 Yamasaki K, Edington HD, McClosky C, Tzeng E, Lizonova A, Kovesdi I, Steed DL, Billiar TR (1998) Reversal of impaired wound repair in iNOS-deficient mice by topical adenoviral-mediated iNOS gene transfer. *J Clin Invest* 101: 967–971

54 Bachmaier K, Neu N, Pummerer C, Duncan GS, Mak TW, Matsuyama T, Penninger JM (1997) iNOS expression and nitrotyrosine formation in the myocardium in response to inflammation is controlled by the interferon regulatory transcription factor 1. *Circulation* 96: 585–591

55 McInnes IB, Leung B, Wei XQ, Gemmell CC, Liew FY (1998) Septic arthritis following *Staphylococcus aureus* infection in mice lacking inducible nitric oxide synthase. *J Immunol* 160: 308–315

56 McCafferty D-M, Sihota E, Muscara MN, Wallace JL, Sharkey KA, Kubes P (2000)

Spontaneously developing chronic colitis in IL-10/iNOS-double deficient mice. *Am J Physiol* 279: 690–699

57 Ikeda M, Ikeda IL, Takahashi M, Shimada K, Minota S, Kano S (1996) Nitric oxide inhibits intercellular adhesion molecule-1 expression in rat mesangial cells. *J Am Soc Hephrol* 7: 2213–2218

58 Khan BV, Harrison DG, Olbrych MT, Alexander RW, Medford RM (1996) Nitric oxide regulates vascular cell adhesion molecule-1 gene expression and redox-sensitive transcriptional events in human vascular endothelial cells. *Proc Natl Acad Sci USA* 93: 9114–9119

59 Tsao PS, Buitrago R, Chan JR, Cooke JP (1996) Fluid flow inhibits endothelial adhesiveness Nitric oxide and transcriptional regulation of VCAM-1. *Circulation* 94: 1682–1689

60 Binion DG, Fu S, Ramanujam KS, Chai YC, Dweik RA, Drazba JA, Wade JG, Ziats NP, Erzurum SC, Wilson KT (1998) iNOS expression in human intestinal microvascular endothelial cells inhibits leukocyte adhesion. *Am J Physiol* 275: G592–G603

61 Spiecker M, Darius H, Kaboth K, Hubner F, Liao JK (1998) Differential regulation of endothelial cell adhesion molecule expression by nitric oxide donors and antioxidants. *J Leukoc Biol* 63: 732–739

62 Yao J, Schoecklmann HO, Prols F, Gauer S, Sterzel RB (1998) Exogenous nitric oxide inhibits mesangial cell adhesion to extracellular matrix components. *Kidney Int* 53: 598–608

63 Kawachi S, Cockrell A, Laroux FS, Gray L, Granger DN, van der Heyde HC, Grisham MB (1999) Role of inducible nitric oxide synthase in the regulation of VCAM-1 expression in gut inflammation. *Am J Physiol* 277: G572–G576

64 Brown CR, Reiner SL (1999) Development of lyme arthritis in mice deficient in inducible nitric oxide synthase. *J Infect Dis* 179: 1573–1576

65 Shin WS, Hong YH, Peng HB, De Caterina R, Libby P, Liao JK (1996) Nitric oxide attenuates vascular smooth muscle cell activation by interferon-γ. The role of constitutive NF-κB activity. *J Biol Chem* 271: 11317–11324

Nitric oxide regulation of lymphocyte function

Rosemary A. Hoffman[1] and Henri R. Ford[2]

[1]University of Pittsburgh, Department of Surgery, W1545 Bioscience Tower, 200 Lothrop Street, Pittsburgh, PA 15213, USA; [2]Children's Hospital of Pittsburgh, Pittsburgh, PA 15213, USA

Introduction

Similar to other biological systems where the effect of nitric oxide (NO) has been examined, paradoxical findings on the effects of NO on lymphocyte function have been reported. The most paradoxical effect may be that on the one hand, NO can inhibit apoptosis, a major mechanism of down-regulation of the immune response. In this capacity, NO would serve as a facilitator of the immune response, promoting survival of effector lymphocyte populations. Yet, NO also has been shown to inhibit lymphocyte proliferation and promote apoptosis and thus effectively prevent amplification of the immune response. Therefore, the challenge in the study of the effect of NO on lymphocytes is to determine under which circumstances NO acts as a facilitator *versus* an inhibitor of the immune response.

The usual variables can be invoked to explain the dichotomies observed when the effect of NO on lymphocyte function is examined. Widely diverse populations of lymphocytes, from natural killer lymphocytes to B lymphocytes to CD4+ and CD8+ T cells have been exposed to NO and functions evaluated. The lymphoid populations exposed to NO were derived from various species, providing another source of variation. T lymphocytes with widely divergent ontogeny and function such as T cells bearing either a αβ or a γδ T cell-receptor have been studied. Another important variable is the maturational state of the T cell, ranging from the immature thymocyte, to the naïve mature T cell, to the activated T cell and finally, to subpopulations of activated T cells such as T helper 1 *versus* T helper 2. Studies have also been performed using transformed lymphocytes such as T- and B-cell tumor lines. The caveat in interpreting these studies is whether the NO effect is modulated due to the myriad of physiological changes associated with cellular transformation. Nevertheless, the apparent inconsistencies in experimental results observed in different studies examining the effect of NO on lymphocyte function may not be so paradoxical when all the variables are taken into account.

While all of these concerns are important, another crucial variable is probably not the cellular target as much as the source, amount, and duration of the exposure of the lymphocyte to NO. The amount of NO to which the lymphocyte is exposed might be determined by whether NO is produced from one of the constitutive NOS enzymes which produce lesser amounts of NO compared to the greater amounts of NO produced over a longer period of time by the inducible NOS enzyme. While NK cells have been shown to express iNOS, T and B lymphocytes do not, although some controversy exists in this area of NO research. Transformed T- and B-cell lines seem to be positive for iNOS while normal human peripheral blood T and B lymphocytes express the constitutive eNOS isoform [1]. The effects attributable to the small amount of NO produced by this isoform may be *via* an amplification mechanism such as elevation of cGMP.

Intracellular events that ensue upon engagement of a cytokine with its receptor or the T-cell receptor with its target antigen are certainly influenced by concomitant exposure to NO, even to small amounts of NO that could be produced by the constitutive NOS isoforms. Many studies examine events associated with activation of the lymphocyte by interaction with an antigen presenting cell (APC) relative to the NO produced by the antigen presenting cell. It is important to realize that during the primary immune response in particular, lymphocyte activation and NO production by the APC are not coincident events. Cytokines produced by activated T cells such as interferon γ (IFNγ), are potent inducers of NO in many cell types, but this cytokine is not produced until after the initial T-cell signaling events associated with antigen recognition have taken place. In this scenario, NO would be viewed as a down-regulator of the immune response, preventing further expansion of lymphocytes in response to antigen. Thus, further amplification of the immune response would be prevented by an APC that has been induced to make NO by lymphocytes that have already undergone one round of activation and cell division. However, if a lymphocyte encounters an APC that has been primed to upregulate NO production, such as in an inflammatory site, activation of the lymphocyte would be inhibited, even in a primary immune response. This chapter will review the intracellular signaling pathways in the lymphocyte that are modulated by NO exposure *in vitro* and summarize how NO appears to be functioning *in vivo* in various animal models of disease.

Nitric oxide induction/inhibition of lymphocyte apoptosis

The induction of apoptosis is an important mechanism in the deletion of autoreactive T cells in the thymus as well as in the periphery. Fehsel et al. [2] were the first to show that NO donors in high concentration could induce apoptosis in thymocytes and mature T lymphocyte lines. Hortelano et al. [3] demonstrated that NO is highly efficient at inducing mitochondrial permeability transition in thymocytes, thereby causing the liberation of apoptogenic factors from mitochondria that can induce nuclear apoptosis in isolated nuclei *in vitro*. Inhibitors of mitochondrial permeability transition such as bongkrekic acid and a cyclophilin D-binding cyclosporin A derivative, N-methyl-Val-4-cyclosporin A, prevent the mitochondrial as well as all post-mitochondrial signs of apoptosis induced by NO, including nuclear DNA fragmentation and exposure of phosphatidyl serine residues on the cell surface. Recently, we have demonstrated that NO induces apoptosis in thymocytes *via* a *p53* and *bax* dependent pathway (manuscript submitted). Furthermore, apoptosis in thymocytes exposed to SNAP is accompanied by activation of caspase-1, not caspase-3. We showed that caspase-1 could reliably cleave the inhibitor of caspase-activated deoxyribonuclease (ICAD), and lead to DNA fragmentation. This phenomenon was blocked by a known caspase-1 inhibitor, Ac-YVAD-cho, but not by a caspase-3 inhibitor Ac-DEVD-cho. We also showed that thymocytes from caspase-1 knockout mice were not susceptible to NO-induced apoptosis [4].

Nitric oxide has also been implicated in thymocyte apoptosis *in vivo*. Expression of iNOS was detected in the corticomedullary junction and medulla of fetal thymi. The levels of iNOS mRNA became maximal around gestational day 18, and then declined after birth. Tai et al. [5] demonstrated that NO, which is generated in association with TCR stimulation in the thymus, functions to induce deletion of double positive (CD4+8+) thymocytes, especially when the TCR is triggered. Furthermore, NO leads to DNA fragmentation in CD4+8+, but not single positive thymocytes stimulated with anti-CD3. Bras et al. [6] detailed a somewhat different response when apoptosis was monitored in BALB/c mice that received an injection of the superantigen, staphylococcal enterotoxin B (SEB), with and without administration of the NO donor, isosorbide dinitrate (ISO). Administration of NO delayed the deletion of peripheral T cells activated by the superantigen and decreased apoptosis was seen in splenocytes obtained from ISO treated mice. Similarly, in the thymus, the decrease in double positive thymocytes was not as severe in mice treated with the NO donor and a more rapid recovery of the double positive thymocytes was observed in ISO treated mice. Therefore, in contrast to previous work detailing the pro-apoptotic effects of NO, these investigators provided evidence of the anti-apoptotic effect of NO *in vivo*.

Various *in vitro* studies have delineated the mechanism of the anti apoptotic effect of NO. Mannik et al. [7] showed that Fas induced apoptosis could be inhibited in various human leukocyte lines by adding an NO synthesis inhibitor to the cultured cells, indicating that basal expression of NO inhibited apoptosis. Subsequently, these authors demonstrated that S-nitrosylation of the catalytic site cysteine in caspase-3 zymogens became de-nitrosylated upon activation of the Fas apoptotic pathway. These studies, along with others [8–11], detailed the inhibitory effect of NO on the activity of caspases activated during apoptosis in various cell types. In a similar vein, Genaro et al. [12] demonstrated that culture of human peripheral blood B cells in the presence of NO delays apoptosis and that NO also can rescue B cells from antigen induced cell death. NO prevented the drop in Bcl-2 expression, providing a link between NO signaling and this anti-apoptotic molecule. However,

Okuda et al. [13] were unable to demonstrate that NO could delay apoptosis in cultured mouse splenic T lymphocytes, but demonstrated that high concentrations of NO induced apoptosis in these cells, similar to the effect seen upon exposure of thymocytes to NO.

However, using human T blasts and a mouse T-cell hybridoma, Williams et al. [14] showed that activation induced cell death was blocked by inhibition of NO synthesis, but that apoptosis induced by triggering Fas R or by dexamethasone was not affected by iNOS inhibitors. T-cell receptor signaling increased nitrotyrosine specific staining in these cells indicating that NO may play a role in the apoptotic cell death of mature T lymphocytes. Thus, this study provided evidence that NO is not always protective against apoptosis in T cells and that under certain circumstances, NO could promote apoptosis in mature T lymphocytes. A novel mechanism whereby NO could promote apoptosis in T lymphocytes was described by Allione et al. [15] using normal human peripheral blood T cells and several T-cell tumor lines. Exposure of these cells to an NO donor resulted in a population of cells that expressed high levels of both IFNγR chains, R1 and R2, and is in contrast to unexposed cells which expressed high levels of IFNγR1 and almost no IFNγR2. These NO exposed cells, upon subsequent exposure to IFNγ, underwent apoptosis due to the increased expression of IFNγR2. This study indicates that NO exposure can prime lymphocytes to undergo apoptosis upon subsequent exposure to IFNγ, providing a mechanism whereby NO can indirectly facilitate lymphocyte apoptosis and control of the immune response.

Nitric oxide and NK cell, γδ T-cell function

In contrast to rodent NK cells, human peripheral blood NK cells can be induced to express only endothelial NOS and not iNOS [16]. This finding is in contrast to uterine NK cells (see below). Human peripheral blood NK cells produce NO upon interaction with target cells or triggering with anti CD16 mAb, and inhibition of NO synthesis resulted in enhanced apoptosis triggered by CD16. The mechanism of NO induced inhibition was due to decreased production of tumor necrosis factor α (TNFα), associated with the decreased DNA binding activity of the transcription factor NF-AT (nuclear factor activation T cells). Another T-cell population shown to be rescued from apoptosis by NO is the γδ T cell, which, similar to the human peripheral blood NK cell has been shown to express eNOS and not iNOS [17]. Exposure of γδ T cells to CD95 crosslinking in the presence of a NO donor prevents apoptosis through a cGMP dependent mechanism. Subsequently, Sciorati et al. [18] showed that NO provided by a NO producing macrophage or by a NO donor interfered with intracellular accumulation of ceramide, and thus caspase activation in the γδ T cell. Thus in human peripheral blood NK cells and γδ T cells, both of which express eNOS, apoptosis is inhibited by NO.

Peroxynitrite induced apoptosis

Peroxynitrite is a potent oxidizing and nitrating agent produced by the reaction of nitric oxide with superoxide. The tyrosine residue in some proteins becomes nitrosylated, inhibiting subsequent phosphorylation reactions. Brito et al. [19] demonstrated that exposure of human peripheral blood T cells to peroxynitrite resulted in inhibition of activation-induced protein tyrosine phosphorylation and apoptosis was induced. These investigators also demonstrated that apoptotic death was facilitated by NO only when T cells were stimulated *via* the T-cell receptor and not when stimulated by PMA and ionomycin, indicating that the phosphorylation events associated with engagement of the T-cell receptor were the target of peroxynitrite. Virag et al. [20] have proposed that peroxynitrite plays a role in the negative selection process in the thymus by promoting thymocyte apoptosis. This apoptotic process was seen only in a narrow concentration range of peroxynitrite since higher concentrations of peroxynitrite resulted in ATP depletion and the activation of caspase-3, an energy requiring process, was prevented.

Nitric oxide mediated inhibition of lymphocyte proliferation

Although the initial description of NO mediated inhibition of lymphocyte proliferation was published 10 years ago [21, 22], the details of this inhibitory mechanism are still unknown in lymphocytes as well as in other cell types. The inhibition of proliferation could occur on several levels such as inhibition of a signal transduction pathway after T-cell receptor stimulation, or by inhibition of cytokine synthesis, or by inhibition of utilization of a cytokine such as IL-2, which is a major stimulator of lymphocyte proliferation. Berendji et al. [26] have examined the mechanism of NO induced inhibition of IL-2 mRNA expression in EL4-6.1, a mouse T-cell lymphoma which can be induced to make IL-2 upon stimulation with IL-1β. NO, derived from the NO donor SNOC (S-nitrosocysteine), prevented the DNA binding of the zinc finger transcription factor, Sp1. This NO mediated inhibition was seen only if NO was present during the first 30 min of stimulation of the cells with IL-1β. In contrast, NO did not inhibit the binding of the transcription factor NFAT (nuclear factor of activation T cells), indicating some specificity for zinc finger transcription factors.

Roozendaal [23] demonstrated a differential effect of NO on cytokine synthesis by human T lymphocytes stimulated with anti CD3/CD28 mAb. In the presence of NO donor compounds, IFNγ, IL-4 and IL-5, but not IL-2 secretion were inhibited. However, 24 h of pretreatment of T cells with NO donors resulted in inhibition of IFNγ secretion, but little inhibitory effect on IL-4 and -5 secretion, indicating that the effects of NO on IFNγ secretion were longer lasting than the effect on IL-4 and -5 secretion. The inhibition of IFNγ secretion mediated by NO was dependent on elevations in cGMP. Similarly, using phytohemagglutinin/PMA stimulated Jurkat T cells exposed to an NO donor, Benbernou et al. [24] showed that IFNγ mRNA expression was inhibited while IL-10 mRNA expression was enhanced. As for the effect of NO on activated T lymphocytes, van der Veen. [25] demonstrated that the proliferation of activated T helper 1 and T helper 2 clones exposed to NO producing macrophages was equally inhibited. The inhibition of proliferation was not accompanied by apoptosis nor was production of IFNγ (TH1 cytokine) and IL-5 (TH2 cytokine) affected.

In contrast to the NO induced inhibition of IL-2 synthesis described by Berendji et al. [26], NO has also been shown to affect IL-2 utilization. Bingissen et al. [27] have demonstrated that the inhibition of Concanavalin A stimulated rat T lymphocytes by NO is accompanied by decreased anti-phosphotyrosine staining of cell lysates treated with NO donors, specifically the tyrosine phosphorylation of Jak3 and Stat 5 (signal transducer and activator transcription), known to be involved in IL-2 receptor signaling.

Facilitation of the immune response by nitric oxide

In contrast, NO has also been shown to be an intracellular signaling molecule that is required for the production of the cytokine, IFNγ in NK cells. Diefenbach et al. [28] have shown that production of IFNγ by IL-12 stimulated NK cells was inhibited in the presence of an NO synthesis inhibitor. NOS-2 activity was required for the tyrosine auto-phosphorylation and activation of Jak2, which in turn trans-phosphorylates Tyk2, resulting in the tyrosine phosphorylation of Stat 4 which regulates IL-12 signaling in NK cells.

Another example of the promotion of the immune response by NO comes from the studies of Cefone et al. [29] who demonstrated that IL-2 stimulated rat NK cells were induced to express iNOS and that NO was required for optimal IFNγ production as well as DNA fragmentation and lysis of sensitive tumor target cells. Additionally, acquisition of the cytotoxic molecule perforin was shown to be significantly reduced in uterine NK cells in iNOS$^{-/-}$ *versus* wild type mice even though the migration and proliferation of the uterine NK cells was independent of NO [30]. These studies provide evidence showing that NO can function as an intracellular signaling molecule facilitating production of cytokines or other molecules that are critical for various physiological processes.

Mechanisms of action of nitric oxide in disease states

In order to ultimately make use of our knowledge of the mechanism of action of NO to alleviate disease severity or progression, it is important to examine the role of NO in various animal models of disease. Various autoimmune disease processes as well as models of infection with a pathogen have been examined in the context of the role that NO plays in the disease processes.

NO has been shown to participate in the destruction of islets in the progression to diabetes by several mechanisms. Macrophages present in the inflammatory infiltrate produce IL-1β, which can induce NO synthesis by β cells in the pancreas [31], and exposure of β cells to NO can result in upregulation of Fas receptor, which facilitates their destruction [32]. Recently, Gurlo et al. [33] have shown that the interaction of CD8+ T cells recovered from diabetic mice with the inflammatory macrophage infiltrate and the β cells results in destruction of the islet in a IFNγ and NO dependent manner. Production of IFNγ by the CD8+ T cells might stimulate NO production by the macrophages resulting in islet destruction.

In contrast, in a model of autoimmune uveitis, administration of IL-12 downregulated the disease process in susceptible strains of mice [34]. Since this disease is mediated by T helper 1-like T cells and IL-12 promotes the TH1 response by increasing IFNγ production, the hypothesis was that IL-12 administration would exacerbate the disease process. The mechanism responsible for the decreased severity of disease due to IL-12 administration was found to be increased IFNγ production, which in turn increased NO production, which in turn induced apoptotic deletion of antigen reactive T cells. This NO induced apoptosis was found to be due in part to downregulation of the anti-apoptotic protein, Bcl-2. Similarly, in a model of experimental encephalomyelitis in Lewis rats, administration of IL-4 resulted in improved clinical scores which was found to be due to enhanced proliferation of DC that produced NO, again leading to apoptosis of autoreactive T cells [35].

In models of infection, the paradoxical role of NO is very evident in that NO production by cells that have phagocytosed the invading organism exerts a cytostatic/cytotoxic effect on the invading organism. However, the NO produced might also serve to downregulate the acquired immune response needed for resolution of the infectious process by inhibition of lymphocyte proliferation and induction of apoptosis in the antigen reactive T cell. To this end, James et al. [36] demonstrated that although iNOS−/− mice developed an enhanced type 1 immune response after vaccination with attenuated *Schistosoma mansoni* cercariae, characterized by enhanced levels of parasite specific IgG2a antibody levels and enhanced mRNA for IFNγ and TNFα, these mice displayed reduced resistance to the challenge infection. Therefore, even though a less robust TH1 response was elicited in iNOS sufficient mice in response to *Schistosoma mansoni* vaccination, NO was required for optimal protection. Similarly, iNOS−/− mice were more susceptible to herpes simplex virus infection even though enhanced TH1-like response was also seen in these virally infected mice [37].

Several models of infection have shown that the NK cell plays a pivotal role in the resolution of the infection. As described above, Diefenbach et al. [28] have shown that NK cell production of IFNγ induced by IL-12, which requires the participation of NO, prevents the spreading of *Leishmania* parasites that is necessary for successful resolution of the infection. In a model of *Salmonella typhimurium* infection in mice, Schwacha et al. [38] demonstrated that NK cells in the splenocyte preparation were the source of the IFNγ, which was ultimately responsible for the NO synthesis and decreased immune responses displayed by the splenocytes from the infected mice.

In a model of *Trypanosoma cruzi* infection, Martins et al. [39] demonstrated that IFNγ plays a dual role in the induction of apoptosis in that this cytokine upregulated CD95 and CD95 ligand expression as well as increased NO synthesis and subsequent apoptosis of spleen cells. This apoptotic process was thought to serve as a control of the immune response and thus prevent deleterious inflammatory reactions.

Nitric oxide in HIV infection

HIV-1 infection is associated with enhanced nitrogen oxide metabolites in the serum and *in vitro* infection of human macrophages with HIV-1 or stimulation with envelope gp120 glycoprotein results in nitric oxide production [40, 41]. Nitric oxide produced by HIV-1 infected monocytes/macrophages may result in the suppression of the immune response as seen in other infectious processes [42]. Mossalayi and colleagues demonstrated that peripheral blood mononuclear cells from patients with AIDS were more susceptible to NO induced apoptosis when cells from patients with a low CD4+ T-cell count were compared to patients or controls with a normal CD4+ T-cell count [43]. Furthermore, addition of an NO synthesis inhibitor to the mononuclear cells resulted in enhanced cell survival, indicating that NO was participating in the apoptotic process.

In order to elucidate a mechanism for the enhanced serum IgE levels seen in HIV-1 infected patients, Dugas et al. [44] exposed human PBMCs to IL-4 and glycoprotein gp120. IgE production was assessed in the presence and absence of an NO synthesis inhibitor and the results indicated that inhibition of NO synthesis resulted in significantly decreased IgE levels. The mechanism of this enhanced antibody production was that low amounts of NO protected the B cells from apoptosis and thus more B cells participated in antibody production. These results indicate that in HIV-1 infection NO can function as an inhibitor of the immune response by promotion of CD4+ T cell-apoptosis and yet also function as a promoter of an immune response by protecting B cells from programmed cell death.

Nitric oxide as a regulator of lymphocyte migration

Interactions between circulating leukocytes and vascular endothelial cells control normal recirculation and migration of cells as well as emigration of cells into sites of inflammation. NO has been shown to play an important role in leukocyte adhesion to endothelium and inhibition of NO synthesis can result in patterns of leukocyte adhesion characteristic of an acute inflammatory response [45]. Hickey reported that iNOS-deficient mice have enhanced leukocyte-endothelium interactions in endotoxemia [46]. The rolling and adherence of lymphocytes in NOS inhibitor-treated rats were significantly increased in post-capillary venules of Peyer's patches [47]. This increased lymphocyte-endothelial cell interaction resulting from inhibition of NO synthesis was prevented by anti-α4-integrin antibody as well as anti-P-selectin antibody. Using a culture model of human umbilical vein endothelial cells and human peripheral blood monocytes, Adams et al. [48] showed that addition of L-arginine resulted in decreased adhesion of the monocytes while addition of L-NMMA resulted in increased monocyte adhesion. The addition of L-arginine also resulted in decreased expression of ICAM-1 and VCAM-1. Similarly, Qian et al. [49] showed that Ad.nNOS gene therapy in the rabbit carotid artery rapidly and substantially reduced both ICAM-1 and VCAM-1 expression as well as lymphocyte and monocyte infiltration. However, Cartwright et al. [50] showed that NO donors did not alter the cell surface expression of VCAM-1, ICAM-1, or E-selectin on an endothelial cell line. Recently, Austrup and colleagues have shown that T-cell subpopulations can be preferentially recruited to inflammatory sites due to the expression of P and E selectin molecules on TH1, but not TH2 cells [51]. Modulation of this recruitment process by NO may influence the accumulation of TH1 cells at an inflammatory site.

Conclusion

It is clear from studies on the effects of NO on lymphocyte function that this molecule is an important modulator of the immune response. An important new concept is that NO can play a necessary role in the intracellular signal transduction pathways to facilitate production of the cytokine IFNγ and perhaps other molecules. In some lymphoid populations, exposure to NO seems to increase the intensity of the immune response and in other systems, NO exposure results in the attenuation of the immune response due to inhibition of proliferation and/or induction of apoptosis. These paradoxical *in vitro* observations are paralleled by certain *in vivo* observations, in particular the immune response of iNOS$^{-/-}$ mice to a pathogenic challenge. In this system, enhancement of a TH1-like response, with increased IFNγ synthesis and IgG2a antibody synthesis in iNOS$^{-/-}$ *versus* wild type mice is accompanied by an inferior clinical outcome. More experimentation is needed in order to exploit the powerful effects of NO on the immune response to successfully alleviate disease processes.

References

1　Reiling N, Kröncke R, Ulmer A J, Gerdes J, Flad HD, Hauschildt S (1996) Nitric oxide synthase: expression of the endothelial, CA2+/calmodulin-dependent ioform in human B and T lymphocytes. *Eur J Immunol* 26: 511–516

2　Fehsel K, Kroncke KD, Meyer KL, Huber H, Wahn V, Kolb-Bachofen V (1995) Nitric oxide induces apoptosis in mouse zhymocytes. *J Immunol* 155: 2858–2865

3　Hortelano S, Dallaporta B, Zamzami N, Hirsch T, Susin SA, Marzo I, Bosca L, Kroemer G (1997) Nitric oxide induces apoptosis *via* triggering mitochondrial permeability transition. *FEBS Lett* 410: 373–377

4　Zhou X, Gordon SA, Kim YM, Hoffman RA, Chen Y, Zhang XR, Simmons RL, Ford HR (2000) Nitric oxide induces thymocyte apoptosis *via* a caspase-1-dependent mechanism. *J Immunol* 165: 1252–1258

5　Tai X G, Toyo-oka K, Yamamoto N, Yashiro Y, Mu J, Hamaoka T, Fujiwara H (1997) Expression of an inducible type of nitric oxide (NO) synthase in the thymus and involvement of NO in deletion of TCR-stimulated double-positive thymocytes. *J Immunol* 158: 4696–4703

6　Brás A, Rodriguez-Borlado L, Gonzalez-Garcia A, Martinez AC (1997) Nitric oxide regulates clonal expansion and activation-induced cell death triggered by staphylococcal enterotoxin B. *Infect Immun* 65: 4030–4037

7　Mannick JB, Miao XQ, Stamler JS (1997) Nitric oxide inhibits Fas-induced apoptosis. *J Biol Chem* 272: 24125–24128

8　Dimmeler S, Haendeler J, Nehls M, Zeiher AM (1997) Suppression of apoptosis by nitric oxide *via* inhibition of interleukin-1beta-converting enzyme (ICE)-like and cysteine protease protein (CPP)-32-like proteases. *J Exp Med* 185: 601–607

9　Li J, Billiar T, Talanian RV, Kim YM (1997) Nitric oxide reversibly inhibits seven members of the caspase family *via* S-nitrosylation. *Biochem Biophys Res Commun* 240: 419–424

10　Kim YM, Talanian RV, Billiar T (1997) Nitric oxide inhibits apoptosis by preventing increases in caspase-3-like activity *via* two distinct mechanisms. *J Biol Chem* 272: 31138–31148

11　Kim YM, de Vera ME, Watkins SC, Billiar T (1997) Nitric oxide protects cultured rat hepatocytes from TNFα-induced apoptosis by inducing heat shock protein 70 expression. *J Biol Chem* 272: 1402–1411

12　Genaro AM, Hortelano S, Alvarez A, Martinez C, Bosca L (1995) Splenic B lymphocyte programmed cell death is prevented by nitric oxide release through mechanisms involving sustained Bcl-2 levels. *J Clin Invest* 95: 1884–1890

13　Okuda Y, Sakoda S, Shimaoka M, Yanagihara T (1996) Nitric oxide induces apoptosis in mouse splenic T lymphocytes. *Immunol Lett* 52: 135–138

14　Williams MS, Noguchi S, Henkart PA, Osawa Y (1998) Nitric oxide synthase plays a signaling role in TCR-triggered apoptotic death. *J Immunol* 161: 6526–6531

15　Allione A, Bernabei P, Bosticardo M, Ariott S, Forni G, Novelli F (1999) Nitric oxide suppresses human T lymphocyte proliferation through IFN-γ-dependent and IFN-γ-independent induction of apoptosis. *J Immunol* 163: 4182–4191

16   Furuke K, Burd PR, Horvath-Arcidiacono JA, Hori K, Mostowski H, Bloom ET (1999) Human NK cells express endothelial nitric oxide synthase, and nitric oxide protects them from activation-induced cell death by regulating expression of TNF-α. *J Immunol* 163: 1473–1480

17   Sciorati A, Rovere P, Ferrarini M, Heltai S, Manfredi AA, Clementi E (1997) Autocrine nitric oxide modulates CD95-induced apoptosis in gamma delta T lymphocytes. *J Biol Chem* 272 (37): 23211–23215

18   Sciorati C, Rovere P, Ferrarini M, Paolucci C, Heltai S, Vaiani R, Clementi E, Manfredi AA (1999) Generation of nitric oxide by the inducible nitric oxide synthase protects γδ T cells from *Mycobacterium tuberculosis*-induced apoptosis. *J Immunol* 163: 1570–1576

19   Brito C, Naviliat M, Tiscornia AC, Vuillier F, Gualco G, Dighiero G, Radi R, Cayota A M (1999) Peroxynitrite inhibits T lymphocyte activation and proliferation by promoting impairment of tyrosine phosphorylation and peroxynitrite-drive apoptotic death. *J Immunol* 162: 3356–3366

20   Virag L, Scott GS, Cuzzocrea S, Marmer D, Salzman AL, Szabo C (1998) Peroxynitrite-induced thymocyte apoptosis: the role of caspases and poly (ADP-ribose) synthetase (PARS) activation. *Immunol* 94: 345–355

21   Hoffman RA, Langrehr JM, Billiar T, Curran RD, Simmons RL (1990) Alloantigen-induced activation of rat splenocytes is regulated by the oxidative metabolism of L-arginine. *J Immunol* 145: 2220–2226

22   Albina JE, Abate JA, Henry WL Jr (1991) Nitric oxide production is required for murine Resident peritonealmacrophages to suppress mitogen-stimulated T cell proliferation. Role of IFN-gamma in the induction of the nitric oxide-synthesizing pathway. *J Immunol* 147: 144–148

23   Roozendaal R, Vellenga E, Postma DS, De Monchy JGR, Kauffman HF (1999) Nitric oxide selectively decreases interferon-γ expression by activated human T lymphocytes *via* a cGMP-independent mechanism. *Immunol* 98: 393–399

24   Benbernou N, Esnault S, Shin HCK, Fekkar H, Guenounou M (1997) Differential regulation of IFN-γ, IL-10 and inducible nitric oxide synthase in human T cells by cyclic AMP-dependent signal transduction pathway. *Immunol* 91: 361–368

25   van der Veen RC, Dietlin TA, Gray JD, Gilmore W (2000) Macrophage-derived nitric oxide inhibits the proliferation of activated T helper cells and is induced during antigenic stimulation of resting T cells. *Cell Immunol* 199: 43–49

26   Berendji D, Kolb-Bachofen V, Zipfel PF, Skerka C, Carlberg C, Kroncke KD (1999) Zinc finger transcription factors as molecular targets for nitric oxide-mediated immunosuppression: inhibition of IL-2 gene expression in murine lymphocytes. *Molecular Medicine* 5: 721–730

27   Bingisser RM, Tilbrook PA, Holt PG, Kees UR (1998) Macrophage-derived nitric oxide

regulates T cell activation *via* reversible disruption of the Jak3/STAT5 signaling pathway. *J Immunol* 160: 5729–5734

28 Diefenbach A, Schindler H, Rollinghoff M, Yokoyama WM, Bogdan C (1999) Requirement for type 2 NO synthase for IL-12 signaling in innate immunity. *Science* 284: 951–955

29 Langrehr JM, Hoffman RA, Demetris AJ, Lee KKW, Neuhaus P, Wren SM, Ildstad ST, Schraut WH (1992) Evidence that indefinite survival of small bowel allografts achieved by a brief course of cyclosporine or FK506 is not due to systemic hyporesponsiveness. *Transplantation* 54: 505–510

30 Burnett TG, Hunt JS (2000) Nitric oxide synthase-2 and expression of perforin in uterine NK cells. *J Immunol* 164: 5245–5250

31 Corbett JA, Wang JL, Sweetland MA, Lancaster JrJR, McDaniel ML (1992) Interleukin 1β induces the formation of nitric oxide by β-cells purified from rodent islets of Langerhans. *J Clin Invest* 90: 2384–2391

32 Ruan X, Pereda A, Stassi DL, Zeidner D, Summers RG, Jackson M, Shivakumar A, Kakavas S, Staver MJ, Donadio S et al (1997) Acyltransferase domain substitutions in erythromycin polyketide synthase yield novel erythromycin derivatives. *J Bacteriol* 179: 6416–6425

33 Gurlo T, Kawamura K, von Grafenstein H (1999) Role of inflammatory infiltrate in activation and effector function of cloned islet reactive nonobese diabetic CD8[+] T cells: involvement of a nitric oxide-dependent pathway. *J Immunol* 163: 5770–5780

34 Tarrant TK, Silver P, Wahlsten JL, Rizzo LV, Chan CC, Wiggert B, Caspi RR (1997) Interleukin 12 protects from a T helper type 1-mediated autoimmune disease, experimental autoimmune uveitis, through a mechanism involving Interferon γ, nitric oxide, and apoptosis. *J Exp Med* 189: 219–230

35 Xu LY, Huang YM, Yang JS, Van Der Meide PH, Levi M, Wahren B, Link H, Xiao BG (1999) Dendritic cell-derived nitric oxide is involved in IL-4-induced suppression of experimental allergic encephalomyelitis (EAE) in Lewis rats. *Clin Exp Immunol* 118: 115–121

36 James SL, Cheever A W, Caspar P, Wynn TA (1998) Inducible nitric oxide synthase-deficient mice develop enhanced type 1 cytokine-associated cellular and humoral immune responses after vaccination with attenuated *Schistosoma mansoni* cercariae but display partially reduced resistance. *Infect Immun* 66: 3510–3518

37 MacLean A, Wei X-Q, Huang FP, Al-Alem UAH, Chan WL, Liew FY (1998) Mice lacking inducible nitric-oxide synthase are more susceptible to herpes simplex virus infection despite enhanced Th1 cell responses. *J Gen Virol* 79: 825–830

38 Schwacha MG, Meissler JJ, Eisenstein TK (1998) *Salmonella typhimurium* infection in mice induces nitric oxide-mediated immunosuppression through a natural killer cell-dependent pathway. *Infect Immun* 66: 5862–5866

39 Martins GA, Vieira LQ, Cunha FQ, Silva JS (1999) Gamma interferon modulates CD95 (Fas) and CD95 ligand (Fas-L) expression and nitric oxide-induced apoptosis during the

acute phase of *Trypanosoma cruzi* infection: a possible role in immune response control. *Infect Immun* 67: 3864–3871

40 Bukrinsky MI, Nottet HSLN, Schmidtmayerova H, Dubrovsky L, Flanangan CR, Mullins ME, Lipton SA, Gendelman HE (1995) Regulation of nitric oxide synthase activity in human immunodeficiency virus type 1 (HIV-1)-infected monocytes: implications for HIV-associated neurological disease. *J Exp Med* 191: 735–745

41 Baldeweg T, Sooranna S, Das I, Catalan J, Cazzard B (1996) Serum nitrite concentration suggests a role for nitric oxide in AIDS. *AIDS* 10: 451–452

42 Torre D, Ferrario G (1996) Immunological aspects of nitric oxide in HIV-1 infection. *Medical Hypotheses* 47: 405–407

43 Mossalayi MD, Becherel PA, Debré P (1999) Critical role of nitric oxide during the apoptosis of peripheral blood leukocytes from patients with AIDS. *Molecular Medicine* 5: 812–819

44 Dugas N, Dereuddre-Bosquet N, Goujard C, Dormont D, Tardieu M, Delfraissy JF (2000) Role of nitric oxide in the promoting effect of HIV Type 1 infection and of gp120 envelope glycoprotein on interleukin 4-induced IgE production by normal human mononuclear cells. *AIDS Research and Human Retroviruses* 16: 251–258

45 Kubes P, Suzuki M, Granger DN (1991) Nitric oxide: An endogenous modulator of leukocyte adhesion. *Proc Natl Acad Sci USA* 88: 4651–4655

46 Hickey MJ, Sharkey KA, Sihota EG, Reinhardt PH, MacMicking JD, Nathan C, Kubes P (1997) Inducible nitric oxide synthase-deficient mice have enhanced leukocyte-endothelium interactions in endotoxemia. *FASEB J* 11: 955–964

47 Hokari R, Miura S, Fujimori H, Tsuzuki Y, Shigematsu T, Higuchi H, Kimura H, Kurose I, Serizawa H, Suematsu M et al (1998) Nitric oxide modulates T-lymphocyte migration in Peyer's patches and villous submucosa of rat small intestine. *Gastroenterology* 115: 618–627

48 Adams MR, Jessup W, Hailstones D, Celermajer DS (1997) L-arginine reduces human monocyte adhesion to vascular endothelium and endothelial expression of cell adhesion molecules. *Circulation* 95: 662–668

49 Qian H, Neplioueva V, Shetty GA, Channon KM, George SE (1999) Nitric oxide synthase gene therapy rapidly reduces adhesion molecule expression and inflammatory cell infiltration in carotid arteries of cholesterol-fed rabbits. *Circulation* 99: 2979–2982

50 Cartwright JE, Whitley GStJ, Johnstone AP (1997) Endothelial cell adhesion molecule expression and lymphocyte adhesion to endothelial cells: effect of nitric oxide. *Exp Cell Res* 235: 431–434

51 Austrup F, Vestweber D, Borges E, Lohning M, Brauer R, Herz U, Renz H, Hallmann R, Scheffold A, Radbruch A et al (1997) P-and E-selectin mediate recruitment of T-helper-1 but not T-helper-2 cells into inflamed tissues. *Nature* 385: 81–83

Role of nitric oxide and reactive oxygen species in arthritis

Salvatore Cuzzocrea

Institute of Pharmacology, School of Medicine, University of Messina, Torre Biologica, Policlinico Universitario, Via C. Valeria, Gazzi, 98100 Messina, Italy

Oxygen radical generation in rheumatic diseases

Production of nitric oxide (NO)

The free radical nitric oxide (NO) is synthesized from the guanidino group of L-arginine by a family of enzymes termed NO synthases (NOS). Three isoforms have been described and cloned: endothelial cell NOS (ecNOS, or type 3), brain NOS (bNOS, nNOS, or type 1), and inducible macrophage type NOS (iNOS, or type 2). The cytotoxic effects of NO (in high local concentrations) involve the inhibition of key mitochondrial Fe-S enzymes, including NADH:ubiquinone oxidoreductase, NADH:succinate oxidoreductase, and aconitase [1]. cGMP-independent activation by NO of other enzymes, such as cyclooxygenase, has also been described. This action may be related to the reaction of NO with the iron-heme center at the active site of the enzyme [2]. Administration of NOS inhibitors reduces blood flow to most organs.

Many inflammatory conditions are associated with production of comparatively large amounts of NO, produced by iNOS, with consequent cytotoxic effects. iNOS, first identified in macrophages, can be expressed in essentially any cell type. Although constitutive expression of iNOS has been localized to the kidney, the intestine, and the bronchial epithelia, iNOS is expressed typically in response to immunological stimuli and produces nanomoles, rather than picomoles, of NO. Once produced in high local concentrations, NO may act as a cytostatic and cytotoxic molecule for fungal, bacterial, helminthic, and protozoal organisms as well as tumor cells. Induction of iNOS can be inhibited by numerous agents, including glucocorticoids, thrombin, macrophage deactivation factor, tumor growth factor beta, platelet-derived growth factor, IL-4, IL-8, IL-10, and IL-13. Induction of iNOS may have either toxic or protective effects. Factors that appear to dictate the consequences of iNOS expression include the type of insult, the tissue type, the level and duration of iNOS expression, and probably the redox status of the tissue. Much attention has focused on the toxicity of iNOS. For example, induction of iNOS in endothelial cells produces endothelial injury [3].

Nitric Oxide and Inflammation, edited by Daniela Salvemini, Timothy R. Billiar and Yoram Vodovotz
© 2001 Birkhäuser Verlag Basel/Switzerland

Induction of iNOS has been shown to inhibit cellular respiration in macrophages and vascular smooth muscle cells; these processes can lead to cell dysfunction and cell death. The notion that arthritis is associated with overproduction of NO is hardly novel: enhanced formation of NO in serum and synovial fluid samples from patients with rheumatoid arthritis (RA) and osteoarthritis (OA) arthritis was first demonstrated in early studies [4]. This finding has been confirmed and extended by the measurement of evaluation of iNOS expression in the joint of arthritic rats (Fig. 1A) [5]. Beneficial effects of NOS inhibitors in arthritis include a reduction of the symptom [6], protection against the loss of body weight [9], and protection against joint injury [7].

In more recent studies, selective inhibitors for iNOS have been tested in models of osteoarthritis and were found to exert beneficial effects. For example, N-iminoethyl-l-lysine (L-NIL), a high selective iNOS inhibitor, has been shown to reduce the progression of experimental osteoarthritis [8]. Mercaptoalkylguanidines represent another novel class of iNOS inhibitors [9], which, however, also have an important additional independent pharmacological action related to inhibition of peroxynitrite-induced oxidations [10]. Mercaptoethylguanidine (MEG), a member of this class of compounds, has marked protective effects in rodent models of arthritis [11].

It is well known that during arthritis the inflammatory cascades are characterized by increased cytokine production, leukocyte adhesion molecule expression, and neutrophil infiltration into tissues. To determine if induced NO participated in proinflammatory signaling following resuscitation, two approaches were undertaken [12]. First, rats subjected to arthritis received the iNOS inhibitor N-iminoethyl-Llysine (NIL). Second, the responses of iNOS knockout mice to arthritis were compared to responses of wild-type mice with the same genetic background [13]. In both instances, the lack of iNOS was associated with a marked reduction in the arthritis progression [11, 13]. These studies indicated that NO can pay a key role in arthritis. With the many known targets for NO and peroxynitrite, this finding is perhaps not surprising. However, a potentially unique aspect of NO-mediated signaling in arthritis is the associated redox stress. It is possible under conditions of reduced antioxidant capacity that NO or a reaction product, such as peroxynitrite, activates intracellular redox-sensitive signaling pathways. Further, nitrogen-based radicals most likely represent only one of the oxidant species that participate in oxidant signaling in arthritis.

Figure 1
Staining for iNOS (A), nitrotyrosine (B), and for PARS (C) at 35 days following collagen-induced arthritis. Original magnification: × 125. Figure is representative of at least three experiments performed on different experimental days.

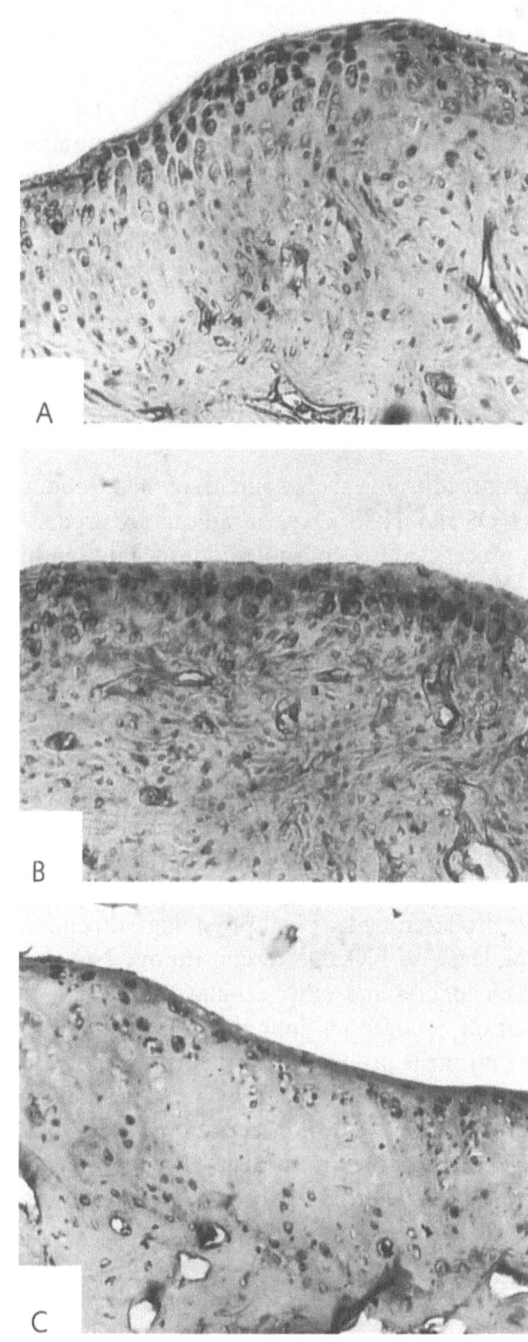

The role of iNOS-derived NO (or peroxynitrite) as an amplifier of the inflammatory response is now also supported by the following observations: inhibition of iNOS suppresses TNF production in the delayed phase of allergic encephalomyelitis [14]; inhibition of iNOS suppresses IL-1, collagenase, and stromelysin production in arthritis [15, 16]; inhibition of iNOS suppresses interferon γ (IFNγ) production in a murine model of leishmaniasis [17]; and the expression of certain chemokines is suppressed in the absence of iNOS in zymosan-induced peritonitis [18]. Thus, a picture of a pathway is evolving that contributes to tissue damage both directly *via* the formation of peroxynitrite, with its associated toxicities, and indirectly through the amplification of the inflammatory response. The participation of iNOS ranges from an amplifier and terminal mediator of tissue injury (e.g., in various forms of inflammation, see above), to cytoprotective or anti-inflammatory roles.

Production of peroxynitrite (ONOO⁻)

As already indicated, sources of NO production during arthritis include both ecNOS and iNOS. Oxygen radicals are produced in abundance during inflammatory process. Sources of superoxide include xanthine oxidase and NADPH oxidase, as well as various metabolic and signaling pathways. Simultaneous generation of nitric oxide and superoxide favors the production of a toxic reaction product, peroxynitrite anion [19] (Fig. 2). It is important to point out that, under certain conditions, NOS can produce both precursors of peroxynitrite (NO and superoxide). Such conditions cannot be found under normal circumstances, but can occur during L-arginine depletion. Low levels of arginine might be expected following resuscitation with crystalline solutions [20]. Under low cellular arginine concentrations, NOS produces both NO and superoxide, and the resulting generation of peroxynitrite can contribute to cytotoxicity. This mechanism has been confirmed in neuronal cultures, as well as in macrophages that express iNOS [21]. Small amounts of peroxynitrite are produced under basal physiological conditions, since most cells are exposed to low levels of NO due to constitutive NO production, and also superoxide from mitochondria and other cellular sources are always produced [22]. It is probable that the endogenous antioxidant systems are sufficient to neutralize such low-level peroxynitrite production, which is, therefore, not cytotoxic. It may be important to note that, although peroxynitrite is generally considered as a cytotoxic molecule, peroxynitrite in low concentrations, in the presence of intact antioxidant systems, has been proposed to mediate physiological effects. For instance, a low concentration of peroxynitrite has been shown to inhibit neutrophil adhesion [23].

Under these conditions, peroxynitrite is likely to form NO adducts with glucose, thiols, and other species [24] which, in turn, can act as NO donors, activating guanylyl cyclase [24]. Currently, little information is available regarding these "physiological" roles of peroxynitrite, while the evidence for the roles of peroxyni-

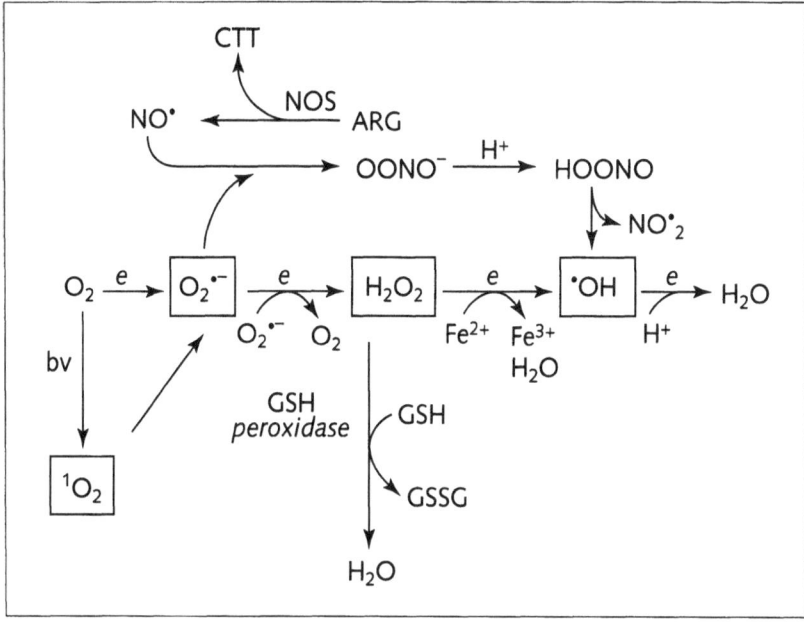

Figure 2

Free radicals and reactive oxygen intermediates considered in this review. The three electron (e) reduction of oxygen (O_2) generates the highly toxic hydroxyl radical (.OH); intermediates in this process include the superoxide anion radical ($O_2^{-\cdot}$) and the non-radical species hydrogen peroxide (H_2O_2). The $O_2^{-\cdot}$ is enzymatically converted to H_2O_2 by a widely distributed family of enzymes known as superoxide dismutase (SOD). Transition metals, e.g., Fe^{2+} generate the . OH via the Fenton reaction. Singlet oxygen, an activated form of O_2, also is a toxic agent. H_2O_2 is metabolized to non-toxic products by GSH peroxidase; in the process reduced glutathione (GSH) is converted to oxidized glutathione (GSSG). Nitric oxide synthase (NOS) generates nitric oxide (NO) which can degrade into more reactive radicals. These interactions are explained in the text.

trite in pathophysiological conditions is expanding. Although there are a number of experimental difficulties related to delineation of the actual role of peroxynitrite in arthritis and other pathophysiological conditions, theoretical considerations strongly favor the production of peroxynitrite when NO and superoxide are produced simultaneously, because the reaction of these two species is nearly diffusion-controlled. In fact, the reaction of superoxide with NO is the only reaction that outcompetes the reaction of superoxide with superoxide dismutase [19].

Although chemical considerations favor the production of peroxynitrite, the actual demonstration of the presence or production of peroxynitrite in pathophysiological conditions is far from straightforward. The finding that peroxynitrite is produced during inflammation is not surprising, in light of the previous evidence for the over-production of oxygenderived free radicals. The formation of nitrotyrosine staining as an indication of "increased nitrosative stress", and peroxynitrite formation has recently been demonstrated in the joint of rats subjected to arthritis (Fig. 1B) [26].

Thus, multiple lines of evidence strongly suggest that peroxynitrite is produced in arthritis. Specific peroxynitrite scavengers could help further delineate the role of peroxynitrite in inflammation. Therefore, the evidence implicating the role of per-oxynitrite in a given pathophysiological condition can only be indirect. However, recently Salvemini et al. using a specific class of peroxynitrite decomposition cayta-lyst have demonstrated that peroxynitrite play a role in acute inflammation [27]. Therefore, it is likely that additional interactions of oxygen- and nitrogen-derived free radicals also contribute to the inflammatory cell injury. Peroxynitrite induces the oxidation of sulfhydryl groups and thioethers and the nitration and hydroxyla-tion of aromatic compounds, such as tyrosine, tryptophan, and guanine.

These reactions, when occurring during the reaction of peroxynitrite with vari-ous enzymes of the cell, can markedly suppress the catalytic activity of these enzymes. For instance, peroxynitrite has been shown to inhibit manganese superox-ide dismutase, tyrosine hydroxylase, membrane sodium/potassium ATP ase, mem-brane sodium channels mitochondrial and cytosolic aconitase, and a number of crit-ical enzymes in the mitochondrial respiratory chain, as well as NOS [19]. While per-oxynitrite inactivates many enzymes, the catalytic activity of some enzymes is actually enhanced by peroxynitrite a primary example being cyclooxygenase. In addition to the interactions of peroxynitrite with proteins, an important interaction of peroxynitrite occurs with nucleic acids. Two main types of reactions have been described: DNA base modifications and DNA single strand breakage. In addition to direct cytotoxic effects, an indirect pathway of peroxynitrite-induced cellular injury has also been proposed. The generation of peroxynitrite, either intracellularly or extracellularly, has been shown to trigger DNA single strand breakage and activa-tion of the nuclear enzyme poly (ADP-ribose) synthetase (PARS). The PARS path-way activation generally lead to cell death *via* the necrotic pathway (Fig. 3). This is the pathway affected by pharmacological inhibitors of PARS [28]. On the other hand, peroxynitrite can also lead to cell death *via* the apoptotic pathway. PARS, however, does not play a role in this latter process, since inhibition of PARS does not appear to prevent peroxynitrite-induced apoptosis [29]. Recent investigations tested the effects of pharmacological inhibitors of PARS in rodent model of arthri-tis. In a murine model of potassium peroxochromate-induced arthritis, the mice treated with the PARS inhibitor nicotinamide showed a significant reduction of arthritis development [30]. Similar to the protective effect of PARS inhibitor, the NO synthase inhibitor, MEG, also prevents the development of arthritis [11]. A number of recent observations suggest that PARS activation plays a role in the oxidant injury in various forms of inflammation. In fact PARS activation was found in the joint of arthritic rats (Fig. 1C). The blockade of neutrophil recruitment associated

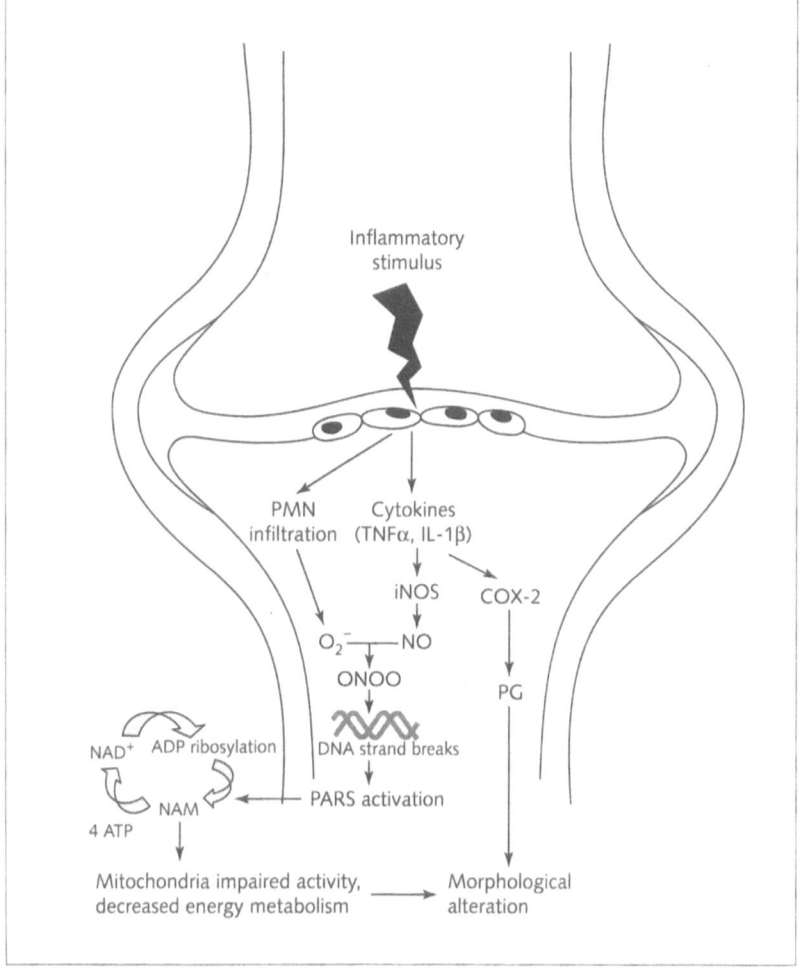

Figure 3
Suggested mode of activation of poly (ADP-ribose) synthetase.

with PARS inhibition, coupled with a direct cytoprotective effect of PARS inhibition, protects against oxidant injury [31] and may explain the antiinflammatory effects seen with inhibition of PARS. Furthermore, recent studies have demonstrated the PARS$^{-/-}$ mice developed less arthritis when compared with PARS$^{+/+}$ mice [32]. Based on these studies, it has been proposed that inhibition of PARS represents a novel strategy for anti-inflammatory therapy under conditions of oxidant stress.

Antioxidant defences

Endogenous antioxidant

In 1974, McCord [33] pointed out that superoxide dismutase (SOD, the enzyme that dismutes superoxide into hydrogen peroxide) was an intracellular protein; the levels in the bovine synovial fluids (SFs) that he tested were detectable, but quite low. As it became apparent that ROS generation might be phlogistic, i.e., proinflammatory, it was then rather obvious to start looking at scavenger levels in various disease states. Clearly, if SOD protection was diminished, e.g. in RA, either in cells or outside, then a scenario for inflammatory and destructive process would be established. Blake et al. studied eight human RA SFs and found no detectable SOD and only trivial amounts of catalase [34]; thus there would be no barrier to the action of O_2^- on HA, for example. However, Igari et al. [35] depolymerised the SFs with hyaluronidase first and then measured SOD in both serum and joint aspirate, comparing RA to OA. In this study, SOD acted like an acute phase reactant. The SOD level was four times higher in RA SF than in OA (but not significantly higher in serum), and SF SOD correlated with disease class and C-reactive protein (CRP) level.

The only study of SF using a non-arthritic control group was that of Marklund et al. [36] involving patients with RA, reactive arthritis, and meniscal injury. Only in the RA group was a statistically significant decrease in SF SOD level found, coincident with a substantial increase in total protein content (probably creating a dilution factor). Ceruloplasmin has long been recognized as an acute phase reactant and is a contributor to the enhanced antioxidant capacity of RA serum [37] where its complicated biochemical reactivity is intimately linked to the availability of trace metals such as iron and copper. The major intracellular pool of SOD in the circulation is in the erythrocytes; red cell SOD was found not to be different from normal in 50 patients with RA [38], and to be lower than normal in a different study [39]. In PMNs, the reports include increased [40], decreased [41], and normal [42] neutrophil SOD content in RA.

It would be naïve to think that the root of RA lies in neutrophilic SOD. There is also extensive literature on reduced levels of selenium in RA, especially in red blood cells. Se is a component of glutathione peroxidase, a scavenger of peroxides that can also be viewed as part of the natural antioxidant armamentarium. D-Penicillamine is an interesting drug in the oxygen radical context, because low molecular weight complexes of copper and D-penicillamine have themselves a stoichiometric (not catalytic) scavenging effect on superoxide [43]. In addition, this drug chelates copper and enhances its urinary excretion, which depletes red cell SOD levels rather substantially [44]. Since D-penicillamine has been accepted as an efficacious agent for RA, one might interpret this fact as evidence that ROS are not crucial mediators of those aspects of RA which are aided by D-penicillamine.

Effects of anti-rheumatics drugs on oxygen radical production or action

It is perhaps no surprise that the largest subtopic in the field of oxygen radicals and inflammation pertains to the effects of drugs on their production and/or action. Because pharmacological agents are the mainstay of the treatment of most arthritic disorders, and because the actual mode of action for most of these compounds is not understood, investigators have been quick to add NSAIDs, steroids, gold compounds, and in fact all of the anti-rheumatics, to ROS systems, both *in vitro* and *in vivo*, expecting to find an inhiltitory effect that can be adduced as a mechanism of action. Given enough drug, most such experiments have been successful; suffice it to say a drug that enhances oxygen radical activity has yet to be found. Some initial studies were done in cell-free systems, adding the drugs *in vitro*. Steroids have profound effects on PMNs, and alter many leukocyte functions. Hydrocortisone and methylprednisolone, when added *in vitro*, suppressed both PMN release of lysosomal enzymes as well as superoxide generation induced by soluble stimuli or opsonized zymosan [45]. Similar results were obtained with phagocytosis of bacteria [46] or latex particles [47]. In a study involving steroid treatment of RA, monocyte superoxide production was reported to be suppressed only after *in vivo* administration, the same agent being ineffective *in vitro* [48]. The authors interpreted this in light of leukocyte traffic and bone marrow egress, which is certainly the most plausible explanation.

Gold compounds have attracted substantial interest from ROS researchers. Davis et al. tested the three common gold preparations *in vitro* [49]. Whereas none of them scavenged O_2 from XO, triethylphosphine gold (auranofin) inhibited PMN O_2^- generation (from FMLP) significantly, especially at 1.5 pg/mL or higher. This was confirmed in several papers [50, 51] with immune complexes and frustrated phagocytosis, and the effect was irreversible by washing. Auranofin was also shown to quench singlet oxygen in a organic solvent system and was proposed as a protector of lipid peroxidation [52]. In an *in vivo* study using injectable gold, a reversal of depressed PMN O_2^-, production after a course of chrysotherapy was reported [53].

In view of the many theories on the mechanism of action of gold, such findings are intriguing. One can argue the contrary point, however, that auranofin is a weak agent in the treatment of RA, and its effect of ROS production may well mean that free radicals have no real importance in the pathogenesis of the disease.

Finally, there are the NSAIDs, where again there have been extensive studies. Abramson et al. [54] noted that ibuprofen and indomethacin had no effect on O_2^- production, neither *in vitro* nor after *in vivo* administration to normal volunteers; however, piroxicarn had a substantial effect on this parameter of PNM function. Different responses were noted to different stimuli, along with disparities with regard to aggregation of lysosomal enzyme secretion, suggesting that PMNs can be activated by multiple pathways and that NSAIDs do not necessarily share common mechanisms of action, a position now rather widely accepted. The piroxicam results led to several studies of that agent in particular; results include a demonstrable (but mild) effect after *in vivo* treatment of RA and OA patients [55]. In addition Aza-propazone, a weak NSAID by standard criteria, had a substantial effect on O_2^- production [56]. Hurst et al. reported that successful second-line therapy with either gold or D-penicillamine resulted in improved monocyte O_2^- generation, along with a rise in serum thiol levels [57]; the result correlated with clinical response rather than with the drug used. Finally, methotrexate and gold showed a trend towards normalization of ROS response in groups of RA patients so treated [58].

Pharmacology of superoxide dismutase mimetic (SODm)

The discovery of the enzymatic action of SOD in 1969 by McCord and Fridovich [59] was widely heralded. Unnoticed in the same year was an abstract about a putative new antiinflammatory protein; the data were so preliminary that the protein (orgotein) was stated not to be an enzyme [60]. One of the major problems in SOD pharmacology has been the short half-life of injected material. The use of polyethylene glycol (PEG)-conjugation to lengthen the half-life of scavenging enzymes has attracted substantial attention. A new approach to extending the half-life of SOD and catalase was reported by Schalkwijk et al. [61]. The proteins were made cationic, i.e. with isoelectric points greater than 8.5, by coupling the amino group of N,N-dimethyl-1,3-propanediamine to free carboxyl groups in the protein, a process referred to as "amidation" by the authors. The amidated proteins retained their catalytic activity, had the same molecular weight as the parent protein, had cationic isoelectric points (IEPs), and when injected into mouse joints, were cleared much more slowly than native molecules. Amidated catalase and horseradish peroxidase had measurable antiinflannnatory effects in a murine arthritis model, whereas amidated SOD was inactive. The cationic proteins were presumed to stick tightly to the multiple fixed anions of cartilage and other joint tissues. Although such an approach might have benefits for local treatment of joint disorders, its applicability to other organs without fixed anionic charges in situ is not readily apparent.

A third new approach to SOD half-life prolongation was reported by Halliwell et al. [60] using state-of-the-art techniques of molecular biology. Based on an analogy between the three-dimensional structures of the native SOD dimer and the folding of immunoglobulin molecules, these authors genetically engineered a series of SOD polymers in a bacterial expression system. One system consisted of two SOD single chains joined end-to-end, and the other was constructed of two SOD monomers linked by an IgA hinge sequence. Obviously, this approach offers the most exciting (as well as the most elegant) potential for development of oxygen scavenger protein preparations for human use.

Two other aspects of SOD pharmacological development are also of interest. First, it has been commented before about the disparity in both half-life and pharmacological effect between CuZn SOD and manganese SOD [61]. Fortunately, the safety data for SOD continues to be quite favorable. The agent has been administered safely to human neonates with no evidence of local allergic hypersensitivity, systemic allergy, or toxicity towards hematologic, hepatic, or renal systems. In a trial of intraarticular bovine CuZn SOD treatment for OA (see below), McIlwain et al. [62] reported that the only drug-related side-effects were minor episodes of skin irritation/itching at the injection site; the authors recommended that in all future trials with this agent, pretreatment skin testing be performed to screen out potentially allergic patients. No major toxicities have been reported elsewhere.

SOD applied in animal models continues to engender both enthusiasm and pessimism. Intraarticular SOD given to rabbits proved to be of no benefit in an immobilization model, [63] and in staphylococcal arthritis, SOD treatment worsened the situation [64], a testimonial perhaps to the time-honored role of oxygen radicals as antimicrobials.

SOD, as a general rule, is of little efficacy in adjuvant disease of rats, although some favorable long-term data for the chronic phase of the disease appeared recently [65]. The McIlwain study is the first protocol for human OA to have been multicenter, blinded, and randomized [63]. Seventy-four patients (out of 139 enrolled) completed a 14-week trial without NSAIDs. The patients received, in the first 3 weeks, injections into the affected knee of SOD and/or placebo in various combinations. As has been observed previously, there were few clinical differences during the first month of the study, but in later time periods, long after the injections had ceased, clinical efficacy (dropout rates, visual analog pain scores, etc.) became apparent. Because SOD is not analgesic, and because inflammation (and especially free radical generation) probably plays only a minor role in the pain of OA, these results are difficult to interpret.

Furthermore, to overcome the limitations associated with native enzyme therapy as therapeutic agents (e.g., solution instability, immunogenicity of non-human enzymes, bell-shaped dose-response curves, high susceptibility to proteolytic digestion) and as pharmacological tools (e.g., they do not penetrate cells or cross the blood-brain barrier, limiting the dismutation of superoxide only to the extracellular space or compartments), Salvemini et al.. have recently developed a series of superoxide dismutase mimetics (SODm) that catalytically remove O_2^-. M40403 is a prototypic example of a stable, low molecular weight, manganese-containing, non-peptidic molecules possessing the function and catalytic rate of native SOD enzymes, but with the advantage of being a much smaller molecule (MW 483 vs. MW 30 000 for the mimetic and native enzyme, respectively) [67]. An important and unique property of these SODm is that they selectively remove superoxide at a high rate without interacting with other reactive species, including nitric oxide, hydrogen peroxide, oxygen or hydroxyl radicals [68]. Also, SODm are not deactivated by $ONOO^-$ or hydrogen peroxide (Riley, unpublished results), an added advantage over the native Mn SOD enzyme that is nitrated and deactivated by $ONOO^-$ [69].

Recently, M40403 has been tested in an animal model of arthritis (Cuzzocrea et al., unpublished results) and showed beneficial and protective effects. Future studies are needed in order to understand if this new class of SODm can be used as pharmacological tools in arthritis.

References

1   Nathan C (1992) Nitric oxide as a secretory product of mammalian cells. *FASEB J* 30: 51–64

2   Salvemini D, Masferrer JL (1996) Interactions of nitric oxide with cyclooxygenase: *in vitro, ex vivo,* and *in vivo* studies. *Methods Enzymol* 269: 1225

3   Palmer RMJ, Bridge L, Foxwell NA, Moncada (1992) The role of nitric oxide in endothelial cell damage and its inhibition by glucocorticoids. *Br J Pharmacol* 105: 11–12

4   Farrell AJ, Blake DR, Palmer RM, Moncada S (1992) Increased concentrations of nitrite in synovial fluid and serum samples suggest increased nitric oxide synthesis in rheumatic diseases. *Ann Rheum Dis* 51: 1219–1222

5   Cuzzocrea S, Mazzon E, Bevilaqua C, Costantino G, Britti D, Mazzullo G, De Sarro A, Caputi AP (2000) Cloricromene, a coumarine derived, protects against collagen-induced arthritis in Lewis rats. *Br J Pharmacol* 131: 1399–1407

6   Ialenti A, Moncada S, DI Rosa M (1993) Modulation of adjuvant arthritis by endogenous nitric oxide *Br J Pharmacol* 110: 701–706

7   McCartney-Francis N, Allen JB, Mizel DE, Albina JE, Xie QW, Nathan CF, Wahl SM (1993) Suppression of arthritis by an inhibitor of nitric oxide synthase. *J Exp Med* 178: 749–754

8   Pelletier JP, Jovanovic DV, Lascau-Coman V, Fernandes JC, Manning PT, Connor JR, Currie MG, Martel-Pelletier J (2000) Selective inhibition of inducible nitric oxide synthase reduces progression of experimental osteoarthritis *in vivo*: possible link with the reduction in chondrocyte apoptosis and caspase 3 level. *Arthritis Rheum* 43: 1290–1299

9   Southan GJ, Zingarelli B, O'Connor M, Salzman AL, Szabò C (1996) Spontaneous rearrangement of aminoalkylguanidines into mercaptoalkylguanidines – a novel class of nitric oxide synthase inhibitors with selectivity towards the inducible isoform. *Br J Pharmacol* 117: 619–632

10 Szabò C, Ferrer-Sueta G, Zingarelli B, Southan GJ, Salzman AL, Radi R (1997) Mercaptoethylguanidine and related guanidine nitric oxide synthase inhibitors react with peroxynitrite and protect against peroxynitrite-induced oxidative damage. *J Biol Chem* 272: 9030–9036

11 Brahn E, Banquerigo ML, Firestein GS, Boyle DL, Salzman AL, Szabo C (1998) Collagen induced arthritis: reversal by mercaptoethylguanidine, a novel antiinflammatory agent with a combined mechanism of action. *J Rheumatol* 25: 1785–1793

12 Hierholzer C, Harbrecht B, Menezes JM, Kane J, MacMicking J, Nathan CF, Peitzman

AB, Billiar TR, Tweardy DJ (1998) Essential role of induced nitric oxide in the initiation of the inflammatory response after hemorrhagic shock. *J Exp Med* 187: 917–928

13 McInnes IB, Leung B, Wei XQ, Gemmell CC, Liew FY (1998) Septic arthritis following *Staphylococcus aureus* infection in mice lacking inducible nitric oxide synthase. *J Immunol* 160: 308–315

14 Brenner T, Brocke S, Szafer F, Sobel RA, Parkinson JF, Perez DH, Steinman L (1997) Inhibition of nitric oxide synthase for treatment of experimental autoimmune encephalomyelitis. *J Immunol* 158: 2940–2946

15 Pelletier JP, Jovanovic D, Fernandes JC, Manning P, Connor JR, Currie MG, Di Battista JA, Martel-Pelletier J (1998) Reduced progression of experimental osteoarthritis *in vivo* by selective inhibition of inducible nitric oxide synthase. *Arthritis Rheum* 41: 1275–1286

16 Brahn E, Banquerigo ML, Firestein GS, Boyle DL, Salzman AL, Szabo C (1998) Collagen-induced arthritis: reversal by mercaptoethylguanidine, a novel anti-inflammatory agent with a combined mechanism of action. *J Rheumat* 25: 1785–1793

17 Diefenbach A, Schindler H, Donhauser N, Lorenz E, Laskay T, MacMicking J, Rollinghoff M, Gresser I, Bogdan C (1998) Type 1 interferon (IFNalpha/beta) and type 2 nitric oxide synthase regulate the innate immune response to a protozoan parasite. *Immunity* 8: 77–87

18 Ajuebor MN, Viràg L, Flower RJ, Perretti M, Szabò C (1998) Role of inducible nitric oxide synthase in the regulation of neutrophil migration in symosan-induced inflammation: relationship to IL-10 and chemokine production. *Immunology* 95: 625–630

19 Beckman IS, Koppenol WH (1996) Nitric oxide, superoxide, and peroxynitrite: the good, the bad, and ugly. *Am J Physiol* 271: CI424–CI437

20 Angele MK, Smail N, Wang P, Cioffi WG, Bland KI, Chaudry IH (1998) L-arginine restores the depressed cardiac output and regional perfusion after trauma-hemorrhage. *Surgery* 124: 394–401

21 Xia Y, Dawson VL, Dawson TM, Snyder SH, Zweier JL (1996) Nitric oxide synthase generates superoxide and nitric oxide in arginine-depleted cells leading to peroxynitrite-mediated cellular injury. *Proc Natl Acad Sci USA* 93: 6770–6774

22 Nohl H (1994) Generation of superoxide radicals as byproduct of cellular respiration. *Ann Biol Clin* 52: 199–204

23 Lefer DJ, Scalia R, Campbell B, Nossuli T, Hayward R, Salamon M, Grayson J, Lefer, AM (1997) Peroxynitrite inhibits leukocyte-endothelial interactions and protects against ischemia-reperfusion injury in rats. *J Clin Invest* 99: 684–691

24 Moro MA, Darley-Usmar VM, Lizasoain I, Su Y, Knowles RG, Radomski MW, Moncada S (1995) The formation of nitric oxide donors from peroxynitrite. *Br J Pharmacol* 116: 1999–2004

25 Mayer B, Schrammel A, Klatt P, Koesling D, Schmidt K (1995) Peroxynitrite-induced accumulation of cyclic GMP in endothelial cells and stimulation of purified soluble guanylyl cyclase: Dependence on glutathione and possible role of S-nitrosation. *J Biol Chem* 270: 17355–17360

26   Cuzzocrea S, McDonald MC, Mota-Filipe H, Mazzon E, Costantino G, Britti D, Mazzullo G, Caputi AP, Thiemermann C (2000) Beneficial effects of tempol, a membrane-permeable radical scavenger, in a rodent model of collagen-induced arthritis. *Arthritis Rheum* 43: 320–328

27   Salvemini D, Wang ZQ, Stern MK, Currie MG, Misko TP (1998) Peroxynitrite decomposition catalysts: therapeutics for peroxynitrite-mediated pathology. *Proc Natl Acad Sci USA* 95: 2659–2663

28   Virag L, Salzman AL, Szabò C (1998) Poly (ADP-ribose) synthetase activation mediates mitochondrial injury during oxidant-induced cell death. *J Immunol* 161: 3753–3759

29   Szabò C, Cuzzocrea S, Zingarelli B, O'Connor M, Salzman AL (1997) Endothelial dysfunction in endotoxic shock: importance of the activation of poly (ADP ribose) synthetase (PARS) by peroxynitrite. *J Clin Invest* 100: 723–735

30   Miesel R, Kurpisz M, Kroger H (1995) Modulation of inflammatory arthritis by inhibition of poly(ADP ribose) polymerase. *Inflammation* 19: 379–87

31   Szabò C, Dawson VL (1998) Role of poly (ADP-ribose) synthetase in inflammation and ischaemia-reperfusion. *Trends Pharmacol Sci* 19: 287–298

32   Szabo C, Virag L, Cuzzocrea S, Scott GS, Hake P, O'Connor MP, Zingarelli B, Salzman A, Kun E (1998) Protection against peroxynitrite-induced fibroblast injury and arthritis development by inhibition of poly(ADP-ribose) synthase. *Proc Natl Acad Sci USA* 95: 3867–3872

33   McCord JM (1974) Free radicals and inflammation: Protection of synovial fluid by superoxide dismutase. *Science* 185: 529–531

34   Blake DR, Hall ND, Treby DA et al (1981) Protection against superoxide and hydrogen peroxide in synovial fluid from rheumatoid patients. *Clin Sci* 61: 483–486

35   Igari T, Kaneda H, Horiuchi S et al (1982) A remarkable increase of superoxide dismutase activity in synovial fluid of patients with rheumatoid arthritis. *Clin Orthopaedics* 162: 282–287

36   Marklund SL, Bjelle A, Elmqvist LG (1986) Superoxide dismutase isoenzymes of the synovial fluid in rheumatoid arthritis and in reactive arthritides. *Ann Rheum Dis* 45: 847–851

37   Gutteridge JMC, Hill C, Blake DR (1984) Copper stimulated phospholipid membrane peroxidation: Antioxidant activity of serum and synovial fluid from patients with rheumatoid arthritis. *Clin Chim Acta* 139: 85–90

38   Scudder P, Stocks J, Dormandy TL (1976) The relationship between erythrocyte superoxide dismutase activity and erythrocyte copper levels in normal subjects and in patients with rheumatoid arthritis. *Clin Chim Acta* 69: 397–403

39   Imadaya A, Terasawa K, Tosa H et al (1988) Erythrocyte antioxidant enzymes are reduced in patients with rheumatoid arthritis. *J Rheumatol* 15: 1628–1631

40   Youssef AAR, Baron DN (1983) Leucocyte superoxide dismutase in rheumatoid arthritis. Ann Rheum Dis 42: 558–562

41   Rister M, Bauermeister K (1982) Superox-Dismutase und Superox-Radikal-Freisetzung bei juveniler rheumatoider Arthritis. *Klin Wochenschr* 60: 561–565

42 Pasquier C, Mach PS, Raichvarg D et al (1984) Manganese containing superoxide dismutase deficiency in polymorphonuclear leukocytes of adults with rheumatoid arthritis. *Inflammation* 8: 27–32

43 Greenwald RA (1981) Effects of oxygen derived free radicals on connective tissue macromolecules: inhibition by copper penicillamine complex. *J Rheumatol* 8: 9–13

44 Marklund SI, Ek B, Steen L (1984) Effect of long-term penicillamine therapy on erythrocyte CuZn superoxide dismutase activity. *Scand J Lab Invest* 44: 13–17

45 Goldstein IM, Roos D, Weissmann G et al (1976) Influence of corticosteroids on human polyrnorphonuclear leukocyte function *in vitro. Inflammation* 1: 301–315

46 Fuenfer MM, Carr EA, Polk HC (1979) The effect of hydrocortisone on superoxide production by leukocytes. *J Surg Res* 27: 29–35

47 Bell AL, Hurst NP, Nuki G (1986) Effect of corticosteroid therapy on blood monocyte superoxide generation in rheumatoid arthritis: studies *in vitro* and *ex vivo. Br J Rheumatol* 25: 366–371

48 Davis P, Johnston C, Miller CL et al (1983) Effects of gold compounds on the function of phagocytic cells. *Arthritis Rheum* 26: 82–86

49 Roisman FR, Walz DT, Finkelstein AE (1983) Superoxide radical production by human leukocytes; exposed to immune complexes: inhibitory action of gold compounds. *Inflammation* 7: 355–362

50 Walz DT, Dimartino MJ, Griswold DE et al (1983) Biologic actions and pharmacokinetic studies of auranofin. *Am J Med* 75: 90–108

51 Corey EJ, Mehrotra MM, Khan AU (1987) Antiarthritic gold compounds effectively quench electronically excited singlet oxygen. *Science* 236: 68–69

52 Bertouch JV, Johnston C, Davis P (1987) Reversal of depressed neutrophil superoxide production in Felty's syndrome after gold therapy. *J Rheumatol* 14: 52–54

53 Abramson S, Edelson H, Kaplan H et al (1984) The inactivation of the polymorphonuclear leukocyte by nonsteroidal anti-inflammatory drugs. *Inflammation* 8: S103–S107

54 Biemond P, Swaak AJG, Penders JMA et al (1986) Superoxide production by polymorphonuclear leukocytes in rheumatoid arthritis and osteoarthritis: *in vivo* inhibition by the anti-rheumatic drug piroxicam due to interference with the activation of the NADPH-oxidase. *Ann Rheum Dis* 45: 249–255

55 Mackin WM, Rakich SM, Marshall CL (1986) Inhibition of rat neutrophil functional responses by azapropazone, an anti-gout drug. *Biochem Pharmacol* 35: 917–922

56 Hurst NP, Bell AL, Nuki G (1986) Studies of the effect of d-penicillamine and sodium aurothiomalate therapy on superoxide anion production by monocytes from patients with rheumatoid arthritis: evidence for *in vivo* stimulation of monocytes. *Ann Rheum Dis* 45: 37–43

57 Al Balla S, Johnston C, Davis P (1990) The *in vivo* effect of nonsteroidal antiinflammatory drugs, gold sodium thiomalate and methotrexate on neutrophil superoxide radical generation. *Clin Exp Rheum* 8: 41–45

58 McCord JM, Fridovich I (1969) Superoxide dismutase: an enzymic function for erythrocuprein (hemocuprein). *J Biol Chem* 244: 6049–6055

59 Huber W, Schulte TL, Carson S et al (1968) Some chemical and pharmacologic properties of a novel antiinflammatory protein. *Toxicol Appl Pharmacol* 12: 308

60 Schwalwijk J, van den Berg WB, van de Putte L et al (1985) Cationization of catalase, peroxidase, and superoxide dismutase. *J Clin Invest* 76: 198–205

61 Hallewell RA, Laria I, Tabrizi A et al (1989) Genetically engineered polymers of human CuZn superoxide dismutase. *J Biol Chem* 264: 5260–5268

62 Greenwald RA (1985) Therapeutic benefits of oxygen radical scavenger treatments remain unproven. *J Free Radicals Biol Med* 1: 173–177

63 McIlwain H, Silverfield JC, Cheatum DE et al (1989) Intra-articular orgotein in osteoarthritis of the knee: a placebo controlled efficacy, safety, and dosage comparison. *Am J Med* 87: 295–300

64 Neumuller J, Gialamas J, Hoger H et al (1986) Einflus von Superoxid-Dismutase (SOD) auf ein Arthrosemodell beim Kaninchen. *Zeit Rheumatol* 45: 312–318

65 Linhart WE, Zadravac S, Esterbauer H et al (1989) Staphilococcal arthritis – Effects of superoxide dismutase on infected knee joints of rabbits. *Free Radicals Res Commun* 7: 325–333

66 Vaille A, Jadot G, Elizagaray A (1990) Antiinflammatory activity of various superoxide dismutases; on polyarthritis in the Lewis rat. *Biochem Pharmacol* 39: 247–255

67 Salvemini D, Wang ZQ, Zweier JL, Samouilov A, Macarthur H, Misko TP, Currie MG, Cuzzocrea S, Riley D (1999) Synzymes: potent non-peptidic agents against superoxide-driven tissue injury. *Science* 286: 304–306

68 Riley DP, Henke SL, Lennon PJ, Weiss RH, Neumann WL, Rivers WJ, Aston KW, Sample KR, Ling CS, Shieh JJ, Busch DH, Szulbinski W (1996) Synthesis, characterization and stability of manganese (II) C-substituted 1,4,7,10,13-Pentaazacyclopentadecane complexes exhibiting superoxide dismutase activity. *Inorg Chem* 35: 5213–5231

69 Yamakura F, Taka H, Fujimura T, Murayama K (1998) Inactivation of human manganese-superoxide dismutase by peroxynitrite is caused by exclusive nitration of tyrosine 34 to 3-nitrotyrosine. *J Biol Chem* 273: 14085–14089

Role of nitric oxide in chronic gut inflammation

Matthew B. Grisham[1], Shigeyuki Kawachi[1], F. Stephen Laroux[1], Laura Gray[1], Jason Hoffman[1] and Henri van der Heyde[2]

[1]Department of Molecular and Cellular Physiology and [2]Department of Microbiology and Immunology, Louisiana State University Health Sciences Center, 1501 Kings Highway, P.O. Box 33932, Shreveport, LA 71130-3932, USA

Introduction

The inflammatory bowel diseases (IBD; Crohn's disease, ulcerative colitis) are chronic, idiopathic inflammatory disorders of the intestine and/or colon character- ized by rectal bleeding, severe diarrhea, abdominal pain, fever and weight loss. His- tologic examination of biopsies obtained from patients with active episodes of IBD reveal the infiltration of large numbers of leukocytes such as polymorphonuclear leukocytes (PMNs), monocytes, and lymphocytes into the intestinal interstitium. Extensive mucosal and/or transmural injury and dysfunction including edema, loss of goblet cells, decreased mucous production, crypt cell hyperplasia, erosions and ulcerations, accompany this inflammatory infiltrate. Despite several years of intense investigation, the etiology and specific pathogenetic mechanisms responsible for IBD remain poorly defined. Recent experimental and clinical studies suggest that the initiation and pathogenesis of these diseases are multi-factorial involving interac- tions among genetic, environmental and immune factors [1]. Regardless of exactly how these interactions ultimately promote chronic gut inflammation, it is becoming increasingly apparent that the immune system plays a crucial role in disease patho- genesis. Because the inflammation is localized primarily to the intestinal tract in IBD, investigators have focused on the intestinal lumen as the site for the antigenic trigger. Indeed, the chronic relapsing nature of IBD coupled to the fact that a large percentage of patients with Crohn's disease will experience recurrence of the disease following surgical resection of the bowel, suggests that the antigen or antigens that initiate and perpetuate this disease are part of the normal gut flora. Different etio- logic theories have been proposed to account for this apparent mucosal immune sys- tem activation, however, data obtained from numerous experimental studies suggest that chronic gut inflammation may result from a dysregulated immune response to components of the normal gut flora [2]. For example, several groups of investiga- tors have shown that targeted deletion of certain genes known to be important in regulating the inflammatory response or immune manipulation in mice induces chronic colitis in these animals [3]. Furthermore, the colonic inflammation observed

Nitric Oxide and Inflammation, edited by Daniela Salvemini, Timothy R. Billiar and Yoram Vodovotz
© 2001 Birkhäuser Verlag Basel/Switzerland

in virtually all of these animal models is dependent upon the presence of normal gut flora. Animals raised under germ-free conditions either fail to develop disease or develop much milder forms of colitis [3]. These studies have lead investigators to suggest that bacterial/immune interactions in individuals with defects in their immune system may represent an important pathophysiological mechanism for the development of IBD in humans.

Co-incident with the extensive inflammation and tissue injury is the enhanced expression of the inducible isoform of nitric oxide synthase (iNOS; NOS 2) and the sustained overproduction of the free radical nitric oxide (NO) [4–21]. Because NO is known to modulate the inflammatory response, there is increasing interest in defining the role that NO may play in the pathophysiology of IBD. This review will discuss some of the basic concepts related to the initiation and regulation of chronic gut inflammation and summarize the current state-of-knowledge on the role that NO may play in modulating the inflammatory response.

Immune activation and gut inflammation

The intestinal mucosal interstitium is continuously exposed to large amounts of exogenous (i.e. dietary) and endogenous (e.g. bacteria) antigens. Fortunately, the mucosal immune system has evolved efficient mechanisms to distinguish between potentially pathogenic bacterial, parasitic, viral and dietary antigens from non-pathologic antigens and resident gut flora. In addition to being able to respond to specific antigens, the mucosal immune system is able to choose the appropriate effector functions to deal with each pathogen. Specific subsets of CD4$^+$ T lymphocytes play a major role in mediating and regulating these effector functions *in vivo* and are called T helper (Th) cells. Activated Th1 cells secrete interleukin-2 (IL-2), interferon γ (IFNγ) and lymphoxin-α (LT), whereas Th2 cells produce IL-4, IL-5, IL-6, IL-9, IL-10 and IL-13. A number of different studies have shown that Th1 cells are primarily involved in cell mediated immunity (CMI) which is mounted against certain infectious agents such as intracellular bacteria, fungi and protozoa. This protective immune response involves not only activation of Th1 cells and the subsequent release of their cytokines, but also Th1 cytokine-mediated activation of intestinal macrophages and other phagocytic leukocytes to release additional pro-inflammatory cytokines such as tumor necrosis factor α (TNFα), IL-1β, IL-6, IL-8, IL-12, IL-18. Dysregulation of this normally protective response has been hypothesized to be importantly involved in the pathogenesis of IBD [1, 2]. Cell-mediated immunity is the major protective mechanism by which the intestinal mucosa defends against invading pathogenic organisms (Fig. 1).

Activation of the intestinal immune system involves the co-ordinated and highly specific interactions among a variety of different cell types. The first step in the immune response to antigen is the uptake, processing and presentation of antigen

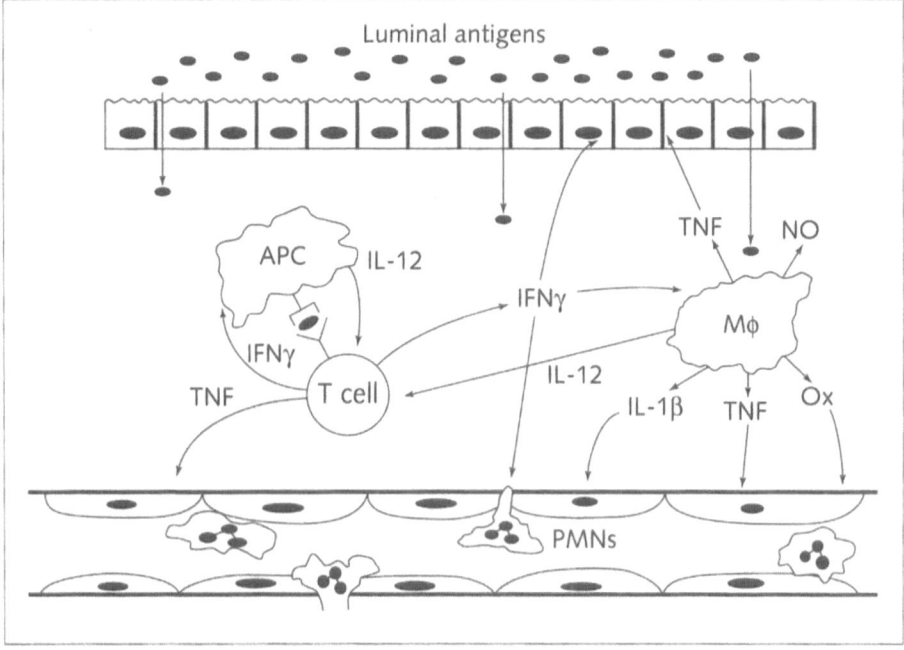

Figure 1
Cell-mediated immunity (CMI) in the intestine and colon. Antigen presenting cells (APCs) process and present luminal antigens that continuously gain access to the mucosal interstitium. T cell/APC interactions activate T cells to produce IL-2 and IFNγ which activate tissue macrophages to release a variety of pro-inflammatory cytokines and mediators including TNFα, IL-1β, IL-12, nitric oxide (NO) and reactive oxygen species (Ox). IL-12 feeds back onto the effector T cells to induce Th1 differentiation. Th1- and macrophage-derived cytokines and mediators activate microvascular endothelium to enhance expression of adhesion molecules thereby promoting the recruitment of phagocytic leukocytes such as PMNs. The net result is the destruction of invading pathogens. Uncontrolled CMI may result in tissue injury.

by antigen presenting cells (APCs) such as dendritic cells, macrophages and possibly endothelial cells. Antigen recognition by a Th precursor subset of CD4+ T lymphocytes involves the specific interaction between the T-cell receptor (TCR) and the antigen presented on the surface of the APC by its major histocompatability complex class II (MHC II) (Fig. 1). This antigen specific interaction activates the lymphocytes to synthesize and release IFNγ and IL-2. IL-2 promotes the clonal expansion of T cells and enhances the function of helper T cells and B cells, whereas IFNγ interacts with and activates APCs and macrophages to produce IL-12. IL-12 feeds back onto the T cells to enhance further production of IFNγ and promotes the differentiation of these T cells to Th1 cells producing even larger amounts of IFNγ and IL-2. IFNγ can also activate endothelial cells and enhance endothelial cell adhesion molecule (ECAM) expression on the post-capillary venular endothelium. In addition, IFNγ-activated macrophages produce large amounts of pro-inflammatory cytokines such as TNFα, IL-1β, IL-6, IL-8 and IL-12 as well as reactive oxygen and nitrogen metabolites (e.g. superoxide, hydrogen peroxide, nitric oxide). All of these mediators are thought to be important in recruiting and activating phagocytic leukocytes such as PMNs and monocytes/macrophages for the efficient destruction of the invading pathogens. Because many of these Th1 and macrophage-derived cytokines may possess potent pro-inflammatory activity *in vivo*, failure to down-regulate production of these mediators may lead to severe inflammatory tissue injury. Indeed, active IBD is associated with the local overproduction of many of these pro-inflammatory cytokines [1].

The potential for immune system activation to lead to local and even systemic injury suggests that healthy individuals possess cellular mechanisms to limit the immune response and in some cases completely suppress it. It is thought that this is accomplished by the action of additional subsets of CD4+ T cells called regulatory T cells (Tr1) and Th3 cells. Tr1 and Th3 cells are thought to suppress or limit intestinal CMI by the synthesis and release of large amounts of the cytokines IL-10 and transforming growth factor β (TGFβ). Both of these cytokines are known to down-regulate Th1- and macrophage-derived cytokine synthesis [2] (Fig. 2). Recent evidence suggests that both Tr1 and Th3 cells possess T cell receptors (TCRs) that are specific for the same antigens as are the TCRs of the Th1 effector T cells they regulate. These observations suggest that the presence of these regulatory cells within the intestinal and/or colonic interstitium will effectively regulate the immune response to luminal antigens thereby limiting inflammatory tissue injury and dysfunction (Fig. 2).

Not surprisingly, animals rendered deficient in IL-10 or TGFβ or lack the appropriate regulatory cell responses develop chronic gut inflammation. Numerous studies have identified three major groups of immune-based rodent models of IBD [3]. The first group consists of mice with alterations in T-cell subsets and T-cell selection including the TCRα or TCRβ deficient mice, MHC class II-deficient mice, SCID mice reconstituted with CD4+, CD45RB^high T cells, human CD3ε transgenic mice reconstituted with T cell depleted F1 bone marrow cells and HLA-B27 transgenic rats. A second group of mice that develop spontaneous and chronic colitis includes animals with targeted gene deletion of IL-2, IL-10 and TGFβ. Finally, genetically engineered mice deficient in certain signaling proteins such as $G_{\alpha i2}$ develop spontaneous and chronic colitis. It has been suggested that most, if not all, of the genetically-engineered or immune manipulated mouse models of IBD develop chronic colitis as a result of a lack of appropriate downregulation of normal cell mediated immunity to luminal antigens.

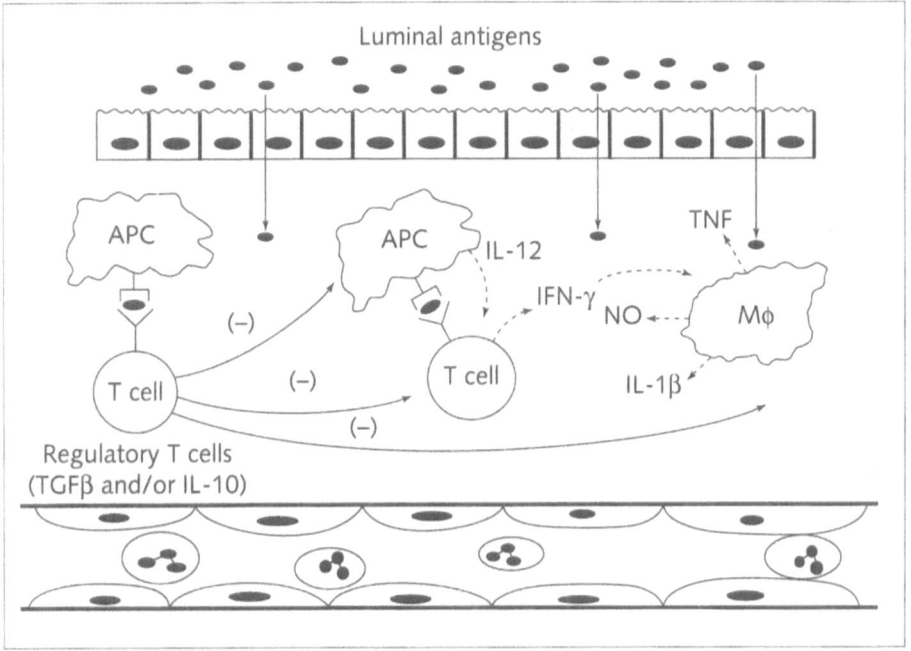

Figure 2
Regulation of intestinal immune response to luminal antigens. Interaction of regulatory CD4+ T cells (Tr1 and/or Th3 subsets) with APCs activates these leukocytes to release IL-10 and TGFβ. These cytokines inhibit Th1 activation as well as Th1-dependent activation of tissue macrophages. These regulatory cytokines also inhibit the activation of the venular endothelium within the mucosa thereby downregulating the intestinal inflammatory response.

The importance of certain cytokines such as TNFα as mediators of chronic gut inflammation is apparent in a number of recent clinical studies where investigators have demonstrated that administration of antibodies specific for TNFα attenuates Crohn's disease (reviewed in [22]). As mentioned previously, many of the Th1 and macrophage-derived cytokines are potent inducers of a number of different genes thought to play important roles in the inflammatory response. One such gene is iNOS. The role that iNOS-derived NO plays in modulating gut inflammation is currently under active investigation. Although a number of recent studies demonstrate that NO may play a important role in mediating some of the pathophysiology associated with chronic gut inflammation, there is an equally impressive number of publications suggesting that NO may either play no role, or may be a protective mediator that limits the extent and severity of intestinal and/or colonic inflammation. An understanding of some of the basic concepts involved in regulation of the inflammatory response may prove useful in ultimately defining the role of NO in the pathophysiology of IBD.

Regulation of chronic gut inflammation

It is well appreciated that Th1 and macrophage-derived cytokines such as TNFα, TNFβ (lymphotoxin-α), IFNγ or IL-1β, either alone or in combination induce inflammation *in vivo*. The mechanisms by which this diverse group of pro-inflammatory agents promotes cytokine synthesis, leukocyte adhesion and iNOS expression *in vivo* is not clear, however, recent *in vitro* data suggest that cytokine-receptor interaction may activate the nuclear transcription factor-kappa B (NF-κB). NF-κB is a ubiquitous transcription factor and pleiotropic regulator of numerous inflammatory and immune responses [23]. Once activated, NF-κB translocates to the nucleus of the cell where it binds to its consensus sequence on the promoter-enhancer region of different genes, thereby activating the transcription of genes known to be important in the immune and inflammatory responses (Fig. 3). For example, NF-κB appears to regulate the transcription of several different cytokines (IL-1β, IL-2, IL-6, IL-8, IL-12, TNFα), certain ECAMs such as intercellular adhesion molecule-1 (ICAM-1), vascular cell adhesion molecule-1 (VCAM-1), E-selectin and mucosal addressin cell adhesion molecule-1 (MAdCAM-1) as well as iNOS (NOS 2) and the inducible isoform of cyclo-oxygenase (COX 2). NF-κB belongs to the Rel family of transcription factors where members share a region of about 300 amino acids known as the Rel homology domain. The heterodimeric NF-κB is composed of p50 and p65 subunits and is normally sequestered in the cytoplasm associated with its inhibitor IκB. A large number of different bacterial and viral products, cytokines and lipid mediators activate NF-κB. It is unlikely that each of these stimuli activates the cytoplasmic NF-κB-IκB complex *via* completely different pathways. Indeed, there is a growing body of experimental data to suggest that many, if not all, of these stimuli activate multiple signaling pathways, which converge to enhance reactive oxygen metabolism within the cell [24, 25]. This has been shown for the NF-κB activators TNF, IL-1, lipopolysaccharide, phorbol esters, UV light, γ radiation, anti-IgM, okadaic acid and anti-CD28. Further supporting this concept is the recognition that certain lipophilic, membrane-permeable oxidants, such as H_2O_2 and oxidant producing xenobiotics (e.g. menendione) active NF-κB as well. The identity of the specific intracellular source(s) for this enhanced oxidative metabolism has (have) not been identified, however prostaglandin synthase, xanthine oxidase, mitochondria, NADPH oxidase and cytochrome P-450 are likely candidates. Sources of exogenous oxidants *in vivo* that could activate NF-κB include activated phagocytic leukocytes (e.g. PMNs, monocytes, macrophages, eosinophils). Furthermore, NF-κB activation has been shown to be inhibited, *in vitro*, by a wide variety of structural-

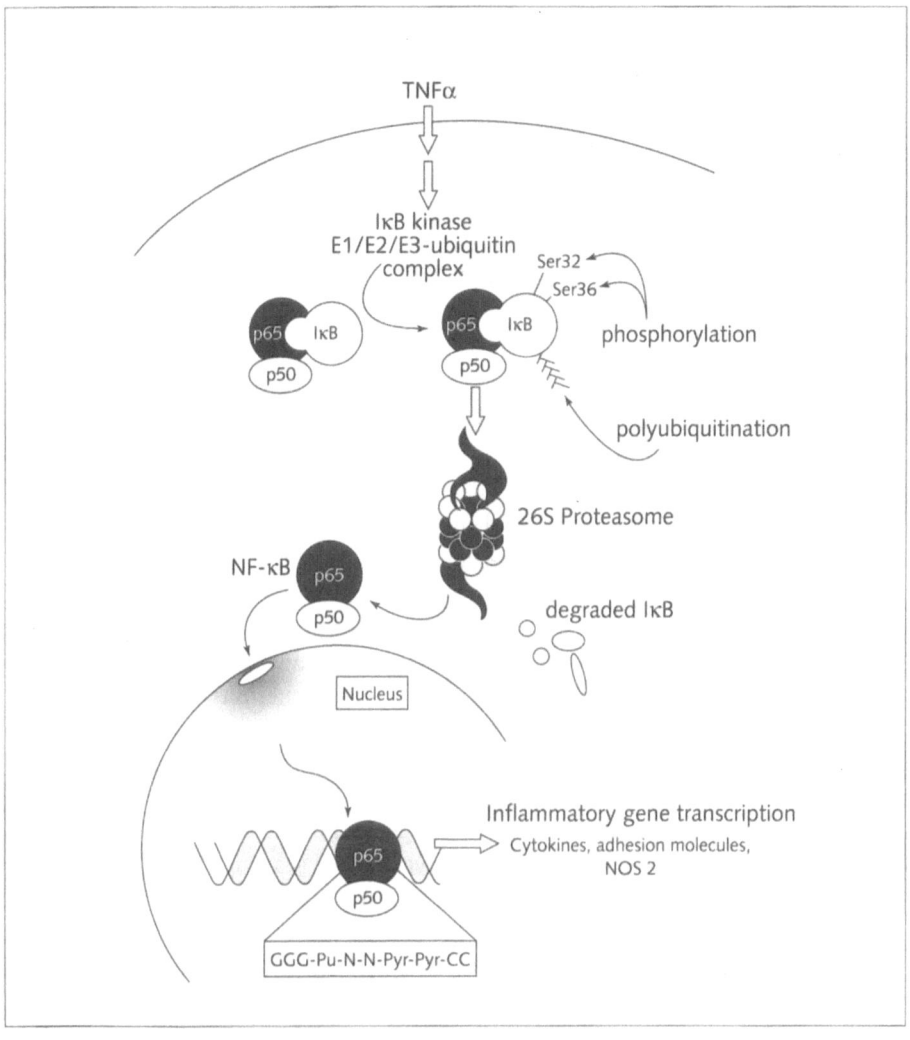

Figure 3
TNFα induced activation of nuclear transcription factor kappa B (NF-κB). Cytokine-receptor interaction initiates multiple signaling pathways that converge to enhance intracellular reactive oxygen metabolism. These oxidants directly or indirectly activate one or more IκB kinases and ubiquitinating enzymes resulting in the phosphorylation and polyubiquitination of IκB. The 26S proteasome complex selectively degrades the post-translationally modified IκB thereby liberating the transcriptionally active p50/p65 heterodimer. This transcription factor is transported into the nucleus where it binds to its consensus sequence in the promoter/ enhancer region upstream of different genes where it activates the transcription of a variety of genes known to be important in the inflammatory response such as endothelial cell adhesion molecules (ECAMs) and cytokines as well as iNOS and COX2.

ly diverse enzymatic or non-enzymatic antioxidants or free radical scavengers such as SOD, catalase, GSH peroxidase, N-acetylcysteine, vitamin E derivatives, α-lipoic acid and certain dithiocarbamates. Indeed, it is intriguing to speculate that the observed protective effects of antioxidants in various models of GI inflammation (e.g. peptic ulcer disease, ischemia/reperfusion, transplantation) may be due more to inhibition of NF-κB activation than inhibition of oxidant-induced toxicity.

The mechanisms by which oxidants activate NF-κB have not been defined. This intracellular oxidative stress is thought to then activate *via* several intermediate reactions, one or more redox-sensitive kinases which specifically phosphorylate IκB. Once phosphorylated, IκB is selectively ubiquinated and then degraded *via* the non-lysosomal, ATP-dependent 26S proteolytic complex. Thus, the 26S proteasome represents an important step in the activation of NF-κB. Inhibition of the proteasome pathway using selective, yet structurally distinct inhibitors, blocks cytokine induction of ICAM-1, E-selectin and VCAM-1 with resultant alterations in adhesion of PMNs and lymphocytes to endothelial monolayers. Findings from our laboratory indicate that inhibition of NF-κB using a selective proteasome inhibitor attenuates colonic VCAM-1 expression and the chronic granulomatous colitis induced in female Lewis rats *via* a single subserosal injection of peptidoglycan/polysaccharide (PG/PS) [26]. In addition, Neurath and coworkers have demonstrated that antisense oligonucleotides specific for the p65 subunit of NF-κB is effective at inhibiting the colonic inflammation observed in two different models of colitis [27]. Taken together, these data suggest that NF-κB activation and its subsequent transcriptional activation of a multitude of inflammatory genes is crucial for the development of chronic gut inflammation. These data also suggest that the anti-adhesive and anti-inflammatory properties of antioxidants, free radical scavengers and proteasome inhibitors may be due to their abilities to inhibit the activation of NF-κB.

Role of nitric oxide as a modulator of chronic colitis

One of the most consistent findings in both experimental and human IBD is the upregulation of iNOS and overproduction of NO [4–20, 26, 28–54]. Nitric oxide is a particularly interesting mediator in that it possesses both anti-inflammatory as well as pro-inflammatory properties. For example, NO has been shown to possess potent anti-inflammatory activity due to its ability to attenuate adhesion and recruitment of leukocytes in postcapillary venules exposed to different acute inflammatory stimuli such as ischemia and reperfusion (I/R), oxidized low density lipoproteins (oxLDL), or reactive oxygen metabolites [55]. One explanation that has been offered to explain the anti-adhesion properties of NO relates to the ability of this molecule to rapidly interact with and decompose superoxide (O_2^-). Since O_2^- reacts with NO three times faster than with superoxide dismutase, it has been proposed that NO may act as a physiological scavenger of O_2^-. This possibility is supported by studies demonstrating that NO donors are only effective in inhibiting leukocyte-endothelial cell adhesion in models of inflammation wherein SOD is also anti-adhesive

A second mechanism by which NO may attenuate leukocyte adhesion during the acute inflammatory response, involves modulation of ECAM expression. It has been reported that NO inhibits the activation of NF-κB *in vitro* in cultured cells [56, 57]. Furthermore, it has been shown that exogenous NO donors induce the expression and/or stabilization of IκB thereby maintaining NF-κB in its inactive ternary complex [58–63]. Recent work from our laboratory suggests that iNOS-derived NO may play a role in regulating ECAM expression *in vivo* in acute but not chronic gut inflammation [36]. We found that intraperitoneal injection of 10 μg/kg TNFα enhanced VCAM-1 expression by approximately two-fold in the colon and cecum of iNOS-deficient (iNOS$^{-/-}$) mice compared to TNF-injected wild type mice. Injection of wild type mice with 25 μg/kg TNF enhanced further VCAM-1 expression by approximately two-fold compared to wild type mice injected with 10 μg/kg TNF, however, VCAM-1 expression was not enhanced further in any gastrointestinal organ system in iNOS$^{-/-}$ mice. In a second series of experiments, we found that continuous inhibition of iNOS using oral administration of L-NIL did not alter the enhanced levels of VCAM-1 expression in the colon, nor did it alter the severity of colonic inflammation in SCID mice reconstituted with CD4$^+$, CD45RB^{high} T cells. We conclude that iNOS may regulate VCAM-1 expression in acute inflammation, however, this effect is modest and tissue specific and occurs only when VCAM-1 expression is submaximal. Inducible NOS does not appear to modulate VCAM-1 expression in an immune model of chronic colitis.

The role of iNOS-derived NO in IBD remains the subject of considerable controversy and active debate. Several studies have demonstrated, using a variety of different NOS inhibitors that NO may promote, attenuate or have little effect on gut inflammation and injury. The reasons for these conflicting results are not at all clear, however, inhibitor selectivity, timing of administration (prophylactic vs. therapeutic) and/or type of intestinal inflammation (acute vs. chronic) have been suggested as possible reasons. For example, it has been shown that prophylactic administration of non-selective NOS inhibitors such as N^G-nitro-L-arginine methyl ester (L-NAME) or N^G-monomethyl-L-arginine (L-NMMA) attenuates the colonic injury and inflammation observed in chemical-induced, self-limiting models of colitis such as the trinitrobenzene sulfonic acid/ethanol or acetic acid models [35, 39, 45]. These data are difficult to interpret because L-NAME or L-NMMA are known to inhibit the constitutive endothelial NOS (eNOS) as well as iNOS. This is an important consideration because inhibition of eNOS is known to promote vasoconstriction with the concomitant reduction in blood flow. Since the delivery of leukocytes and inflammatory mediators is blood flow-dependent, a reduction in blood flow could account for some or all of the anti-inflammatory effects of L-NAME. In addition, NO has been suggested to promote angiogenesis thereby contributing to the neovascularization and hyperemia known to be associated with colitis [64–66]. Inhibition of new vessel growth would attenuate the hyperemic effect and reduce blood flow to the involved colon thereby limiting delivery of leukocytes and inflammatory mediators to the injured tissue.

Aminoguanidine (AG), on the other hand, is reported to be 30–40 times more selective for iNOS than eNOS, however, it does have additional pharmacologic activities such as acting as a histaminase inhibitor. We have recently demonstrated that prophylactic or therapeutic administration of AG attenuates gut inflammation in two different models of immune-based chronic colitis [30, 33]. The mechanisms by which the sustained overproduction of iNOS-derived NO promotes chronic gut inflammation, or more precisely the mechanisms by which NOS inhibitors attenuate experimental colitis have not been clearly delineated. There are several possibilities. First, NO has been implicated as a mediator for the enhanced microvascular permeability induced by IL-2 [67, 68]. Increases in vascular permeability could account for the edema and tissue dysfunction observed during acute flares of IBD. Another potentially important mechanism by which iNOS-derived NO may promote IBD is *via* its ability to modulate COX-2 dependent production of prostaglandins [67]. Other mechanisms include NO-dependent promotion of chemotaxis of certain leukocytes, production of proinflammatory mediators such as IL-8 or TNF and lymphocyte activation [69]. Furthermore, NO may rapidly interact with certain reactive oxygen species such as O_2^- to yield the potent oxidant $ONOO^-$ [70]. Because of the large influx of phagocytic leukocytes such as PMNs, monocytes and macrophages, it has been suggested that iNOS-derived NO could promote chronic gut inflammation by reacting with leukocyte-derived O_2^- to form $ONOO^-$ which in turn upregulate cytokine and/or ECAM expression and injure the tissue. The question of whether $ONOO^-$ is actually formed *in vivo* remains the subject of vigorous debate. Indeed, there is little direct evidence that implicates $ONOO^-$ in the pathophysiology of any inflammatory disorder [70–75]. In fact, the only evidence suggesting that $ONOO^-$ may be formed in chronically inflamed tissue has been the detection of 3-nitrotyrosine, the nitrated derivative thought to be produced by the interaction between $ONOO^-$ and tyrosine [76]. Recent reports demonstrating that leukocyte-associated peroxidases such as myeloperoxidase catalyze the H_2O_2-dependent nitration of tyrosine to form 3-nitrotyrosine in a $ONOO^-$ independent reaction casts considerable doubt on validity of the use of 3-nitrotyrosine as a specific "footprint" for $ONOO^-$ formation *in vivo* [77–79]. In fact, these data question whether $ONOO^-$ is produced at all in inflamed tissue.

The recent development of the highly selective iNOS inhibitors such as L-N[6]-(iminoethyl)-lysine (L-NIL) without additional pharmacological activities as well as mice renderred deficient in iNOS has allowed investigators to more accurately explore the role of iNOS in different models of colonic inflammation. The results of these studies have however cast considerable doubt on the role of iNOS-derived NO as an important mediator in gut inflammation. Miller and coworkers have demonstrated that adminstration of either L-NIL or AG to monkeys with established distal bowel inflammation is ineffective in attenuating colitis [47]. We have demonstrated that continuous oral administration of L-NIL to SCID reconstituted with CD45RB[high] T cells for 4 weeks fails to retard the development or attenuate the severity of the colitis produced in these animals [36]. Finally, McCafferty et al. have reported that chemically induced colonic injury and inflammation was not attenuated in mice deficient in iNOS [80]. Indeed, restitution and repair in these mutant mice was significantly delayed compared to their wild type controls suggesting an important role for iNOS-derived NO in epithelial cell proliferation.

Summary

The recent development of genetically engineered and immune-manipulated mice that develop spontaneous and chronic colitis has made it possible to investigate the various molecular, cellular and immunological mechanisms responsible for the inflammation and tissue injury observed in these models of IBD. One of the most consistant and dramatic findings in both experimental and human IBD is enhanced expression of iNOS and the overproduction of NO. The role that iNOS-derived NO plays in the pathophysiology of IBD remains to be elucidated. Although earlier work using nonimmune, erosive models of colonic inflammation and nonselective inhibitors of NOS suggested that NO may act as a pro-inflammatory mediator, more recent studies using immune-based models in both rodents and nonhuman primates suggest that iNOS may not play an important role in intiating and/or perpetuating distal bowel inflammation. In fact, the upregulation of iNOS may actually represent a protective response designed to promote epithelial cell restitution and repair in the injured gut. Obviously, more work is needed in this area to finally answer, one way or the other, the question of whether iNOS-derived NO is involved in the pathogenesis of IBD.

Acknowledgements
Some of the work reported in this chapter was supported by grants from the NIH (DK47663), The Crohns and Colitis Foundation of America, the Feist Foundation and the Arthritis Center of Excellence.

References

1   Fiocchi C (1998) Inflammatory bowel disease: etiology and pathogenesis. *Gastroenterology* 115: 182–205
2   Powrie F (1995) T cells in inflammatory bowel disease: protective and pathogenic roles. *Immunity* 3: 171–174

3   Elson CO, Sartor RB, Tennyson GS, Riddell RH (1995) Experimental models of inflammatory bowel disease. *Gastroenterology* 109: 1344–1367

4   Boughton-Smith NK, Evans SM, Hawkey CJ, Cole AT, Balsitis M, Whittle BJ, Moncada S (1993) Nitric oxide synthase activity in ulcerative colitis and Crohn's disease. *Lancet* 342: 338–340

5   Godkin AJ, De Belder AJ, Villa L, Wong A, Beesley JE, Kane SP, Martin JF (1996) Expression of nitric oxide synthase in ulcerative colitis. *Eur J Clin Invest* 26: 867–872

6   Ikeda I, Kasajima T, Ishiyama S, Shimojo T, Takeo Y, Nishikawa T, Kameoka S, Hiroe M, Mitsunaga A (1997) Distribution of inducible nitric oxide synthase in ulcerative colitis. *Am J Gastroenterol* 92: 1339–1341

7   Iwashita E, Miyahara T, Hino K, Tokunaga T, Wakisaka H, Sawazaki Y (1995) High nitric oxide synthase activity in endothelial cells in ulcerative colitis. *J Gastroenterol* 30: 551–554

8   Iwashita E, Iwai A, Sawazaki Y, Matsuda K, Miyahara T, Itoh K (1998) Activation of microvascular endothelial cells in active ulcerative colitis and detection of inducible nitric oxide synthase. *J Clin Gastroenterol* 27 Suppl 1: S74–S79

9   Iwashita E (1998) Greatly increased mucosal nitric oxide in ulcerative colitis determined *in situ* by a novel nitric oxide-selective microelectrode. *J Gastroenterol Hepatol* 13: 391–395

10 Kimura H, Miura S, Shigematsu T, Ohkubo N, Tsuzuki Y, Kurose I, Higuchi H, Akiba Y, Hokari R, Hirokawa M, Serizawa H, Ishii H (1997) Increased nitric oxide production and inducible nitric oxide synthase activity in colonic mucosa of patients with active ulcerative colitis and Crohn's disease. *Dig Dis Sci* 42: 1047–1054

11 Kimura H, Hokari R, Miura S, Shigematsu T, Hirokawa M, Akiba Y, Kurose I, Higuchi H, Fujimori H, Tsuzuki Y, Serizawa H, Ishii H (1998) Increased expression of an inducible isoform of nitric oxide synthase and the formation of peroxynitrite in colonic mucosa of patients with active ulcerative colitis. *Gut* 42: 180–187

12 Lundberg JO, Herulf M, Olesen M, Bohr J, Tysk C, Wiklund NP, Morcos E, Hellstrom PM, Weitzberg E, Jarnerot G (1997) Increased nitric oxide production in collagenous and lymphocytic colitis. *Eur J Clin Invest* 27: 869–871

13 Middleton SJ, Shorthouse M, Hunter JO (1993) Increased nitric oxide synthesis in ulcerative colitis. *Lancet* 341: 465–466

14 Rachmilewitz D, Stamler JS, Bachwich D, Karmeli F, Ackerman Z, Podolsky DK (1995) Enhanced colonic nitric oxide generation and nitric oxide synthase activity in ulcerative colitis and Crohn's disease. *Gut* 36: 718–723

15 Reynolds PD, Middleton SJ, Hansford GM, Hunter JO (1997) Confirmation of nitric oxide synthesis in active ulcerative colitis by infra-red diode laser spectroscopy. *Eur J Gastroenterol Hepatol* 9: 463–466

16 McLaughlan JM, Seth R, Vautier G, Robins RA, Scott BB, Hawkey CJ, Jenkins D (1997) Interleukin-8 and inducible nitric oxide synthase mRNA levels in inflammatory bowel disease at first presentation. *J Pathol* 181: 87–92

17 Zhang XJ, Thompson JH, Mannick EE, Correa P, Miller MJ (1998) Localization of

inducible nitric oxide synthase mRNA in inflamed gastrointestinal mucosa by *in situ* reverse transcriptase-polymerase chain reaction. *Nitric Oxide* 2: 187–192

18 Whittle BJ (1997) Nitric oxide – a mediator of inflammation or mucosal defence [see comments] Eur. *J Gastroenterol* Hepatol 9: 1026–1032

19 Tomita R, Tanjoh K (1998) Role of nitric oxide in the colon of patients with ulcerative colitis. *World J Surg* 22: 88–91

20 Singer II, Kawka DW, Scott S, Weidner JR, Mumford RA, Riehl TE, Stenson WF (1996) Expression of inducible nitric oxide synthase and nitrotyrosine in colonic epithelium in inflammatory bowel disease. *Gastroenterology* 111: 871–885

21 Rachmilewitz D, Eliakim R, Ackerman Z, Karmeli F (1998) Direct determination of colonic nitric oxide level – a sensitive marker of disease activity in ulcerative colitis. *Am J Gastroenterol* 93: 409–412

22 Sandborn WJ, Hanauer SB (1999) Antitumor necrosis factor therapy for inflammatory bowel disease: a review of agents, pharmacology, clinical results, and safety. *Inflamm Bowel Dis* 5: 119–133

23 Baeuerle PA, Baltimore D (1996) NF-kappa B: ten years after. *Cell* 87: 13–20

24 Flohe L, Brigelius-Flohe R, Saliou C, Traber MG, Packer L (1997) Redox regulation of NF-kappa B activation. *Free Radic Biol Med* 22: 1115–1126

25 Schreck R, Rieber P, Baeuerle PA (1991) Reactive oxygen intermediates as apparently widely used messengers in the activation of the NF-kappa B transcription factor and HIV-1. *EMBO J* 10: 2247–2258

26 Conner EM, Brand S, Davis JM, Laroux FS, Palombella VJ, Fuseler JW, Kang DY, Wolf RE, Grisham MB (1997) Proteasome inhibition attenuates nitric oxide synthase expression, VCAM-1 transcription and the development of chronic colitis. *J Pharmacol Exp Ther* 282: 1615–1622

27 Neurath MF, Pettersson S, Meyer zum Buschenfelde KH, Strober W (1996) Local administration of antisense phosphorothioate oligonucleotides to the p65 subunit of NF-kappa B abrogates established experimental colitis in mice. *Nat Med* 2: 998–1004

28 Zingarelli B, Szabo C, Salzman AL (1999) Reduced oxidative and nitrosative damage in murine experimental colitis in the absence of inducible nitric oxide synthase. *Gut* 45: 199–209

29 Aiko S, Grisham MB (1995) Spontaneous intestinal inflammation and nitric oxide metabolism in HLA-B27 transgenic rats. *Gastroenterology* 109: 142–150

30 Aiko S, Fuseler J, Grisham MB (1998) Effects of nitric oxide synthase inhibition or sulfasalazine on the spontaneous colitis observed in HLA-B27 transgenic rats. *J Pharmacol Exp Ther* 284: 722–727

31 Asfaha S, Bell CJ, Wallace JL, MacNaughton WK (1999) Prolonged colonic epithelial hyporesponsiveness after colitis: role of inducible nitric oxide synthase. *Am J Physiol* 276: G703–G710

32 Ferretti M, Gionchetti P, Rizzello F, Venturi A, Stella P, Corti F, Mizrahi J, Miglioli M, Campieri M (1997) Intracolonic release of nitric oxide during trinitrobenzene sulfonic acid rat colitis. *Dig Dis Sci* 42: 2606–2611

33   Grisham MB, Specian RD, Zimmerman TE (1994) Effects of nitric oxide synthase inhibition on the pathophysiology observed in a model of chronic granulomatous colitis. *J Pharmacol Exp Ther* 271: 1114–1121

34   Harren M, Schonfelder G, Paul M, Horak I, Riecken EO, Wiedenmann B, John M (1998) High expression of inducible nitric oxide synthase correlates with intestinal inflammation of interleukin-2-deficient mice. *Ann NY Acad Sci* 859: 210–215

35   Hogaboam CM, Jacobson K, Collins SM, Blennerhassett MG (1995) The selective beneficial effects of nitric oxide inhibition in experimental colitis. *Am J Physiol* 268: G673–G684

36   Kawachi S, Cockrell A, Laroux FS, Gray L, Granger DN, van der Heyde HC, Grisham MB (1999) Role of inducible nitric oxide synthase in the regulation of VCAM-1 expression in gut inflammation. *Am J Physiol* 277: G572–G576

37   MacNaughton WK, Lowe SS, Cushing K (1998) Role of nitric oxide in inflammation-induced suppression of secretion in a mouse model of acute colitis. *Am J Physiol* 275: G1353–G1360

38   Miampamba M, Sharkey KA (1999) Temporal distribution of neuronal and inducible nitric oxide synthase and nitrotyrosine during colitis in rats. *Neurogastroenterol Motil* 11: 193–206

39   Miller MJ, Sadowska-Krowicka H, Chotinaruemol S, Kakkis JL, Clark DA (1993) Amelioration of chronic ileitis by nitric oxide synthase inhibition. *J Pharmacol Exp Ther* 264: 11–16

40   Miller MJ, Thompson JH, Zhang XJ, Sadowska-Krowicka H, Kakkis JL, Munshi UK, Sandoval M, Rossi JL, Eloby-Childress S, Beckman JS (1995) Role of inducible nitric oxide synthase expression and peroxynitrite formation in guinea pig ileitis. *Gastroenterology* 109: 1475–1483

41   Miller MJ, Sandoval M (1999) Nitric Oxide III A molecular prelude to intestinal inflammation. *Am J Physiol* 276: G795–G799

42   Neilly PJ, Gardiner KR, Rowlands BJ (1996) Experimental colitis is ameliorated by inhibition of nitric oxide synthase activity. *Gut* 38: 475

43   Obermeier F, Kojouharoff G, Hans W, Scholmerich J, Gross V, Falk W (1999) Interferon-gamma (IFN-gamma)- and tumour necrosis factor (TNF)-induced nitric oxide as toxic effector molecule in chronic dextran sulphate sodium (DSS)-induced colitis in mice. *Clin Exp Immunol* 116: 238–245

44   Pfeiffer CJ, Qiu BS (1995) Effects of chronic nitric oxide synthase inhibition on TNB-induced colitis in rats. *J Pharm Pharmacol* 47: 827–832

45   Rachmilewitz D, Karmeli F, Okon E, Bursztyn M (1995) Experimental colitis is ameliorated by inhibition of nitric oxide synthase activity. *Gut* 37: 247–255

46   Ribbons KA, Zhang XJ, Thompson JH, Greenberg SS, Moore WM, Kornmeier CM, Currie MG, Lerche N, Blanchard J, Clark DA (1995) Potential role of nitric oxide in a model of chronic colitis in rhesus macaques. *Gastroenterology* 108: 705–711

47   Ribbons KA, Currie MG, Connor JR, Manning PT, Allen PC, Didier P, Ratterree MS,

Clark DA, Miller MJ (1997) The effect of inhibitors of inducible nitric oxide synthase on chronic colitis in the rhesus monkey. *J Pharmacol Exp Ther* 280: 1008–1015

48 Seago ND, Clark DA, Miller MJ (1995) Role of inducible nitric oxide synthase (iNOS) and peroxynitrite in gut inflammation. *Inflamm Res* 44 (Suppl 2): S153–S154

49 Seo HG, Takata I, Nakamura M, Tatsumi H, Suzuki K, Fujii J, Taniguchi N (1995) Induction of nitric oxide synthase and concomitant suppression of superoxide dismutases in experimental colitis in rats. *Arch Biochem Biophys* 324: 41–47

50 Southey A, Tanaka S, Murakami T, Miyoshi H, Ishizuka T, Sugiura M, Kawashima K, Sugita T (1997) Pathophysiological role of nitric oxide in rat experimental colitis. *Int J Immunopharmacol* 19: 669–676

51 Yamada T, Sartor RB, Marshall S, Specian RD, Grisham MB (1993) Mucosal injury and inflammation in a model of chronic granulomatous colitis in rats. *Gastroenterology* 104: 759–771

52 Miller MJ, Thompson JH, Liu X, Eloby-Childress S, Sadowska-Krowicka H, Zhang XJ, Clark DA (1996) Failure of L-NAME to cause inhibition of nitric oxide synthesis: role of inducible nitric oxide synthase. *Inflamm Res* 45: 272–276

53 Miller MJ, Chotinaruemol S, Sadowska-Krowicka H, Kakkis JL, Munshi UK, Zhang XJ, Clark DA (1993) Nitric oxide: the Jekyll and Hyde of gut inflammation. *Agents Actions* 39 (Spec No): C180–C182

54 Mourelle M, Vilaseca J, Guarner F, Salas A, Malagelada JR (1996) Toxic dilatation of colon in a rat model of colitis is linked to an inducible form of nitric oxide synthase. *Am J Physiol* 270: G425–G430

55 Grisham MB, Granger DN, Lefer DJ (1998) Modulation of leukocyte-endothelial interactions by reactive metabolites of oxygen and nitrogen: relevance to ischemic heart disease. *Free Radic Biol Med* 25: 404–433

56 De Caterina R, Libby P, Peng HB, Thannickal VJ, Rajavashisth TB, Gimbrone MA Jr, Shin WS, Liao JK (1995) Nitric oxide decreases cytokine-induced endothelial activation Nitric oxide selectively reduces endothelial expression of adhesion molecules and proinflammatory cytokines. *J Clin Invest* 96: 60–68

57 Khan BV, Harrison DG, Olbrych MT, Alexander RW, Medford RM (1996) Nitric oxide regulates vascular cell adhesion molecule 1 gene expression and redox-sensitive transcriptional events in human vascular endothelial cells. *Proc Natl Acad Sci USA* 93: 9114–9119

58 Peng HB, Rajavashisth TB, Libby P, Liao JK (1995) Nitric oxide inhibits macrophage-colony stimulating factor gene transcription in vascular endothelial cells. *J Biol Chem* 270: 17050–17055

59 Peng HB, Libby P, Liao JK (1995) Induction and stabilization of I kappa B alpha by nitric oxide mediates inhibition of NF-kappa B. *J Biol Chem* 270: 14214–14219

60 Peng HB, Spiecker M, Liao JK (1998) Inducible nitric oxide: an autoregulatory feedback inhibitor of vascular inflammation. *J Immunol* 161: 1970–1976

61 Spiecker M, Peng HB, Liao JK (1997) Inhibition of endothelial vascular cell adhesion

molecule-1 expression by nitric oxide involves the induction and nuclear translocation of IkappaBalpha. *J Biol Chem* 272: 30969–30974

62   Spiecker M, Darius H, Kaboth K, Hubner F, Liao JK (1998) Differential regulation of endothelial cell adhesion molecule expression by nitric oxide donors and antioxidants. *J Leukoc Biol* 63: 732–739

63   Spiecker M, Liao JK (1999) Assessing induction of I kappa B by nitric oxide. *Methods Enzymol* 300: 374–388

64   Montrucchio G, Lupia E, de Martino A, Battaglia E, Arese M, Tizzani A, Bussolino F, Camussi G (1997) Nitric oxide mediates angiogenesis induced *in vivo* by platelet-activating factor and tumor necrosis factor-alpha. *Am J Pathol* 151: 557–563

65   Papapetropoulos A, Garcia-Cardena G, Madri JA, Sessa WC (1997) Nitric oxide production contributes to the angiogenic properties of vascular endothelial growth factor in human endothelial cells. *J Clin Invest* 100: 3131–3139

66   Papapetropoulos A, Desai KM, Rudic RD, Mayer B, Zhang R, Ruiz-Torres MP, Garcia-Cardena G, Madri JA, Sessa WC (1997) Nitric oxide synthase inhibitors attenuate transforming-growth-factor-beta 1-stimulated capillary organization *in vitro*. *Am J Pathol* 150: 1835–1844

67   Clancy RM, Amin AR, Abramson SB (1998) The role of nitric oxide in inflammation and immunity. *Arthritis Rheum* 41: 1141–1151

68   Stichtenoth DO, Frolich JC (1998) Nitric oxide and inflammatory joint diseases. *Br J Rheumatol* 37: 246–257

69   Lander HM (1997) An essential role for free radicals and derived species in signal transduction. *FASEB J* 11: 118–124

70   Grisham MB, Jourd'Heuil D, Wink DA (1999) Nitric oxide I Physiological chemistry of nitric oxide and its metabolites: implications in inflammation. *Am J Physiol* 276: G315–G321

71   Pfeiffer S, Mayer B (1998) Lack of tyrosine nitration by peroxynitrite generated at physiological pH. *J Biol Chem* 273: 27280–27285

72   Miles AM, Bohle DS, Glassbrenner PA, Hansert B, Wink DA, Grisham MB (1996) Modulation of superoxide-dependent oxidation and hydroxylation reactions by nitric oxide. *J Biol Chem* 271: 40–47

73   Miles AM, Gibson MF, Kirshina M, Cook JC, Pacelli R, Wink D, Grisham MB (1995) Effects of superoxide on nitric oxide-dependent N-nitrosation reactions. *Free Radic Res* 23: 379–390

74   Wink DA, Cook JA, Kim SY, Vodovotz Y, Pacelli R, Krishna MC, Russo A, Mitchell JB, Jourd'Heuil D, Miles AM, Grisham MB (1997) Superoxide modulates the oxidation and nitrosation of thiols by nitric oxide-derived reactive intermediates Chemical aspects involved in the balance between oxidative and nitrosative stress. *J Biol Chem* 272: 11147–11151

75   Jourd'Heuil D, Miranda KM, Kim SM, Espey MG, Vodovotz Y, Laroux S, Mai CT, Miles AM, Grisham MB, Wink DA (1999) The oxidative and nitrosative chemistry of

the nitric oxide/superoxide reaction in the presence of bicarbonate. *Arch Biochem Biophys* 365: 92–100

76   Beckman JS, Koppenol WH (1996) Nitric oxide, superoxide, and peroxynitrite: the good, the bad, ugly. *Am J Physiol* 271: C1424–C1437

77   Eiserich JP, Hristova M, Cross CE, Jones AD, Freeman BA, Halliwell B, van der Vliet A (1998) Formation of nitric oxide-derived inflammatory oxidants by myeloperoxidase in neutrophils. *Nature* 391: 393–397

78   Eiserich JP, Cross CE, Jones AD, Halliwell B, van d V (1996) Formation of nitrating and chlorinating species by reaction of nitrite with hypochlorous acid A novel mechanism for nitric oxide-mediated protein modification. *J Biol Chem* 271: 19199–19208

79   van d V, Eiserich JP, Halliwell B, Cross CE (1997) Formation of reactive nitrogen species during peroxidase-catalyzed oxidation of nitrite A potential additional mechanism of nitric oxide-dependent toxicity. *J Biol Chem* 272: 7617–7625

80   McCafferty DM, Mudgett JS, Swain MG, Kubes P (1997) Inducible nitric oxide synthase plays a critical role in resolving intestinal inflammation. *Gastroenterology* 112: 1022–1027

Nitric oxide and inflammatory disorders of the skin

Richard Weller[1] and Victoria Kolb-Bachofen[2]

[1]Department of Dermatology, University of Edinburgh, EH3 9YW, UK; [2]Immunobiology Research Group, Medical Faculty, Heinrich-Heine-Universität, P.O. Box 101007, 40001 Düsseldorf, Germany

Skin structure

The skin is the largest organ in the human body, and serves a variety of protective functions to shield the body from physical insults such as ultraviolet radiation, heat and cold. It is the first line of defence against foreign micro-organisms, with both innate defence features and adaptive immunity *via* presentation of antigens. Physical injuries must be repaired and remodelled, and growth has to occur in a co-ordinated manner.

The skin consists of two layers, an ectodermally derived epidermis, and a mesodermally derived dermis with underlying subcutaneous fat. The dermis contains fibroblasts and the structural proteins collagen and elastin together with the skin vasculature and nervous system, sweat glands, hair root papillae and muscles.

The commonest cells in the epidermis are keratinocytes. These arise from dividing stem cells at the basement membrane, and over a period of about 2 weeks move upwards, gradually becoming flattened and dehydrated and losing their nucleus, finally to be shed at the surface as cornified squames. Langerhans cells are the professional antigen presenting cells of the skin and *via* their dendritic processes form a spider-web-like network throughout the lower half of the epidermis, thus allowing for effective immune surveillance. After antigen encounter they migrate to the regional skin draining lymph nodes.

Melanocytes are neuroectodermally derived and located along the basal epidermis. They produce melanosomes, containing the photo-protective pigment melanin which is distributed to the surrounding keratinocytes.

Psoriasis

Psoriasis is a hyperproliferative skin disease characterised by a generally thickened epidermis with incompletely differentiated keratinocytes, dermal infiltration by neu-

Nitric Oxide and Inflammation, edited by Daniela Salvemini, Timothy R. Billiar and Yoram Vodovotz
© 2001 Birkhäuser Verlag Basel/Switzerland

trophils and activated T lymphocytes, and dermal angio-proliferation. The aetiology of psoriasis is incompletely understood, but an interaction between skin homing T lymphocytes and keratinocytes in a genetically susceptible individual is suspected. Elevated levels of the Th1 cytokines IL-2, IFNγ, IL-1β, TNFα and particularly IL-8 are found in lesional psoriatic skin, and it must thus be considered an inflammatory disease. It is therefore no wonder that inducible nitric oxide synthase (iNOS) is expressed in lesional psoriatic skin [1–3]. Expression of iNOS mRNA and protein is found either in basal keratinocytes at the tips of rete ridges, or in focal clusters in the suprabasal keratinocytes [1, 4], and in the dermal capillary endothelial cells [2, 5]. NO itself is measurable at the surface of the psoriatic plaque at up to 100 times the concentration of non-psoriatic skin [6].

In cultured human keratinocytes iNOS expression is induced within 24 h after cytokine challenge. Interestingly, with these cells, no single cytokine will lead to iNOS expression, in contrast to observations with other cells of epithelial origin such as hepatocytes. iNOS expression is induced only with combinations of either IL-1β and TNFα, or else IL-8 with IFNγ [1, 3]. In addition to the cytokine milieu, expression of iNOS in cultured keratinocytes appears also to be dependent on the stage of keratinocyte differentiation [7].

IL-8 receptor mRNA expression closely correlates both temporally and spatially with iNOS mRNA in psoriatic skin, suggesting a paracrine or autocrine pathway involved in leukocyte recruitment and keratinocyte activation [1]. Moreover, in a melanoma cell line, IL-8 production itself appears to be regulated by NO [8].

The role of NO in psoriasis is not yet fully understood. The concentration of serum nitrite and nitrate, stable oxidation products of NO, have been shown to correlate with the clinical severity of psoriasis [9], although measurements of NO at the surface of the psoriatic plaque show that it is the erythema of the psoriatic plaque and not the indurations or scaling which correlates with the NO production (R. Weller, unpublished data). Effective treatments of this disease, such as corticosteroids [6] and retinoids [10] inhibit iNOS expression, while other equally effective treatments like ultraviolet radiation [11] and anthralin increase iNOS expression. NO's effects on keratinocytes is concentration dependent. In primary keratinocyte cultures, NO has biphasic effects, encouraging proliferation at low concentrations, and differentiation at higher concentrations [12].

Langerhans cells, the professional antigen presenting cells of the skin, express iNOS when activated [13], and it has been suggested that dysregulated production of NO by Langerhans cells may play a role in triggering psoriasis [14]. However, in face of the overwhelming evidence that NO in psoriatic skin is produced predominantly by the much more numerous keratinocytes, and the lack of direct proof for iNOS expressing Langerhans cells in psoriatic skin [15, 16], most researchers argue against a dominant role for iNOS-expressing Langerhans cells as a trigger in this disease.

Type I hypersensitivity

Acute urticaria is an IgE dependent disease in which the CD23 receptor is clustered *via* binding of repetitive antigens to mast cells with resultant degranulation and histamine release. Although Th1 cytokines are the predominant inducers of iNOS in keratinocytes, an IgE dependent pathway has also been described. Ligation of the low affinity IgE receptor (CD23) expressed on IL-4 primed keratinocytes will induce iNOS, TNFα and IL-6 expression [17], a process which can be inhibited by IL-10 [18]. However, whether iNOS expression is a direct consequence of CD23 clustering or rather mediated indirectly *via* induction of Th1 cytokines is, so far, an open question. Biopsies from acutely affected skin indeed show co-localization of iNOS, the proinflammatory cytokines TNFα and IL-6, as well as CD23 within keratinocytes [19]. Nonetheless, the role of iNOS expression in disease manifestation remains to be elucidated.

Ultraviolet radiation

Ultraviolet radiation (UVR) has multiple effects on the skin. It induces a biphasic erythema, with an initial vasodilatation after a few minutes, and a delayed and more marked vasodilatation after 8 to 12 h. Langerhans cells are temporarily depleted, as they emigrate to the local draining lymph nodes after UV-challenge. Profound and complex effects on the skin immune system result from prolonged UV exposure. Initial inflammatory effects, such as induction of TNFα release by UVB [20] are followed by both local and systemic immunosuppression, which is characterized by a favouring of Th2- over Th1-type reaction in late responses with, for instance, IL-10 release from keratinocytes.

A hallmark of skin exposed to high doses of UV is the presence of apoptotic keratinocytes [21], referred to as "sunburn cells". At high doses, UV-irradiation induces DNA damage, and the ensuing immunosuppressive effect could potentially limit detection and removal of altered cells, which might in part explain UV induced skin carcinogenesis.

Ultraviolet irradiation of skin stimulates NO release by both constitutive and inducible isoforms of NOS. UVB irradiation of cultured human keratinocytes releases NO within a few minutes (lasting up to 20 min) in a calcium dependent, N^G-monomethyl-L-arginine (L-NMMA) inhibitable manner, and there is a concomitant rise in cyclic GMP [22]. Neuronal NOS (NOS I) has been identified as the isoform responsible [23].

In addition, investigations *in vivo* show that the delayed erythema after UVB is inhibited by L-NMMA [24], and skin biopsies taken 24 h after either UVA or UVB demonstrate iNOS mRNA and protein expression in basal keratinocytes and endothelial cells, which has resolved by 72 h [11].

In endothelial cells UVA will induce apoptosis dependent on the dose of irradiation. Apoptosis is completely inhibited by pre-exposure to exogenous NO from an NO donor, and equally well by endogenous NO synthesis in cells activated to express iNOS prior to UVA challenge. This protective effect correlates with an NO mediated upregulation of Bcl-2 [25]. Interestingly, chemically generated NO will also protect during or immediately after UVA irradiation in both endothelial cells and a keratinocyte cell line by a different mechanism (work in progress).

Skin pigmentation is the best known of all effects of UV on the skin. Melanocytes synthesize melanin which is transferred to surrounding keratinocytes. Conditioned media from irradiated keratinocytes stimulates the melanin producing tyrosinase pathway in melanocytes, and this process is inhibited by NO scavengers [26]. The process can be simulated by exogenous NO donors, and is associated with an increase in cGMP activity, blocking of which also prevents melanogenesis [27]. Thus epidermal pigmentation appears to involve an autocrine pathway in which NO is released from irradiated keratinocytes, diffuses to adjacent melanocytes and *via* the guanylate cyclase, cGMP pathway drives melanogenesis.

In addition to the normal response of healthy skin, a number of dermatoses are induced by UVR. Thus photosensitivity is one of the key characteristics of patients with both cutaneous and systemic lupus erythematosus (LE). Patients suffering from systemic lupus erythematosus (sLE) have been shown to have elevated serum nitrite levels, which correlate with disease activity, and iNOS protein expression was found mainly in vascular endothelial cells [28]. MRL-lpr/lpr mice develop an autoimmune syndrome closely resembling the human SLE, and animals were shown to overexpress iNOS. Treating these mice with iNOS inhibitors will improve their health [29]. However, when crossing the iNOS gene defect into the lpr/lpr background, the failure of iNOS expression will not abolish the SLE-like disease but reduce renal vasculitis [30].

In patients with cutaneous LE (cLE) a key diagnostic tool is the formation of skin lesions after provocation by UVA and/or UVB irradiation. In contrast to healthy volunteers, in cLE patient's skin the kinetics of iNOS appearance after UV exposure are strikingly different, with iNOS appearance being delayed for up to 3 days after irradiation and its expression lasting for the entire duration of the lesional process [31]. These data point to a decisive role for the proper timing of iNOS expression and also for a protective role for this enzyme's activity dependent on strictly regulated timing.

Connective tissue and wound healing

Wound healing and tissue remodelling are complex processes, requiring subtle interactions between different signalling molecules and substrates. The varying effects of NO on cell growth and differentiation and the implications in wound healing are slowly being unravelled. Early *in vitro* work performed by Heck and co-workers in

1992 suggested that inflammatory mediator-stimulated NO production, inhibited keratinocyte growth, and that this effect was antagonised by epidermal growth factor [32]. In keratinocytes, iNOS and GTP-cyclohydrolase I expression were later found to be tightly co-ordinated [33], and the data obtained strongly suggested a regulative role for iNOS-derived NO in gene expression. Indeed, our recently described biphasic effect of NO on keratinocyte growth when cells were maintained for several days at various NO concentrations, points in the same direction. Under these conditions, low concentrations of NO encouraged keratinocyte proliferation, while higher concentrations stimulated keratinocyte differentiation [12]. In contrast, in skin fibroblasts, NO, even at very low concentrations, caused cytostasis, which may reflect differentiation. When applied as a single boost, exogenous NO later results in increased fibroblast proliferation [34].

Cultured human skin fibroblasts were shown to express constitutive NOS, and after activation with IFNγ and LPS also express iNOS [35]. The constitutive NOS also appears to contribute to proper wound healing, as it was shown that fibroblasts from hypertrophic scars, taken from subjects with thermal burns, express lower amounts of constitutive NOS than fibroblasts from uninjured skin [36], but the ability to induce iNOS expression was found to be unchanged .

For effective wound healing the regulation of capillary endothelial cell growth and differentiation is also needed, and indeed, the expression of iNOS has recently been demonstrated in cultured human dermal endothelial cells (huDEC) as well [37]. It was also found that NO will regulate angiogenesis, as inhibition of endothelial NO synthesis favours DNA synthesis and polyamine formation as hallmarks of proangiogenic effects, whereas NO donors will shut down cell division and putrescine synthesis, thus likely allowing for differentiation [38].

Taken together, these complex data all point to a regulative role of iNOS-derived NO in cell growth and differentiation and in situ observations on wounds have all supported this view. Thus it was found that in iNOS deficient mice, wound healing is impaired as compared to wild type mice, and this is reversed by adenoviral iNOS transfection [39]. Evidence for an *in vivo* increase in collagen synthesis mediated by iNOS-synthesised NO comes from experimentally produced wounds in rats. Wounds were transfected with plasmids for iNOS or control genes, by insertion of plasmid bearing sponges. Rats transfected with the active gene produced more collagen than animals transfected with a control gene [40]. Furthermore, in systemic sclerosis, a connective tissue disease characterised by increased collagen synthesis and fibrosis, fibroblasts derived from lesional skin express iNOS [41]. Moreover, a careful immunohistochemical investigation of excised burn wounds at different stages of healing, corroborates the strict spatial and temporal organization of iNOS expression during the healing processes [42].

Since the healing of a wound is a complex process involving both initial accelerated growth and subsequent growth arrest and differentiation, it appears that co-ordinated induction of iNOS and other mediators as well as a timely stop in their

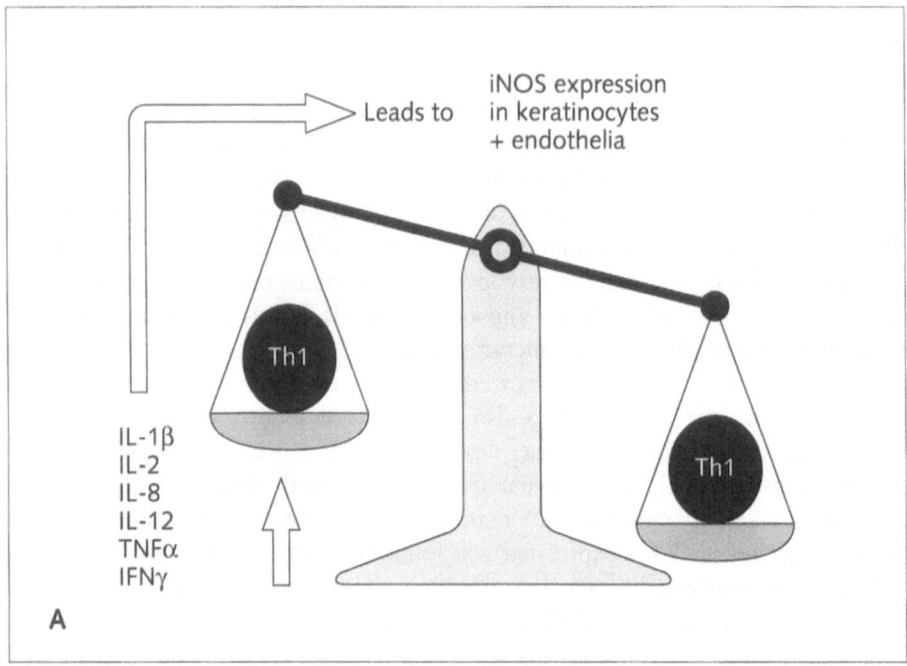

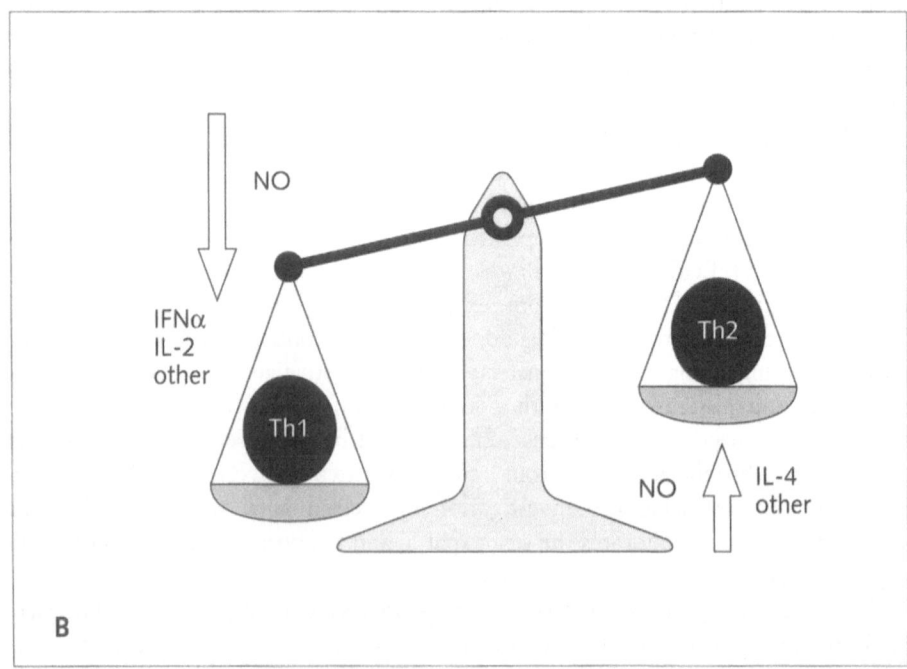

expression is critical in wound repair. Any perturbation of this tightly regulated process will lead to diminished or aberrant wound healing.

Melanoma and cancer

Human melanocytes express NOS III mRNA [43], and both normal and malignant melanocytes show a calcium dependent, non LPS-inducible, NO producing activity [44]. This was higher in malignant melanoma cells and was considered to encourage metastasis and tumour growth by maintaining vasodilator tone in vessels around the melanoma [44]. Murine melanoma cells can be induced to express iNOS with a combination of cytokines. Melanoma cells with the potential to express iNOS do not metastasise when injected into syngeneic mice, whereas metastasising melanocytes cannot be induced to express iNOS [45]. Transfection of a malignant melanoma cell line with an active iNOS gene reduced metastasis after injection into syngeneic mice compared with cells transfected with an inactive iNOS gene [46]. Transfected cells underwent apoptosis. It has also been observed that NO exposed melanocytes become less adherent to extracellular matrix components, and it was suggested that this too may represent a mechanism by which NO exposure reduces tumorigenicity [47].

Conclusion: Multiple protective functions of iNOS-derived NO by helping in skin responses

The expression of iNOS and the ensuing long-term NO synthesis was initially regarded solely as a means of innate immunity to defend against infections. Al-

---

Figure 1

Upper graph: The expression of iNOS in general is an early event during inflammatory responses. Thus, as far as know today, local iNOS expression may be taken as a marker for local inflammatory responses, as all of the inflammatory cytokines – especially when present in combinations will initiate the gene expression of iNOS.

Lower graph: However, once expressed, the enzyme will form NO at higher concentrations and for a prolonged period and this will then downregulate the local response in the mode of a classical feed back inhibition. This downregulation appears to be the consequence of two different actions exerted by NO. Firstly, NO was shown to inhibit the continued expression of IFNγ and block the de novo formation of IL-2. Secondly, NO simultaneously helps in increasing the production of IL-4 and other components thereby establishing a Th2 like reaction. As a probable consequence of this regulatory action, prolonged or extensive iNOS expression, as for instance after excessive sun exposure, might result in a relatively long period of inhibited Th1 like reaction, a situation often termed "immunosuppression".

though this still appears to be one of its tasks, with increasing knowledge of NO's effects on skin function this view now shifts towards a prime role in regulating cellular functions by altering the gene expression pattern in different cell types.

This notion is supported by the increasing data on iNOS expression and its role in wound healing as reviewed above. More importantly, a number of publications directly demonstrate gene products which are under expressional control of NO. It has been shown that VEGF production by keratinocytes is induced by NO [33]. We found that NO, either exogenously applied or endogenously produced, will induce additional bcl-2 expression, thereby modulating apoptotic responses in endothelial cells [25]. Moreover, studying the cytokine expression patterns during immunosuppression resulting from extensive burns has revealed that suppression of proinflammatory cytokine expression is NO-mediated, as iNOS inhibitors will return responses to normal levels [48]. This finding is in full accord with an increasing number of data, all pointing to an immunoregulative effect of NO, as has been reviewed recently [49].

In summary, iNOS expression being a result of proinflammatory, Th1-like reactions will serve to downregulate inflammation by favouring Th2-like responses (Fig. 1) and this may not only explain the immunosuppression following extensive burns, but also the later events after extensive UV-exposure.

How can NO directly influence cellular gene regulation? Several lines of evidence demonstrate that by reaction with transcription factors NO can either enhance or shut down genes depending on the respective DNA-binding proteins necessary for gene activity. Thus, we found that NO will react with zinc-sulphur clusters as they are found in the zinc finger family of transcription factors, leading to zinc release and concomitant loss of DNA-binding [50]. Others have shown that upon S-nitrosylation of cysteine groups at or near active centres, transcription factors will be activated [51] or inactivated [52]. Together with the well known effects of NO on various enzyme activities and its ability to also regulate protein synthesis a complex picture evolves, where NO will influence cellular reactions not only depending on its concentration, but also on the cell type involved as well as its differentiation state.

Learning of these effects in skin cells will not only help us in understanding, diagnosing and treating skin diseases, but will also contribute to our knowledge of normal skin physiology.

References

1   Bruch-Gerharz D, Fehsel K, Suschek C, Michel G, Ruzicka T, Kolb-Bachofen V (1996) A proinflammatory activity of interleukin 8 in human skin: expression of the inducible nitric oxide synthase in psoriatic lesions and cultured keratinocytes. *J Exp Med* 184: 2007–2012

2   Kolb-Bachofen V, Fehsel K, Michel G, Ruzicka T (1994) Epidermal keratinocyte expression of inducible nitric oxide synthase in skin lesions of psoriasis vulgaris. *Lancet* 344: 139

3   Sirsjo A, Karlsson M, Gidlof A, Rollman O, Torma H (1996) Increased expression of inducible nitric oxide synthase in psoriatic skin and cytokine-stimulated cultured keratinocytes. *Br J Dermatol* 134: 643–648

4   Ormerod AD, Weller R, Copeland P, Benjamin N, Ralston SH, Grabowksi P, Herriot R (1998) Detection of nitric oxide and nitric oxide synthases in psoriasis. *Arch Dermatol Res* 290: 3–8

5   Rowe A, Farrell A, Kazmi SH, Bunker CB (1994) Expression of inducible nitric oxide synthase in dermal microvasculature in psoriasis. *Lancet* 344: 1371

6   Weller R, Ormerod A (1997) Increased expression of inducible nitric oxide (NO) synthase. *Br J Dermatol* 136: 136–137

7   Arany I, Brysk MM, Brysk H, Tyring SK (1996) Regulation of inducible nitric oxide synthase mRNA levels by differentiation and cytokines in human keratinocytes. *Biochem Biophys Res Commun* 220: 618–622

8   Andrew PJ, Harant H, Lindley IJD (1995) Nitric oxide regulates IL-8 expression in melanoma cells at the transcriptional level. *Biochem Biophys Res Commun* 214: 949–956

9   Orem A, Aliyazicioglu R, Kiran E, Vanizor B, Cimnocodeit G, Deger O (1997) The relationship between nitric oxide production and activity of the disease in patients with psoriasis. *Arch Dermatol* 133: 1606–1607

10   Becherel PA, Le Goff L, Ktorza S, Chosidow O, Frances C, Issaly F, Mencia-Huerta JM, Debre P, Mossalayi MD, Arock M (1996) CD23-mediated nitric oxide synthase pathway induction in human keratinocytes is inhibited by retinoic acid derivatives. *J Invest Dermatol* 106: 1182–1186

11   Kuhn A, Fehsel K, Lehmann P, Krutmann J, Ruzicka T, Kolb-Bachofen V (1998) Expression of inducible nitric oxide synthase (iNOS) after UV-irradiation in human epidermis (abstract). *J Invest Dermatol* 110: 554

12   Krischel V, Bruch Gerharz D, Suschek C, Kroncke KD, Ruzicka T, Kolb Bachofen V (1998) Biphasic effect of exogenous nitric oxide on proliferation and differentiation in skin derived keratinocytes but not fibroblasts. *J Invest Dermatol* 111: 286–291

13   Qureshi AA, Hosoi J, Xu S, Takashima A, Granstein RD, Lerner EA (1996) Langerhans cells express inducible nitric oxide synthase and produce nitric oxide. *J Invest Dermatol* 107: 815–821

14   Morhenn VB (1997) Langerhans cells may trigger the psoriatic disease process *via* production of nitric oxide. *Immunol Today* 18: 433–436

15   Kolb-Bachofen V, Bruch-Gerharz D (1999) Langerhans cells, nitric oxide, keratinocytes and psoriasis. *Immunol Today* 20: 289

16   McKenzie RC, Weller R (1998) Langerhans cells, keratinocytes, nitric oxide and psoriasis. *Immunol Today* 19: 427–428

17   Becherel PA, Mossalayi MD, Ouaaz F, Le Goff L, Dugas B, Paul-Eugene N, Frances C,

Chosidow O, Kilchherr E, Guillosson JJ et al (1994) Involvement of cyclic AMP and nitric oxide in immunoglobulin E-dependent activation of Fc epsilon RII/CD23⁺ normal human keratinocytes. *J Clin Invest* 93: 2275–2279

18   Becherel PA, Le Goff L, Ktorza S, Ouaaz F, Mencia-Huerta JM, Dugas B, Debre P, Mossalayi MD, Arock M (1995) Interleukin-10 inhibits IgE-mediated nitric oxide synthase induction and cytokine synthesis in normal human keratinocytes. *Eur J Immunol* 25: 2992–2995

19   Becherel PA, Chosidow O, Le Goff L, Frances C, Debre P, Mossalayi MD, Arock M (1997) Inducible nitric oxide synthase and proinflammatory cytokine expression by human keratinocytes during acute urticaria. *J Molec Med* 3: 686–694

20   Walsh LJ (1995) Ultraviolet B irradiation of skin induces mast cell degranulation and release of tumour necrosis factor-alp. *Immunology & Cell Biology* 73: 226–233

21   Henseleit U, Rosenbach T, Kolde G (1996) Induction of apoptosis in human HaCaT keratinocytes. *Arch Dermatol Res* 288: 676–683

22   Deliconstantinos G, Villiotou V, Stravrides JC (1995) Release by ultraviolet B (u.v.B) radiation of nitric oxide (NO) from human keratinocytes: a potential role for nitric oxide in erythema production. *Br J Pharmacol* 114: 1257–1265

23   Kang-Rotondo CH, Major S, Chiang TM, Myers LK, Kang ES (1996) Upregulation of nitric oxide synthase in cultured human keratinocytes after ultraviolet B and bradykinin. *Photodermatol Photoimmunol Photomed* 12: 57–65

24   Warren JB (1994) Nitric oxide and human skin blood flow responses to acetylcholine and ultraviolet light. *FASEB J* 8: 247–251

25   Suschek CV, Krischel V, Bruch-Gerharz D, Berendji D, Krutmann J, Kroncke KD, Kolb-Bachofen V (1999) Nitric oxide fully protects against UVA-induced apoptosis in tight correlation with Bcl-2 up-regulation. *J Biol Chem* 274: 6130–6137

26   Romero-Graillet C, Aberdam E, Clement M, Ortonne JP, Ballotti R (1997) Nitric oxide produced by ultraviolet-irradiated keratinocytes stimulates melanogenesis. *J Clin Invest* 99: 635–642

27   Romero-Graillet C, Aberdam E, Biagoli N, Massabni W, Ortonne JP, Ballotti R (1996) Ultraviolet B radiation acts through the nitric oxide and cGMP signal transduction pathway to stimulate melanogenesis in human melanocytes. *J Biol Chem* 271: 28052–28056

28   Belmont HM, Levartovsky D, Goel A, Amin A, Giorno R, Rediske J, Skovron ML, Abramson SB (1997) Increased nitric oxide production accompanied by the up-regulation of inducible nitric oxide synthase in vascular endothelium from patients with systemic lupus erythematosus. *Arthritis Rheum* 40: 1810–1816

29   Weinberg JB, Granger DL, Pisetsky DS, Seldin MF, Misukonis MA, Mason SN, Pippen AM, Ruiz P, Wood ER, Gilkeson GS (1994) The role of nitric oxide in the pathogenesis of spontaneous murine autoimmune disease: Increased nitric oxide production and nitric oxide synthase expression in MRL-lpr/lpr mice, and reduction of spontaneous glomerulonephritis and arthritis by orally administered N(G)-monomethyl-L-arginine. *J Exp Med* 179: 651–660

30   Gilkeson GS, Mudgett JS, Seldin MF, Ruiz P, Alexander AA, Misukonis MA, Pisetsky

DS, Weinberg JB (1997) Clinical and serologic manifestations of autoimmune disease in MRL-lpr/lpr mice lacking nitric oxide synthase type 2. *J Exp Med* 186: 365–373

31 Kuhn A, Fehsel K, Lehmann P, Krutmann J, Ruzicka T, Kolb Bachofen V (1998) Aberrant timing in epidermal expression of inducible nitric oxide synthase after UV irradiation in cutaneous lupus erythematosus. *J Invest Dermatol* 111: 149–153

32 Heck DE, Laskin DL, Gardner CR, Laskin JD (1992) Epidermal growth factor suppresses nitric oxide and hydrogen peroxide production by keratinocytes. Potential role for nitric oxide in the regulation of wound healing. *J Biol Chem* 267: 21277–21280

33 Frank S, Madlener M, Pfeilschifter J, Werner S (1998) Induction of inducible nitric oxide synthase and its corresponding tetrahydrobiopterin-cofactor-synthesizing enzyme GTP-cyclohydrolase I during cutaneous wound repair. *J Invest Dermatol* 111: 1058–1064

34 Gansauge S, Gansauge F, Nussler AK, Rau B, Poch B, Schoenberg MH, Beger HG (1997) Exogenous, but not endogenous, nitric oxide increases proliferation rates in senescent human fibroblasts. *FEBS Lett* 410: 160–164

35 Wang R, Ghahary A, Shen YJ, Scott PG, Tredget EE (1996) Human dermal fibroblasts produce nitric oxide and express both constitutive and inducible nitric oxide synthase isoforms. *J Invest Dermatol* 106: 419–427

36 Wang R, Ghahary A, Shen YJ, Scott PG, Tredget EE (1997) Nitric oxide synthase expression and nitric oxide production are reduced in hypertrophic scar tissue and fibroblasts. *J Invest Dermatol* 108: 438–444

37 Hoffmann G, Schobersberger W, Rieder J, Smolny M, Seibel M, Fürhapter C, Fritsch P, Sepp N (1999) Human dermal microvascular endothelial cells express inducible nitric oxide synthase *in vitro*. *J Invest Dermatol* 112: 387–390

38 Joshi M, Fuller LR, Batchelor GCL (1999) L-arginine metabolites regulate DNA synthesis and nitric oxide synthase activity in cultured human dermal microvascular endothelial cells – Potential positive and negative regulators of angiogenesis derived from L-arginine. *Cancer Investigation* 17: 235–244

39 Yamasaki K, Edington HDJ, McClosky C, Tzeng E, Lizonova A, Kovesdi I, Steed DL, Billiar TR (1998) Reversal of impaired wound repair in iNOS-deficient mice by topical adenoviral-mediated iNOS gene transfer. J Clin Invest 101: 967–971

40 Thornton FJ, Schaffer MR, Witte MB, Moldawer LL, MacKay SLD, Abouhamze A, Tannahill CL, Barbul A (1998) Enhanced collagen accumulation following direct transfection of the inducible nitric oxide synthase gene in cutaneous wounds. *Biochem Biophys Res Commun* 246: 654–659

41 Yamamoto T, Katayama I, Nishioka K (1998) Nitric oxide production and inducible nitric oxide synthase expression in systemic sclerosis. *J Rheumatol* 25: 314–317

42 Paulsen SM, Wurster SH, Nanney LB (1998) Expression of inducible nitric oxide synthase in human burn wounds. *Wound Repair Regen* 6: 142–148

43 Jackson M, Frame F, Weller R, McKenzie RC (1998) Expression of nitric oxide synthase III (eNOS) mRNA by human skin cells: Melanocytes but not keratinocytes express eNOS mRNA. *Arch Dermatol Res* 290: 350–352

44 Joshi M, Strandhoy J, White WL (1996) Nitric oxide synthase activity is up-regulated in

melanoma cell lines: A potential mechanism for metastases formation. *Melanoma Research* 6: 121–126

45 Dong Z, Staroselsky AH, Qi X, Xie K, Fidler IJ (1994) Inverse correlation between expression of inducible nitric oxide synthase activity and production of metastasis in K-1735 murine melanoma cells. *Cancer Res* 54: 789–793

46 Xie K, Huang S, Dong Z, Juang SH, Gutman M, Xie QW, Nathan C, Fidler IJ (1995) Transfection with the inducible nitric oxide synthase gene suppresses tumorigenicity and abrogates metastasis by K-1735 murine melanoma cells. *J Exp Med* 181: 1333–1343

47 Ivanova K, Le Poole IC, Gerzer R, Westerhof W, Das PK (1997) Effects of nitric oxide on the adhesion of human melanocytes to extracellular matrix components. *J Path* 183: 469–476

48 Masson I, Mathieu J, Nolland XB, De Sousa M, Chanaud B, Strzalko S, Chancerelle Y, Kergonou JF, Giroud J, Florentin I (1998) Role of nitric oxide in depressed lymphoproliferative responses and altered cytokine production following thermal injury in rats. *Cellular Immunology* 186: 121–132

49 Kolb H, Kolb-Bachofen V (1998) Nitric oxide in autoimmune disease: cytotoxic or regulatory mediator? *Immunol Today* 19: 556–561

50 Kröncke KD, Fchsel K, Schmidt T, Zenke FT, Dasting I, Wesener JR, Bettermann H, Breunig KD, Kolb-Bachofen V (1994) Nitric oxide destroys zinc-sulfur clusters inducing zinc release from metallothionein and inhibition of the zinc finger-type yeast transcription activator LAC9. *Biochem Biophys Res Commun* 200: 1105–1110

51 Hausladen A, Privalle CT, Keng T, DeAngelo J, Stamler JS (1996) Nitrosative stress: Activation of the transcription factor OxyR. *Cell* 86: 719–729

52 Nikitovic D, Holmgren A, Spyrou G (1998) Inhibition of AP-1 DNA binding by nitric oxide involving conserved cysteine residues in Jun and Fos. *Biochem Biophys Res Commun* 242: 109–112

Roles of nitric oxide, superoxide, and peroxynitrite in myocardial ischemia-reperfusion injury and ischemic preconditioning

Péter Ferdinandy[1] and Richard Schulz[2]

[1]Department of Biochemistry, Faculty of Medicine, University of Szeged, Dóm tér 9, Szeged, 6720 Hungary; [2]Cardiovascular Research Group, Departments of Pediatrics and Pharmacology, 4-62 Heritage Medical Research Centre, University of Alberta, Edmonton, Alberta T6G 2S2, Canada

Myocardial ischemia-reperfusion and preconditioning

Ischemic heart disease, a major cause of mortality in industrialized countries, is characterized by insufficient blood supply to certain regions of the myocardium which leads to tissue necrosis (infarction). It develops secondary to a variety of disorders such as hypertension, atherosclerosis, dyslipidemia, and diabetes. The treatment of this condition has entered a new era in which mortality can be approximately halved by procedures which allow for the rapid restoration of blood flow (reperfusion), to the ischemic zone of the myocardium. Reperfusion, however, may lead to further complications such as diminished cardiac contractile function (stunning) and arrhythmias. Therefore, development of cardioprotective agents to improve myocardial function, decrease the incidence of arrhythmias, lessen necrotic tissue mass, and delay the onset of necrosis as a result of ischemia-reperfusion is of great clinical importance. The heart was also found to have an inherent ability to adapt to ischemic stress called ischemic preconditioning (PC) [1]. It is a well described adaptive response in which brief exposure of the heart to brief episode(s) of ischemia (PC ischemia) markedly enhances its ability to withstand a subsequent ischemic injury (test ischemia) (see for review see [2]).

Nitric oxide: friend or foe?

There appears to be a controversy in the study of myocardial ischemia-reperfusion injury whether NO plays a protective or detrimental role. Findings from this laboratory and others, and interpretation of the results to date, do not support such a controversy. An understanding of NO, O_2^{-*} and peroxynitrite ($ONOO^-$) biology is necessary to resolve the controversy.

Nitric Oxide and Inflammation, edited by Daniela Salvemini, Timothy R. Billiar and Yoram Vodovotz

Toxicity of NO by reaction with O_2^{-*} to form $ONOO^-$

NO is considered to be one of the biological Jekyll and Hyde molecules: physiologically necessary in small quantities, but potentially toxic in higher concentrations. However, it is now understood that many of the toxic actions of NO are not directly due to NO, but are mediated through $ONOO^-$, the reaction product of NO with O_2^{-*} [3, 4] (Fig. 1).

O_2^{-*} biosynthesis in the heart

Possible sources of O_2^{-*} in the heart are: (i) a NAD(P)H oxidoreductase in coronary artery smooth muscle [5], (ii) xanthine oxidase (XO) and/or xanthine dehydrogenase (XDH) activity [6], (iii) mitochondrial electron transport chain activity, (iv) activated neutrophils, (v) arachidonic acid metabolism, and (vi) autooxidation of certain tissue metabolites.

$ONOO^-$ is stable at alkaline pH, but at pH < 8 it decomposes rapidly upon its protonation to form the unstable intermediate, peroxynitrous acid. This spontaneously decomposes, forming highly reactive oxidant species (Fig. 1).

Understanding the balance between local concentrations of NO, O_2^{-*}, and SOD is critical in understanding NO biology and its potential toxicity in the form of $ONOO^-$ (see [3, 4]). One must consider the competition between NO and SOD for O_2^{-*}. Under normal physiological conditions in vascular endothelium, [NO] is ~ 10 nM, [SOD] is ~1 μM, and:

$$k_{ONOO^-} = (6.7 \times 10^9 \ M^{-1} \ s^{-1}) \ (1 \times 10^{-8} \ M) = 67 \ s^{-1}, \text{ whereas}$$
$$k_{SOD} = (2 \times 10^9 \ M^{-1} \ s^{-1}) \ (1 \times 10^{-6} \ M) = 2000 \ s^{-1}.$$

The ratio of the reaction of O_2^{-*} with NO to form $ONOO^-$ (k_{ONOO^-}) vs. the dismutation of O_2^{-*} by SOD (k_{SOD}) is: 67/2000 = 0.034. The reaction rate of O_2^{-*} to form $ONOO^-$ is only a fraction of the dismutation rate of O_2^{-*} by SOD, and, as a result, very little $ONOO^-$ is formed.

However, at maximal vascular rates of NO production (i.e. which may occur during acute reperfusion of ischemic tissue or during inducible NOS (iNOS) expression), [NO] is ≥ 1 μM, and:

$$k_{ONOO^-} = (6.7 \times 10^9 \ M^{-1} \ s^{-1}) \ (1 \times 10^{-6} \ M) = 6700 \ s^{-1}, \text{ whereas}$$
$$k_{SOD} = (2 \times 10^9 \ M^{-1} \ s^{-1}) \ (1 \times 10^{-6} \ M) = 2000 \ s^{-1}.$$

Therefore the ratio of k_{ONOO^-}/k_{SOD} is: 6700/2000 = 3.4. Thus the formation of $ONOO^-$ will predominate over the dismutation of O_2^{-*}. Under a variety of inflammatory conditions where NO production is upregulated, either by acute increase in

$$O_2^{-*} + NO^* \rightarrow ONOO^- \qquad \text{peroxynitrite}$$
$$k = 6.7 \times 10^9 \; M^{-1} \; sec^{-1}$$

At physiological pH:
$$ONOO^- + H^+ \rightarrow ONO\text{–}OH \qquad \text{peroxynitrous acid}$$

Fates of peroxynitrous acid:
$$ONO\text{–}OH \rightarrow \text{"}^*NO_2 \cdots {}^*OH\text{"} \qquad \textit{homolytic cleavage}$$

$$\begin{array}{c} Cu/Fe \\ ONO\text{–}OH \rightarrow NO_2^+ + OH^- \\ \text{nitronium ion} \end{array} \qquad \textit{heterolytic cleavage}$$

Figure 1
Production and fates of ONOO⁻.

Ca²⁺-dependent endothelial NOS (eNOS) activity *via* changes in shear stress or high $[Ca^{2+}]_i$ as which occurs during acute reperfusion and ischemia, or *via de novo* expression of iNOS in cells or tissues as a result of pro-inflammatory cytokines, one should predict the formation of $ONOO^-$.

Physiological roles of NO in the heart

NO biosynthesis in the heart

Coronary endothelium, endocardial endothelium and cardiomyocytes of the normal heart are all sources of the basal production of NO by a Ca²⁺-dependent eNOS. This serves a number of important physiological roles in the regulation of cardiac function including coronary vasodilation, inhibiting platelet and neutrophil actions, antioxidant effects, modulation of cardiac contractile function, and inhibiting cardiac oxygen consumption [7, 8].

Protective roles of NO in the heart

NO plays protective roles in the heart by: (i) stimulating soluble guanylate cyclase and thus reducing $[Ca^{2+}]_i$ partly through activation of cGMP-dependent protein kinase, (ii) terminating chain propagating lipid radical reactions caused by oxidative stress [9], and (iii) by inhibiting the activation of platelets and neutrophils and their adhesion to the endothelial surface [10, 11]. NO (either *via* NOS activity or through NO donors) protects against the toxic effects of exogenously supplied $ONOO^-$ in the coronary circulation [12] and on platelets [13]. In liposomes subjected to O_2^{-*} and NO generated simultaneously at defined rates, lipid peroxidation was maximal when NO and O_2^{-*} rates were approximately equal, yet it declined when there was an excess of NO generation over O_2^{-*} [9].

Pathophysiology of ONOO⁻ in myocardial ischemia-reperfusion

Stunning (acute injury)

The change in shear stress during reintroduction of flow at reperfusion is a very strong stimulus for NO release from vascular endothelium. Furthermore, the reintroduction of oxygen will drive the formation of NO from L-arginine forwards. The rise in cytoplasmic Ca^{2+} levels that occurs during ischemia stimulates NO formation by eNOS in endothelium and myocytes. Already during ischemia itself the local production of NO in the ischemic myocardium is markedly enhanced [14, 15].

Our lab provided the first evidence that $ONOO^-$ is produced during the acute reperfusion of ischemic hearts and that drugs which inhibit $ONOO^-$ formation or antagonize its toxicity protect the heart from this injury [16, 17]. We developed a novel, simple and effective methodology to detect $ONOO^-$ based on the reaction of $ONOO^-$ with tyrosine to form dityrosine [17]. Rapid generation of $ONOO^-$ during reperfusion of the ischemic heart has also been detected using luminol chemiluminescence in the perfusate and anti-nitrotyrosine labelling of myocardial proteins [18]. We showed that low concentrations of the NOS inhibitor L-NMMA, or a cell permeable SOD mimetic, MnTBAP protected the hearts from ischemia-reperfusion injury [16, 17]. The beneficial effect of L-NMMA fell within a narrow range and was lost at higher concentrations which further reduced coronary flow [17]. Our data also showed that a NO donor, at subvasodilatory concentration, protected hearts from endogenous $ONOO^-$-mediated injury. This study provided the first mechanistic evidence of how either NO donors or NOS inhibitors reduce ischemia-reperfusion injury [17].

Myocardial infarct (late injury, neutrophil dependent)

What is the importance of the neutrophil-independent free radical release during acute reperfusion, as opposed to the neutrophil-dependent reperfusion events which occur several hours later? One very important defect in the heart resulting from acute reperfusion following ischemia is endothelial stunning, which is manifested by a reduced response to endothelium-dependent vasodilators within the first minute of reperfusion [19]. We speculate that this damage is self-inflicted, resulting from the burst of endogenous $ONOO^-$ from the vascular endothelium immediately at reperfusion! This would cause enhanced susceptibility of the endothelial surface to neutrophil and platelet adhesion, platelet aggregation and neutrophil activation, events which are normally inhibited by the physiological production of endothelium-derived NO [10, 11]. Villa et al. [12] showed that bolus injection of $ONOO^-$ into isolated hearts acutely inhibited endothelium-dependent coronary vasodilation. An understanding of the oxidative damage which occurs during acute reperfusion following ischemia is thus crucial to help devise strategies to reduce subsequent neutrophil-mediated damage in the later stages of reperfusion injury. Many *in vivo* studies show that NO donors improve the recovery of mechanical function and/or reduce infarct size following ischemia-reperfusion. Subvasodilatory doses of NO donors [19], L-arginine [20] or agonists of endothelium-derived NO [21] were shown to be protective (see for review [22]). These protective actions of NO include the inhibition of platelet aggregation, attenuation of neutrophil-endothelium interactions and preservation of endothelial function. Myocardial $ONOO^-$ generation has also been show to occur during the neutrophil-dependent phase of ischemia-reperfusion injury, seen 5 h after reperfusion, using an *in vivo* model of regional ischemia in rats [23].

Antioxidants – Which oxidants do they protect against?

The antioxidants of the heart are crucial for maintenance of normal cardiac mechanical function. Unchecked, the highly oxidative heart muscle can potentially be subjected to its own basal production of $O_2^{-\bullet}$ [24], and NO [7]. Mitochondrial MnSOD, cytosolic Cu-Zn SOD, extracellular Cu-Zn SOD, glutathione (GSH), uric acid, and catalase, are but a few of the more important antioxidants. Downregulation of Cu-Zn SOD expression in PC12 cells triggers death by a NO and $ONOO^-$-dependent pathway [25]. A variety of myocardial insults reduce antioxidant levels, for example GSH, whereas oxidized GSH is increased [26]. $ONOO^-$ oxidizes thiols to their disulfides and to higher order oxides [27]. $ONOO^-$ also reacts with GSH to form the nitrosothiol, nitrosoglutathione, a NO donor [12, 28, 29], which accounts for the stimulation of guanylate cyclase by $ONOO^-$ [29]. $ONOO^-$ is a vasodilator [12, 30] and inhibitor of platelet aggregation [13] by this reaction. Thus nature has a built in mechanism to turn Mr. Hyde back into Dr. Jekyll, turning $ONOO^-$, a strong oxidant, back into a NO donor. Hearts with enhanced endogenous GSH levels are less susceptible to ischemia-reperfusion injury [31] and micromolar concentrations of GSH added to the perfusate protects isolated hearts from stunning injury through the reduced formation of $ONOO^-$ at reperfusion [32].

Controversies of $ONOO^-$ in ischemia-reperfusion injury

A report of the protective action of $ONOO^-$ in preventing leukocyte rolling and adherence to the endothelial surface is unfounded [33]. In that study, $ONOO^-$ was mixed with plasma in a syringe before it was applied. Within seconds there would have been no active $ONOO^-$ in the syringe, instead it would have reacted with free and protein-associated thiols, forming NO-donor nitrosothiols which would have mediated the protective effect [33]. A further study showed that the protective actions of direct infusion of $ONOO^-$ into the bloodstream in myocardial ischemia-reperfusion injury was highly concentration dependent, and lost at higher concentrations [34]. In isolated hearts, the $ONOO^-$ donor SIN-1 aggrevated ischemia-reperfusion injury, which was abolished by the co-administration of GSH monoester [35]. Whether $ONOO^-$ in end effect causes damage in the local environment depends upon its concentration, its site of formation, the duration of exposure, and the concentration of antioxidants at that site.

NO is cardioprotective in ischemia-reperfusion injury

A number of *ex vivo* studies using isolated crystalloid-buffer perfused hearts have shown that enhancing NO levels, either by applying NO donors, NO-dependent vasodilators, L-arginine supplementation, angiotensin converting enzyme inhibitors, or pretreating the animal with endotoxin analogues which enhance myocardial iNOS activity, functionally protect the heart from acute stunning injury and/or infarct size development [17, 36–39]. Whether this protective effect is due to the antioxidant properties of NO, lowering $[Ca^{2+}]_i$ *via* guanylate cyclase, or other mechanisms is unclear at the moment.

In vivo studies using eNOS knockout mice enhance the notion that the basal release of NO in the heart is an important endogeneous cardiac protectant, particularly in regards to the prevention of neutrophil sticking and platelet activation. Infarct size in eNOS knockout mice was larger than in the wildtype controls, with higher P-selectin expression and significantly more neutrophils in hearts from eNOS knockout mice [40]. Yang et al. [41] showed that the protective effect of an angiotensin converting enzyme inhibitor in ischemia-reperfusion injury in wildtype mice was lost in the corresponding eNOS knockout mouse. In contrast, an *ex vivo* study showed that the functional recovery of eNOS knockout mouse hearts was improved in comparison to wildtype controls [42], suggesting that NO generated from eNOS contributes to stunning injury seen in early reperfusion.

Inhibition of NO synthase is cardioprotective

Ex vivo studies

Despite evidence that supplementation of NO can protect hearts from ischemia-reperfusion injury, reports that inhibition of NOS can also prevent such injury began to appear. Most importantly, these studies must be examined in regard to the concentration, potency and efficacy of the NOS inhibitor used, as well as to experimental details (i.e. constant flow *versus* constant pressure perfusion, global *versus* low-flow ischemia, etc.). In 1995, we showed that low to moderate inhibitory concentrations of L-NAME (3 µM) or L-NMMA (30 µM, note that L-NMMA is approximately ten-fold less potent than L-NAME) protected isolated working rabbit hearts from stunning injury when given prior to the onset of global, no-flow ischemia, but not at reperfusion, an effect which was reversed in the presence of excess L-arginine [43]. We later showed that the mechanism of cardioprotection by L-NMMA in constant pressure-perfused rat hearts subjected to ischemia-reperfusion was by reducing the formation of ONOO⁻ at reperfusion [17].

Depré et al. [44] showed that L-NMMA at concentrations between 0.001–10 µM significantly protected isolated rabbit hearts perfused at constant flow and subjected to low-flow ischemia. They suggested that the protective effect of L-NMMA was by the enhancement of glycolysis during ischemia, however, they could not exclude a protective effect during reperfusion itself. Another study using constant flow-perfused hearts suggested additional protective effects of L-NAME (30 µM) including the stimulation of adenosine release which occurs only at such high levels of NOS inhibition [45]. A study in isolated rat hearts which used 1 mM L-NAME [18], supermaximal in terms of blocking NO biosynthesis, may have included protective effects unrelated to NOS inhibition, as L-NAME in particular has been shown to be a muscarinic receptor antagonist at concentrations greater than 100 µM [46].

In vivo studies

Essentially there is no study to date which carefully assesses the dose-dependent actions of NOS inhibitors in myocardial ischemia-reperfusion injury *in vivo*. This is an obvious gap in the literature. Studies using high doses of NOS inhibitors (i.e. > IC$_{50}$), which significantly raise mean arterial blood pressure, uniformly provide evidence of a worsened outcome in terms of infarct size or function post ischemia-reperfusion [47, 48]. Interestingly, a study in open-chested rats subjected to only 4 min of regional ischemia and 4 min reperfusion showed that low doses of L-NAME caused a marked reduction in mortality due to ventricular fibrillation. This protective effect was abolished by co-administration of L-arginine and potentiated by co-administration of SOD, suggesting that reperfusion arrythmias may be due to the generation of ONOO⁻ [49].

Myocardial adaptation to ischemia: preconditioning (PC)

Although the effectiveness of ischemic PC might be attenuated in the heart during aging and some disease states such as hyperlipidemia and diabetes, PC confers a remarkable cardioprotection in a variety of species including humans (see for review [2]). PC can be elicited by different sublethal stress signals, such as brief periods of ischemia, hypoxia, rapid electrical pacing, heat stress, or administration of bacterial endotoxin, etc. The cardioprotective effect of PC shows two distinct phases. The early phase is manifested within minutes after the PC stimulus and has a duration of less than 3 h. The late phase is characterized by a slower onset ($\geq$ 20 h) and a duration of up to 72 h. Both phases of PC involve reduction of necrotic tissue mass (infarct size), improvement of cardiac performance and reduction of arrhythmias following ischemia and reperfusion (see for review [2]).

There is considerable debate regarding the cellular mechanism of ischemic PC. NO, oxygen free radicals, and antioxidant enzymes have been suggested to be, and also refuted as, key mediators of PC. The mechanisms of early and late PC seem to be different. Further discrepancies are generally attributed to species differences, different stimuli to induce PC, and different study end-points, i.e. myocardial function, arrhythmias, or infarct size. Understanding the cellular pathways involved in the ischemic adaptation of the myocardium may lead to the development of "PC mimetic" drugs for patients suffering from ischemic heart disease.

NO, O_2^{-*}, and early preconditioning

Vegh at al. demonstrated that 10 mg/kg L-NAME administered both before and after PC abolished the antiarrhythmic effect of PC in a coronary occlusion model of anesthetized, open chest dogs [50]. Bilinska et al. reported that infusion of the NO donor nitroglycerine (500 µM) or SIN-1 (10 µM) for 5 min before coronary occlusion mimicked the antiarrhythmic effect of ischemic PC in isolated rat hearts [51]. Using the electron spin resonance technique to directly measure cardiac NO content we have shown that a decrease in basal cardiac NO content before PC, due to either *in vivo* pretreatment with 1 mg/kg L-nitroarginine [52], experimental hypercholesterolemia [52], or selective depletion of neurotransmitters including NO from cardiac sensory neurons [53] lead to the loss of pacing-induced PC in isolated working rat hearts. However, PC, in turn, markedly decreased the accumulation of NO in heart tissue during subsequent ischemia and reperfusion [15]. In the presence of 4.6 µM L-nitroarginine, a nonvasoactive concentration which reduced basal NO synthesis, PC failed to protect against ischemia-reperfusion and failed to attenuate NO accumulation produced by ischemia-reperfusion [15]. When L-nitroarginine was applied after the PC protocol, the effect of PC on test ischemia-reperfusion and ischemic NO accumulation was not affected [15, 52]. These results prove that intact NO biosynthesis is required for the triggering mechanism of PC and further show that the cardioprotection provided by PC involves a mechanism which decreases the accumulation of NO in the myocardium during ischemia and reperfusion [15]. In accordance with this, Woolfson et al. reported that the limitation of infarct size after inhibition of NO synthesis by L-NAME shares a common mechanism with ischemic PC in rabbit hearts [45]. Furthermore, preliminary studies showed that PC decreases NO synthesis during subsequent ischemia and this is associated with the protective effect of PC in isolated rat hearts [54].

The nature of PC-induced inhibition of NO synthesis is not known. PC may decrease the rate of enzymatic and/or nonenzymatic [55] NO production during ischemia-reperfusion by altering cellular pH and the availability of cofactors and/or arginine for NO synthesis, or may possibly stimulate the formation of endogenous NOS inhibitors [56].

In contrast to the aforementioned studies, Lu et al. [57] reported that 10 mg/kg L-NMMA or L-NAME did not affect the antiarrhythmic effect of PC in anesthetized rats with coronary occlusion/reperfusion. Weselcouch et al. [58] showed that in rat hearts, 30 µM L-NAME did not interfere with the effect of PC on postischemic myocardial function. In these studies, surprisingly, the different NOS inhibitors neither interfered with PC nor the outcome of ischemia-reperfusion without PC. Since NO generation and/or NOS activities were not determined, and only a single dose of NO synthase inhibitors were used in these studies, it is difficult to interpret these negative results.

The possible role for oxygen free radicals in PC was suggested by Tanaka et al. [59] who showed that SOD or the free radical scavenger mercaptopropionyl-glycine were both able to inhibit the protective effect of PC on infarct size in rabbits. Osada et al. [60] reported that the antiarrhythmic effect of PC was lost when the PC ischemia was applied in the presence of both SOD and catalase in isolated rat hearts. Tritto et al. [61] showed that a 5 min infusion of O_2^{-*} generated by purine/xanthine oxidase prior to ischemia-reperfusion resulted in a reduction of infarct size in rabbit hearts, similar to the effect of PC. These studies strongly suggest that the generation of oxygen free radicals during PC stimuli is necessary to trigger the protective machinery of PC. PC, in turn, attenuates the increased free radical synthesis during subsequent ischemia-reperfusion [62]. Others, however, showed using rabbit hearts that PC was not affected by SOD [63].

Taken together, the majority of studies show that NO and oxygen free radicals are both required to elicit PC. Therefore, it is plausible to speculate that formation of ONOO⁻ is an important oxidative stimulus to trigger cellular adaptive mechanisms. PC-induced inhibition of NO and free radical synthesis during subsequent ischemia may lead to decreased $ONOO^-$ formation at reperfusion as part of the cardioprotective mechanism. This hypothesis needs to be tested as the role of $ONOO^-$ in PC has not been studied yet.

NO, O_2^{-*}, and late preconditioning

In a conscious rabbit model of PC with repetitive coronary occlusion/reperfusion, Bolli et al. reported that L-nitroarginine given either during PC or 24 h later abrogated the protective effect of PC and that the selective iNOS inhibitors aminoguanidine or S-methylisothiourea abolished PC only when applied 24 h after PC [64]. They also showed that PC induces an increase in iNOS mRNA levels in the ischemic regions of the rabbit heart, and that this induction is triggered by increased generation of NO during the PC stimulus [65]. Targeted disruption of the iNOS gene in mice led to a complete blockade of late PC [66]. Dexamethasone or selective iNOS inhibitors inhibited the late effect of PC on infarct size in anesthetized rabbits [67] and on arrhythmias in anesthetized dogs [68]. These results suggest a dual role of NO in late PC, as intact NO synthesis by eNOS is necessary to trigger late PC and NO derived from iNOS is a mediator of late protection (see for review [69]).

The involvement of oxygen free radicals in late PC was suggested by Sun et al [70] who showed that a combination of antioxidants (SOD, catalase, mercaptopropionyl-glycine) infused during the PC stimulus completely abolished the late effect of PC on stunning in conscious pigs. Zhou et al. reported that isolated rat myocytes preconditioned with anoxia or with administration of O_2^{-*} both induced late cytoprotection which was characterized by increased MnSOD activity and decreased O_2^{-*} production [71]. Takano et al. demonstrated that i.v. infusion of the NO donors DETA/NO or SNAP induced cardioprotection 24 h later in conscious rabbits and that this effect was lost when they were infused with mercaptopropionyl-glycine [72]. This suggests that the mechanism whereby NO induces PC involves the generation of oxidant species, possibly $ONOO^-$.

Taken together, these results suggest that both NO and oxygen free radicals are necessary to trigger late PC. The initial PC stimulus may lead to deceased free radical production and increased activities of antioxidant enzymes and iNOS during test ischemia. As most of the aforementioned conclusions are based on a pharmacological approach, to elucidate the exact role of NO, O_2^{-*}, and $ONOO^-$ in PC requires further biochemical evidence.

The targets of $ONOO^-$

Research will now focus on the downstream targets of $ONOO^-$-mediated injury in the heart, which are several. These include the polyADP-ribose synthetase, apoptosis, metabolic targets, Ca^{2+} handling proteins [73], matrix metallopro-teinases [74], and others.

Conclusions

In order to understand NO biology, we need to know its relationship with key oxi-dants such as $O_2^{-\bullet}$. The study of $ONOO^-$ in the heart will lead to a better under-standing of basic physiological and pathological mechanisms relevant to cardiac ischemia and reperfusion injury and give new insight to novel therapeutic targets and strategies for its treatment or prevention.

Acknowledgements
Peter Ferdinandy thanks the Hungarian Scientific Research Fund (T029843), Com-mittee for Health Research (ETT 047/98), and the Ministry of Education (1284/1997) for their continuous generosity. Richard Schulz is a Senior Scholar of the Alberta Heritage Foundation for Medical Research. Research in Richard Schulz's laboratory was funded by the Heart and Stroke Foundation of Alberta, NWT and Nunavut.

References

1   Murry C, Jennings R, Reimer K (1986) Preconditioning with ischemia: a delay of lethal cell injury in ischemic myocardium. *Circulation* 74: 1124–1136
2   Ferdinandy P, Szilvassy Z, Baxter GF (1998) Adaptation to myocardial stress in disease states: is preconditioning a healthy heart phenomenon? *Trends Pharmacol Sci* 19: 223–229
3   Beckman JS, Koppenol WH (1996) Nitric oxide, superoxide, and peroxynitrite: the good, the bad and ugly. *Am J Physiol* 271: C1424–C1437
4   Rubbo H, Darley-Usmar V, Freeman B (1996) Nitric oxide regulation of tissue free rad-ical injury. *Chem Res Toxicol* 9: 809–820
5   Mohazzab-H. KM, Kaminski PM, Fayngersh RP, Wolin MS (1996) Oxygen-elicited responses in calf coronary arteries: role of H_2O_2 production *via* NADH-derived super-oxide. *Am J Physiol* 270: H1044–H1053
6   Dupont GP, Huecksteadt TP, Marshall BC, Ryan US, Michael JR, Hoidal JR (1992) Reg-ulation of xanthine dehydrogenase and xanthine oxidase activity and gene expression in cultured rat pulmonary endothelial cells. *J Clin Invest* 89: 197–202
7   Hare JM, Colucci WS (1995) Role of nitric oxide in the regulation of myocardial func-tion. *Prog Cardiovasc Dis* 38: 155–166

8   Xie YW, Wolin MS (1996) Role of nitric oxide and its interaction with superoxide in the suppression of cardiac muscle mitochondrial respiration. *Circulation* 94: 2580–2586

9   Rubbo H, Radi R, Trujillo M, Telleri R, Kalyanaraman B, Barnes S, Kirk M, Freeman BA (1994) Nitric oxide regulation of superoxide and peroxynitrite-dependent lipid peroxidation. *J Biol Chem* 269: 26066–26075

10 Kubes P, Suzuki M, Granger DN (1991) Nitric oxide: an endogenous modulator of leukocyte adhesion. *Proc Natl Acad Sci USA* 88: 4651–4655

11 Radomski MW, Palmer RMJ, Moncada S (1987) The anti-aggregating properties of vascular endothelium: interactions between prostacyclin and nitric oxide. *Br J Pharmacol* 92: 639–646

12 Villa LM, Salas E, Darley-Usmar VM, Radomski MW, Moncada S (1994) Peroxynitrite induces both vasodilatation and impaired vascular relaxation in the isolated perfused heart. *Proc Natl Acad Sci USA* 91: 12388–12387

13 Moro MA, Darley-Usmar VM, Goodwin DA, Read NG, Zamora-Pino R, Feelisch M, Radomski MW, Moncada S (1994) Paradoxical fate and biological action of peroxynitrite in human platelets. *Proc Natl Acad Sci USA* 91: 6702–6706

14 Depré C, Hue L (1994) Cyclic GMP in the perfused rat heart. Effect of ischaemia, anoxia and nitric oxide synthase inhibitor. *FEBS Lett* 345: 241–245

15 Csonka C, Szilvassy Z, Pali T, Blasig IE, Tosaki A, Schulz R, Ferdinandy P (1999) Classic preconditioning decreases the harmful accumulation of nitric oxide during ischemia and reperfusion in rat hearts. *Circulation* 100: 2260–2266

16 Yasmin W, Schulz R (1995) Detection of peroxynitrite after ischemia-reperfusion in isolated hearts. *Circulation* 92: I–563 (abstract)

17 Yasmin W, Strynadka KD, Schulz R (1997) Generation of peroxynitrite contributes to ischemia-reperfusion injury in isolated rat hearts. *Cardiovasc Res* 33: 422–432

18 Wang P, Zweier JL (1996) Measurement of nitric oxide and peroxynitrite generation in the postischemic heart. *J Biol Chem* 271: 29223–29230

19 Siegfried MR, Erhardt J, Rider T, Ma X-L, Lefer AM (1992) Cardioprotection and attenuation of endothelial dysfunction by organic nitric oxide donors in myocardial ischemia-reperfusion. *J Pharmacol Exp Ther* 260: 508–512

20 Weyrich AS, Ma X-L, Lefer A (1992) The role of L-arginine in ameliorating reperfusion injury after myocardial ischemia in the cat. *Circulation* 86: 279–288

21 Richard V, Blanc T, Kaeffer N, Tron C, Thuillez C (1995) Myocardial and coronary endothelial protective effects of acetylcholine after myocardial ischemia and reperfusion in rats: role of nitric oxide. *Br J Pharmacol* 115:1532–1538

22 Grisham MB, Granger DN, Lefer DJ (1998) Modulation of leukocyte-endothelial interactions by reactive metabolites of oxygen and nitrogen: relevance to ischemic heart disease. *Free Rad Biol Med* 25: 404–433

23 Liu P, Hock CE, Nagele R, Wong PY-K (1997) Formation of nitric oxide, superoxide, and peroxynitrite in myocardial ischemia-reperfusion injury in rats. *Am J Physiol* 272: H2327–H2337

24 Boveris A, Chance B (1973) The mitochondrial generation of hydrogen peroxide: gen-

eral properties and effect of hyperbaric oxygen. *Biochem J* 134: 707–716

25   Troy CM, Derossi D, Prochiantz A, Green LA, Shelanski ML (1996) Downregulation of Cu/Zn superoxide dismutase leads to cell death *via* the nitric oxide-peroxynitrite pathway. *J Neurosci* 16: 253–261

26   Janssen M, Koster JF, Bos E, de Jong JW (1993) Malondialdehyde and glutathione production in isolated perfused human and rat hearts. *Circ Res* 73: 681–68

27   Quijano C, Alvarez B, Gatti RM, Augusto O, Radi R (1997) Pathways of peroxynitrite oxidation of thiol groups. *Biochem J* 322: 167–173

28   Cheung P-Y, Schulz, R (1997) Glutathione causes coronary vasodilation *via* a nitric oxide- and soluble guanylate cyclase-dependent mechanism. *Am J Physiol* 273: H1231–H1238

29   Mayer BA, Schrammel A, Klatt P, Koesling D, Schmidt K (1995) Peroxynitrite-induced accumulation of cyclic GMP in endothelial cells and stimulation of purified soluble guanylate cyclase. *J Biol Chem* 270: 17355–17360

30   Wu M, Pritchard KA, Kaminski PM, Fayngersh RP, Hinze H, Wolin MS (1994) Involvement of nitric oxide and nitrosothiols in relaxation of pulmonary arteries to peroxynitrite. *Am J Physiol* 266: H2108–H2113

31   Kirschenbaum LA, Singal P (1993) Increase in endogenous antioxidant enzymes protect hearts against reperfusion injury. *Am J Physiol* 265: H484–H493

32   Cheung P-Y, Wang W, Schulz R (2000) Glutathione protects against myocardial ischemia-reperfusion injury by detoxifying peroxynitrite. *J Mol Cell Cardiol* 32: 1669–1678

33   Lefer DJ, Scalia R, Campbell B, Nossuli T, Hayward R, Salamon M, Grayson J, Lefer AM (1997) Peroxynitrite inhibits leukocyte-endothelial cell interactions and protects against ischemia-reperfusion injury in rats. *J Clin Invest* 99: 684–691

34   Nossuli TO, Hayward R, Jensen D, Scalia R, Lefer AM (1998) Mechanisms of cardioprotection by peroxynitrite in myocardial ischemia and reperfusion injury. *Am J Physiol* 275: H509–H519

35   Ma XL, Lopez BL, Liu G-L, Christopher TA, Ischiropoulos H (1997) Peroxynitrite aggravates myocardial reperfusion injury in the isolated perfused rat heart. Cardiovasc Res 36: 195–204

36   Masini E, Bianchi S, Mugnai L, Gambassi F, Lupini M, Pistelli A, Mannaioni PF (1991) The effect of nitric oxide generators on ischemia reperfusion injury and histamine release in isolated perfused guinea-pig heart. *Agents & Actions* 33: 53–56

37   Schoelkens BA, Linz W (1992) Bradykinin-mediated metabolic effects in isolated perfused rat hearts. *Agents & Actions* 38 (Suppl Pt 2): 36–42

38   Massoudy P, Becker BF, Gerlach E (1995) Nitric oxide accounts for postischemic cardioprotection resulting from angiotensin-converting enzyme inhibition: indirect evidence for a radical scavenger effect in isolated guinea pig heart. J Cardiovasc Pharmacol 25: 440–447

39   Xi L, Jarrett NC, Hess ML, Kukreja RC (1999) Essential role of inducible nitric oxide

synthase in monophosphoryl lipid A-induced late cardioprotection: evidence from pharmacological inhibition and gene knockout mice. *Circulation* 99: 2157–2163

40 Jones SP, Girod WG, Palazzo AJ, Granger DN, Grisham MB, Jourd'Heuil D, Huang PL, Lefer DJ (1999) Myocardial ischemia-reperfusion injury is exacerbated in absence of endothelial cell nitric oxide synthase. *Am J Physiol* 276: H1567–H1573

41 Yang XP, Liu YH, Shesely EG, Bulagannawar M, Liu F, Carretero OA (1999) Endothelial nitric oxide gene knockout mice: cardiac phenotypes and the effect of angiotensin-converting enzyme inhibitor on myocardial ischemia/reperfusion injury. *Hypertension* 34: 24–30

42 Flogel U, Decking UKM, Godecke A, Schrader J (1999) Contribution of NO to ischemia-reperfusion injury in the saline-perfused heart: a study in endothelial NO synthase knockout mice. *J Mol Cell Cardiol* 31: 827–836

43 Schulz R, Wambolt R (1995) Inhibition of nitric oxide synthesis protects the isolated working rabbit heart from ischemia-reperfusion injury. *Cardiovasc Res* 30: 432–439

44 Depré C, Vanoverschelde J-L, Goudemant J-F, Mottet I, Hue L (1995) Protection against ischemic injury by nonvasoactive concentrations of nitric oxide synthase inhibitors in the perfused rabbit heart. *Circulation* 92: 1911–1918

45 Woolfson RG, Patel VC, Neild GH, Yellon DM (1995) Inhibition of nitric oxide synthesis reduces infarct size by an adenosine-dependent mechanism. *Circulation* 91: 1545–1551

46 Buxton ILO, Cheek DJ, Eckman D, Westfall DP, Sanders KM, Keef KD. (1993) N^G-nitro L-arginine methyl ester and other alkyl esters of arginine are muscarinic receptor antagonists. *Circ Res* 72: 387–395.

47 Hoshida S, Yamashita N, Igarashi J, Nishida M, Hori M, Kamada T, Kuzuya T, Tada M (1995) Nitric oxide synthase protects the heart against ischemia-reperfusion injury in rabbits. *J Pharmacol Exp Ther* 274: 413–418

48 Williams M, Taft C, Ramnauth S, Zhao Z-Q, Vinten-Johansen J (1995) Endogenous nitric oxide (NO) protects against ischemia-reperfusion injury in the rabbit. *Cardiovasc Res* 30:79–86

49 Ohoi I, Takeo S (1996) Involvement of superoxide and nitric oxide in the genesis of reperfusion arrhythmias in rats. *Eur J Pharmacol* 306: 123–131

50 Vegh A, Szekeres L, Parratt J (1992) Preconditioning of the ischaemic myocardium; Involvement of the L-arginine nitric oxide pathway. *Br J Pharmacol* 107: 648–652

51 Bilinska M, Maczewski M, Beresewicz A (1996) Donors of nitric oxide mimic effects of ischaemic preconditioning on reperfusion induced arrhythmias in isolated rat heart. *Mol Cell Biochem* 160-161: 265–271

52 Ferdinandy P, Szilvassy Z, Horvath LI, Csont T, Csonka C, Nagy E, Szentgyörgyi R, Nagy I, Koltai M, Dux L (1997) Loss of pacing-induced preconditioning in rat hearts: role of nitric oxide and cholesterol-enriched diet. *J Mol Cell Cardiol* 29: 3321–3333

53 Ferdinandy P, Csont T, Csonka C, Torok M, Dux M, Nemeth J, Horvath LI, Dux L, Szilvassy Z, Jancso G (1997) Capsaicin-sensitive local sensory innervation is involved in pacing-induced preconditioning in rat hearts: role of nitric oxide and CGRP? *Naunyn*

Schmiedebergs Arch Pharmacol 356: 356–363

54 Wang P, Zweier JL (1997) Ischemic preconditioning decreases nitric oxide (NO) formation and NO mediated injury in the postischemic heart. *Circulation* 96 (Suppl 1): 72 (Abstract)

55 Zweier JL, Wang P, Samuilov A, Kuppusamy P (1995) Enzyme-independent formation of nitric oxide in biological tissues. *Nature Med* 1: 804–809

56 Vallance P, Leone A, Calver A, Collier J, Moncada S (1992) Accumulation of an endogenous inhibitor of nitric oxide synthesis in chronic renal failure. *Lancet* 339: 572–575

57 Lu HR, Remeysen P, De Clerck F (1995) Does the antiarrhythmic effect of ischemic preconditioning in rats involve the L-arginine nitric oxide pathway. *J Cardiovasc Pharmacol* 25: 524–530

58 Weselcouch EO, Baird AJ, Sleph P, Grover GJ (1995) Inhibition of nitric oxide synthesis does not affect ischemic preconditioning in isolated perfused rat hearts. *Am J Physiol* 268: H242–H249

59 Tanaka M, Fujiwara H, Yamasaki K, Sasayama S (1994) Superoxide dismutase and N-2-mercaptopropionyl glycine attenuate infarct size limitation effect of ischaemic preconditioning in the rabbit. *Cardiovasc Res* 28: 980–986

60 Osada M, Sato T, Komori S, Tamura K (1991) Protective effect of preconditioning on reperfusion induced ventricular arrhythmias of isolated rat hearts. *Cardiovasc Res* 25: 441–444

61 Tritto I, D'Andrea D, Eramo N, Scognamiglio A, De Simone C, Violante A, Esposito A, Chiariello M, Ambrosio G (1997) Oxygen radicals can induce preconditioning in rabbit hearts. *Circ Res* 80: 743–748

62 Tosaki A, Cordis GA, Szerdahelyi P, Engelman RM, Das DK (1994) Effects of preconditioning on reperfusion arrhythmias, myocardial functions, formation of free radicals, and ion shifts in isolated ischemic/reperfused rat hearts. *J Cardiovasc Pharmacol* 23: 365–373

63 Iwamoto T, Miura T, Adachi T, Noto T, Ogawa T, Tsuchida, Iimura O (1991) Myocardial infarct size-limiting effect of ischemic preconditioning was not attenuated by oxygen free-radical scavengers in the rabbit. *Circulation* 83: 1015–1022

64 Bolli R, Manchikalapudi S, Tang XL, Takano H, Qiu Y, Guo Y, Zhang Q, Jadoon AK (1997) The protective effect of late preconditioning against myocardial stunning in conscious rabbits is mediated by nitric oxide synthase. Evidence that nitric oxide acts both as a trigger and as a mediator of the late phase of ischemic preconditioning. *Circ Res* 81: 1094–1107

65 Jones WK, Flaherty MP, Tang XL, Takano H, Qiu Y, Banerjee S, Smith T, Bolli R (1999) Ischemic preconditioning increases iNOS transcript levels in conscious rabbits *via* a nitric oxide-dependent mechanism. *J Mol Cell Cardiol* 31: 1469–1481

66 Guo Y, Jones WK, Xuan YT, Tang XL, Bao W, Wu WJ, Han H, Laubach VE, Ping P, Yang Z et al (1999) The late phase of ischemic preconditioning is abrogated by targeted disruption of the inducible NO synthase gene. *Proc Natl Acad Sci USA* 96: 11507–11512

67   Imagawa J, Yellon DM, Baxter GF (1999) Pharmacological evidence that inducible nitric oxide synthase is a mediator of delayed preconditioning. *Br J Pharmacol* 126: 701–708

68   Kis A, Vegh A, Papp JG, Parratt JR (1999) Repeated cardiac pacing extends the time during which canine hearts are protected against ischaemia-induced arrhythmias: role of nitric oxide. *J Mol Cell Cardiol* 31: 1229–1241

69   Bolli R, Dawn B, Tang XL, Qiu Y, Ping P, Xuan YT, Jones WK, Takano H, Guo Y, Zhang J (1998) The nitric oxide hypothesis of late preconditioning. *Basic Res Cardiol* 93: 325–338

70   Sun JZ, Tang XL, Park SW, Qiu YM, Turrens JF, Bolli R (1996) Evidence for an essential role of reactive oxygen species in the genesis of late preconditioning against myocardial stunning in conscious pigs. *J Clin Invest* 97: 562–576

71   Zhou X, Zhai X, Ashraf M (1996) Direct evidence that initial oxidative stress triggered by preconditioning contributes to second window of protection by endogenous antioxidant enzyme in myocytes. *Circulation* 93: 1177–1184

72   Takano H, Tang XL, Qiu Y, Guo Y, French BA, Bolli R (1998) Nitric oxide donors induce late preconditioning against myocardial stunning and infarction in conscious rabbits *via* an antioxidant-sensitive mechanism. *Circ Res* 83: 73–84

73   Szabó C (1996) The pathophysiological role of peroxynitrite in shock, inflammation, and ischemia-reperfusion injury. *Shock* 79–88

74   Cheung P-Y, Sawicki G, Wozniak M, Wang W, Radomski M, Schulz R (2000) Matrix metalloproteinase-2 contributes to ischemia-reperfusion injury in the heart. *Circulation* 101: 1833–1839

Nitric oxide and myocarditis

Charles J. Lowenstein and Tomokazu Ohnishi

Division of Cardiology, Department of Medicine, The Johns Hopkins University School of Medicine, 720 Rutland Ave., Baltimore, MD 21205, USA

Introduction

Myocarditis is an inflammatory disease of the heart, usually caused by viral infection. The clinical course of patients with myocarditis is paradoxical. The survival of patients with mild forms of myocarditis is much worse than the survival of patients with severe, fulminant myocarditis. One hypothesis explaining this paradox involves nitric oxide (NO). Perhaps myocarditic patients who produce large amounts of NO clear their viral infections and so survive longer, although they suffer from hemodynamic instability due to excess NO. Conversely, myocarditic patients who generate less NO are hemodynamically stable, but less NO permits greater levels of viral replication, leading to a higher mortality. This review examines the role of NO in myocarditis, focusing on viral myocarditis.

Myocarditis

Although myocarditis is diagnosed in fewer than 5000 patients each year, the true incidence of myocarditis may be much greater. Most cases of idiopathic dilated cardiomyopathy are presumed to be caused by undiagnosed myocarditis [1]. Approximately 5 million people in the United States have dilated cardiomyopathy, and the etiology of up to 30% of dilated cardiomyopathies is never discovered. Subacute myocarditis may be much more common than is suspected; a recent small study reported that 66% of patients with non-structural atrial fibrillation had myocarditis [2].

The two criteria for myocarditis, as defined by a working group of pathologists in Dallas in 1973, are an inflammatory infiltrate and myocyte necrosis [3]. However, the histological severity of myocarditis from endomyocardial biopsy does not correlate well with the clinical course of patients with myocarditis [4–7]. Patients with acute myocarditis have an indistinct onset of myocarditis and are hemodynamically stable. Patients with fulminant myocarditis have a recent distinct onset

Nitric Oxide and Inflammation, edited by Daniela Salvemini, Timothy R. Billiar and Yoram Vodovotz

and are hemodynamically unstable, requiring high doses of vasopressors or left ventricular assist devices. Surprisingly, patients with fulminant myocarditis have an excellent long-term prognosis, in contrast to patients with acute myocarditis, who have a much more dismal prognosis. One study showed that 93% of patients with fulminant myocarditis are alive after 11 years, whereas only 45% of patients with acute myocarditis survive after 11 years [6]. The surprising difference in survival rates may be explained by the nature of the immune response to myocarditis.

The inflammatory infiltrate in the hearts of patients with myocarditis consists of macrophages, natural killer cells, and lymphocytes. The nature of the infiltrating cells, and the activation of these cells, depends in part upon the cause of the myocarditis. Myocarditis can be caused by allergic reactions, drugs, and toxins, but the most common causes of myocarditis are infections, such as bacteria, viruses, fungi, and parasites [1]. Activation of immune cells by infections leads to two immune responses: the innate immune response, an early, rapid, but non-specific response; and the adaptive immune response, a slower but more specific response [8]. One of the components of the innate immune response is the synthesis of nitric oxide [9, 10].

Nitric oxide in viral myocarditis

The most common cause of myocarditis is viral myocarditis. A variety of viruses cause myocarditis, including CMV, EBV, HSV, HIV, and CV (Tab. 1). However, more than 50% of all viral myocarditis is caused by Coxsackievirus (CVB) [11].

Nitric oxide plays a critical role in the host response to viral myocarditis as an anti-viral effector of the innate immune system [10, 12–15]. Nathan and Croen first showed that NO can suppress the replication of HSV and ectromelia virus *in vitro* [16, 17]. Subsequently, a variety of other viruses were shown to induce the inducible nitric oxide synthase (iNOS, or NOS2) in various animals (Tab. 2). NO produced by NOS2 can inhibit viral replication in cells and in animals (Tab. 2) [18–39]. However, further work showed that NO does not inhibit replication of all viruses. In fact, excess NO can be detrimental to the infected host, especially when the virus is resistant to NO [40].

Animal models have been instrumental in understanding the pathogenesis of viral myocarditis. Coxsackievirus B3 (CVB3) causes an acute myocarditis in mice, characterized by viremia between 1–3 days and myocarditis between 5–7 days after infection [41]. Macrophages and natural killer cells, key effector cells of the innate immune response, are necessary to the host response to CVB3. Gaunitt and colleagues showed that inhibition of natural killer cells leads to massive myocyte necrosis and dystrophic calcification of the myocardium [42–44].

Our laboratory and several others have used this murine model to study the role of NO in viral myocarditis [23, 27, 30, 45–56]. Viral infections induce NOS2 in

Table 1 - Causes of myocarditis

Infections	Virus
	Bacteria
	Fungus
	Parasites
Autoimmune	
Drugs	
Toxins	
Eosinophilic	
Giant cell myocarditis	

Table 2 - Viruses that cause myocarditis

Virus	Infection induces NOS2	NO inhibits replication
Coxsackievirus	Yes	Yes
Poliovirus		Yes
Encephalomyocarditis virus		Yes
Cytomegalovirus	Yes	Yes
Varicella zoster virus	Yes	Yes
Epstein-Barr virus	Yes	Yes
Adenovirus		Yes
Arbovirus		
Echovirus		
Rubella virus		
Vaccinia virus		Yes
Respiratory syncytial virus		
Rabies		
Influenza A	Yes	No
Human immunodeficiency virus	Yes	No

infiltrating macrophages 5 days after infection. Although cardiac myocytes can be induced to express NOS2 *in vitro*, cardiac myocytes do not appear to express NOS2 during viral myocarditis. NOS2 levels increase between 5–7 days, and then decrease between 7–15 days after infection.

NO appears to play a critical role in decreasing viral replication in viral myocarditis. Administration of NOS inhibitors such as aminoguanidine to infected animals increases viral titers [30, 46]. Our laboratory showed that Coxsackievirus infection of wild-type mice was limited; in contrast, Coxsackievirus replicated 100-fold more in the hearts of mice that lack the NOS2 alleles [50]. Mice that lack NOS2 also had much more severe histological grades of myocarditis than wild-type mice. Wild-type mice had discrete foci of inflammation scattered throughout the myocardium. In contrast, mice lacking NOS2 had massive areas of myocyte necrosis and dystrophic calcification. These studies suggest that NO plays an important role in the innate immune response to viral myocarditis.

Since NO inhibits the replication of so many different families of viruses, the viral targets of NO are diverse. The precise mechanisms by which NO inhibits viral replication are unclear. Recently, our laboratory identified one of the Coxsackievirus targets of NO [23]. Coxsackieviruses have a single RNA positive-strand genome. After the RNA genome is translated into one large polyprotein, two viral proteases within the polyprotein cleave the polyprotein into its distinct viral polypeptides. These two viral proteases, 2A^{pro} and 3C^{pro}, are cysteine proteases. NO inhibits 3C^{pro} (and probably 2A^{pro} as well), nitrosylating the active site cysteine, inhibiting proteolysis of the large viral polyprotein, and thereby inhibiting viral replication. However, other viral targets of NO may exist as well (Fig. 1).

In summary, NOS2 and NO play a critical role in the host defense against viral myocarditis.

Nitric oxide in bacterial myocarditis

A variety of bacteria can cause myocarditis, including *streptococcus, staphylococcus, pneumococcus, meningococcus, haemophilus, diphtheria, salmonella,* and *tuberculosis* [1]. NO can inhibit the growth of intracellular bacteria such as *Salmonella* and *Mycobacterium tuberculosis* [57–59]. Furthermore, NO also plays a role in the host response to extracellular bacteria such as *Staphylococcus* [60–64]. Unfortunately, bacterial myocarditis is not well studied: bacterial myocarditis is rare, and there are no case reports of NOS2 expression in human bacterial myocarditis. Furthermore, there are no established animal models of bacterial myocarditis. Although there are no data to support this hypothesis, it is theoretically possible that NO plays a role in the host response to bacterial infection of the heart.

Nitric oxide in parasitic myocarditis

Chagas' disease is caused by *Trypanosoma cruzi*, which infects more than 20 million people in Central and South America [65]. Infection with *T. cruzi* is the most common cause of cardiomyopathy and cardiac death in South America. The natural history of Chagas' disease includes acute, latent, and chronic phases. Acute *T.*

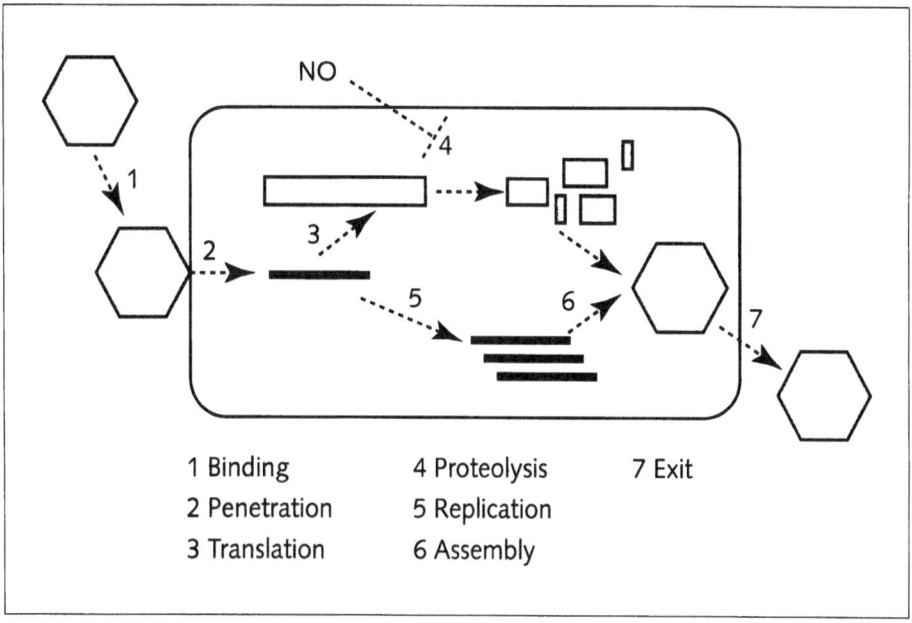

Figure 1
NO Inhibition of Coxsackievirus replication. Nitric oxide synthesized by NOS2 inhibits viral protease activity, blocking processing of the viral polyprotein into polypeptides, thereby inhibiting viral replication.

cruzi infection causes fever, hepatosplenomegaly, and rarely causes acute myocarditis. Parasites are present in the myocardium, provoking an intense inflammatory infiltrate. After the acute infection resolves, the disease enters a latent phase. Chronic Chagas' disease is highly variable, developing in 30–70% of patients within 10–50 years after infection. Chronic Chagas' disease is characterized by focal fibrosis and inflammatory infiltrates of the gastrointestinal tract and most commonly the heart. However, parasites are absent from the heart, suggesting that an autoimmune response may play a role in Chagas' myocarditis.

NO is a component of the host response to *T. cruzi* infection. Acute *T. cruzi* infection induces NOS2 expression in macrophages *in vitro* [66–68]. Monocytes activated with IFNγ and TNFα can destroy the parasite in cultured cells, and L-NMMA inhibits parasite killing [69–71]. NO donors can also inhibit parasite replication *in vitro* [72, 73]. *T. cruzi* infection of mice induces NOS expression and NO levels in the serum and myocardium [72–75]. *T. cruzi* replication is increased in mice in the presence of NOS inhibitors [66, 73]. Finally, mice lacking NOS2 have much higher mortality rates from *T. cruzi* infection than wild-type mice [76].

Serum nitrate levels are higher in patients infected with *T. cruzi* than in controls [77]. Although it has not been shown that NO plays a role in the human immune response to *T. cruzi*, it is interesting to note that the only drugs used to treat *T. cruzi*, Nifurtimox and Benznidamol, are compounds that contain nitro groups. Nifurtimox reduces parasitemia and mortality during the acute phase of Chagas' disease. Although the mechanisms of these drugs are unknown, it is possible that they act in part by generating reactive nitrogen intermediates.

Other protozoa can cause myocarditis. *T. gambiense* and *T. rhodiense* cause African trypanosomiasis, which can lead to a myocarditis [65]. *Toxoplasma gondii* infection can lead to cysts in the brain and the heart. NO may protect the host against infection by these trypanosomes as it does against *T. cruzi* [78–81]. Immunosuppression in infected patients can lead to disseminated infection with severe myocarditis. Perhaps inhibition of nitric oxide plays a role in reactivation of toxoplasmosis.

Metazoan infections rarely cause myocarditis. Echinococcosis can cause cardiac cysts in approximately 1%. *Trichinella spiralis*, the metazoa causing trichinosis, is rarely present in the heart, and the mild myocarditis that can occur is thought to be mediated by an autoimmune host response. The role of NO in these rare cases of myocarditis is also unknown.

Nitric oxide in autoimmune myocarditis

Micro-organisms are rarely identified in the myocardium of patients with myocarditis. When systemic manifestations of an infection are absent, and serological studies of viral infections are negative, it is often assumed that myocarditis is caused by an autoimmune response. Human autoimmune myocarditis is characterized by an inflammatory infiltrate in the myocardium, autoantibodies, and the absence of an identifiable pathogen.

NOS2 is expressed in the hearts of patients with myocarditis [82, 83], and also in the myocardium of patients with dilated cardiomyopathy [83–88]. However, little is known about the mechanisms that lead to induction of NOS2 in human myocarditis, and less is known about the role that NOS2 and NO plays in human cardiomyopathies.

Rodent models have been used to explore the pathogenesis of autoimmune myocarditis. In experimental autoimmune myocarditis, rodents are immunized with purified cardiac myosin. An autoimmune myocarditis develops within 14–28 days, characterized by an inflammatory infiltrate into the myocardium, cardiac myocyte necrosis, and autoantibodies against cardiac antigens, including myosin and the mitochondrial adenine nucleotide transporter.

The role of NO in experimental autoimmune diseases is controversial. Many studies confirm that NOS2 is induced in autoimmune myocarditis [89–93]. NOS2 activity is increased 14 days after immunization, and continues for at least another 14 days [93]. NOS2 is localized in macrophages and cardiac myocytes [89, 91, 93, 94]. Some studies show that NO damages tissue; administration of drugs that inhibit NOS2 or decrease NO production also decrease inflammation and necrosis [89, 91–93]. However, the severity of myocarditis is similar in wild-type mice that express NOS2 and in interferon-regulatory factor-1 (IRF-1) null mice that do not express NOS2 [94]. Although the reasons for this striking discrepancy are unclear, one possibility is that NOS inhibition may have other effects besides NOS2 inhibition. Another possibility is that IRF-1 regulates cardiotoxic pathways other than NOS2.

Nitric oxide in non-infectious myocarditis

The role of NO in myocarditis due to other causes is unclear. Various drugs and toxins can cause myocarditis. Some drugs cause a hypersensitivity reaction, characterized by an eosinophillic infiltrate in the myocardium. Drugs causing hypersensitivity myocarditis include antibiotics (amphotericin B, ampicillin, chloramphenicol, isoniazid, penicillin, streptomycin), anti-hypertensives (hydrochlorothiazide, methyldopa), and anti-psychotics (amitryptiline, carbamezapine, phenytoin). Other compounds can cause myocarditis without eosinophils. Toxins that cause myocarditis include chemotherapeutic agents (adriamycin, cyclophosphamide, fluorouracil), arsenic compounds, paraquat, and cocaine. However, the role of NO in drug and toxin induced myocarditis in unclear.

Giant cell myocarditis is an unusual myocarditis of unknown cause [95, 96]. The hallmark of giant cell myocarditis is multi-nucleated giant cells. Although the identity of the giant cell is unclear, giant cells express monocyte markers. Since activated macrophages can express NOS2 and produce NO, it is possible that giant cells are sources of NO in the myocardium. However, the role NO plays in giant cell myocarditis is unknown.

Nitric oxide and myocardial function

All isoforms of NOS have been identified in the heart. The endothelial NOS (eNOS, or NOS3) is expressed in endothelial cells and cardiac myocytes [97]. The neuronal NOS (nNOS, or NOS1) is located in the sarcoplasmic reticulum of cardiac myocytes [98]. NOS2 is normally absent from the heart, but infectious or autoimmune myocarditis can induce its expression. Since NOS2 is a high-output isoform capable of generating large amounts of NO continuously, myocarditis may lead to higher than normal concentrations of NO within the heart. However, NO has many effects upon cardiac function, so the over-all effect of NO on cardiac function in myocarditis is unclear.

- *NO and vasodilation*

  Excess NO derived from NOS can directly relax vascular smooth muscle, leading to vasodilation. Although an increase in coronary artery blood flow may be beneficial, NOS2 expression and NO production in the heart may also increase vascular permeability, leading to myocardial edema and increased ventricular stiffness [99].

- *NO and cardiac contractility*

  NO can depress cardiac function. Cytokine treatment of isolated strips of cardiac muscle decreases cardiac contractility [100]. Contractility is partially restored with NOS inhibitors. Thus in myocarditis, NO may cause transient left ventricular dysfunction that resolves when inflammation decreases. However, in low concentrations, NO can actually increase cardiac contractility. For example, low doses of NO increase cardiac contractility [101]. NO can also increase myocyte calcium levels by activating L-type calcium release channels and inhibiting the sarcoplasmic reticulum calcium re-uptake channels, which in turn would augment cardiac contractility [102, 103].

- *NO and oxygen consumption*

  NO may plays a protective role in myocarditis as well. NO regulates mitochondria, decreasing mitochondrial respiration and oxygen consumption [104–109]. Furthermore, NO regulates the metabolism of cardiac myocytes, altering the metabolism of glucose and fatty acids [106].

- *NO and apoptosis*

  Apoptotic cardiac myocytes have been identified in human dilated cardiomyopathies, and may occur in myocarditis as well. NO at low concentrations can inhibit apoptosis, in part by inhibition of capspases [110–112]. NOS expression may therefore attenuate apoptotic death in myocarditis.

- *NO and cytotoxicity*

  Several studies suggest that NO contributes to the destruction of cardiac myocytes in myocarditis [89, 91–93]. NO at high concentrations can damage cells, altering protein function by S-nitrosylation, combining with superoxide to form peroxynitrite and other nitrogen oxides which can damage DNA, alter mitochondrial function, disrupt iron-sulfur centers, and deplete glutathione [113].

Thus in addition to its anti-viral properties, NO has many complex effects upon cardiac function, improving cardiac blood flow, protecting cardiac myocytes from apoptosis, regulating myocardial metabolism and decreasing cardiac contractility.

Summary

The role of NO is well established in infectious myocarditis in animals. Infections induce NOS2 expression in inflammatory cells and possibly in cardiac myocytes.

NO then inhibits the replication of pathogens. The role of NO in non-infectious myocarditis is less clear.

NO may have other effects in myocarditis, in addition to inhibiting pathogens. NO at low doses may protect the heart, increasing contractility, decreasing myocardial energy requirements, and blocking apoptosis. However, high levels of NOS2 may lead to excessive concentrations of NO in myocarditis, decreasing cardiac contractility, and directly damaging cells.

NO has not been shown to play a role in human myocarditis. However, production of high concentrations of NO may play an important role in fulminant myocarditis, inhibiting viral replication, but also causing severe hemodynamic instability. In contrast, patients with acute myocarditis may produce less NO, not suppressing cardiac contractility, but also not completely clearing their viral burden. A difference in NO production, in addition to other factors, may account for the excellent prognosis of fulminant myocarditis and the poor prognosis of acute myocarditis.

Acknowledgments

This work was supported in part by grants including NIH P50 HL52315 (CJL), NIH R01 HL5361 (CJL), NIH R01 HL63706 (CJL), and the Ciccarone Center for the Prevention of Heart Disease (CJL).

References

1   Wynne J (1997) The cardiomyopathies and myocarditis. In: ES Braunwald (ed): *Heart disease: a textbook of cardiovascular disease*. 5 ed. WB Saunders, Philadephia 1404–1463

2   Frustaci A, Chimenti C, Bellocci F, Morgante E, Russo MA, Maseri A (1997) Histological substrate of atrial biopsies in patients with lone atrial fibrillation. *Circulation* 96: 1180–1184

3   Aretz HT, Billingham ME, Edwards WD, Factor SM, Fallon JT, Fenoglio JJ Jr, Olsen EG, Schoen FJ (1987) Myocarditis. A histopathologic definition and classification. *Am J Cardiovasc Pathol* 1: 3–14

4   Felker GM, Boehmer JP, Hruban RH, Hutchins GM, Kasper EK, Baughman KL, Hare JM (2000) Echocardiographic findings in fulminant and acute myocarditis. *J Am Coll Cardiol* 36: 227–232

5   Felker GM, Thompson RE, Hare JM, Hruban RH, Clemetson DE, Howard DL, Baughman KL, Kasper EK (2000) Underlying causes and long-term survival in patients with initially unexplained cardiomyopathy. *N Engl J Med* 342: 1077–1084

6   McCarthy RE 3rd, Boehmer JP, Hruban RH, Hutchins GM, Kasper EK, Hare JM,

Baughman KL (2000) Long-term outcome of fulminant myocarditis as compared with acute (nonfulminant) myocarditis. *N Engl J Med* 342: 690–695

7   Felker GM, Hu W, Hare JM, Hruban RH, Baughman KL, Kasper EK (1999) The spectrum of dilated cardiomyopathy. The Johns Hopkins experience with 1,278 patients. *Medicine* (Baltimore) 78: 270–283

8   Medzhitov R, Janeway C Jr (2000) Innate immune recognition: mechanisms and pathways. *Immunol Rev* 173: 89–97

9   Bogdan C, Rollinghoff M, Diefenbach A (2000) The role of nitric oxide in innate immunity. *Immunol Rev* 173: 17–26

10 MacMicking J, Xie QW, Nathan C (1997) Nitric oxide and macrophage function. *Annu Rev Immunol* 15: 323–250

11 Woodruff JF (1980) Viral myocarditis. A review. *Am J Pathol* 101: 425–484

12 Mannick JB (1995) The antiviral role of nitric oxide. *Res Immunol* 146: 693–697

13 Powell KL, Baylis SA (1995) The antiviral effects of nitric oxide. *Trends Microbiol* 3: 81–2

14 Bogdan C (1997) Of microbes, macrophages and nitric oxide. *Behring Inst Mitt* 99: 58–72

15 Reiss CS, Komatsu T (1998) Does nitric oxide play a critical role in viral infections? *J Virol* 72: 4547–4551

16 Karupiah G, Xie QW, Buller RM, Nathan C, Duarte C, MacMicking JD (1993) Inhibition of viral replication by interferon-gamma-induced nitric oxide synthase. *Science* 261: 1445–1448

17 Croen KD 8 (1993) Evidence for antiviral effect of nitric oxide. Inhibition of herpes simplex virus type 1 replication. *J Clin Invest* 91: 2446–2452

18 Xing Z, Schat KA (2000) Inhibitory effects of nitric oxide and gamma interferon on *in vitro* and *in vivo* replication of Marek's disease virus. *J Virol* 74: 3605–3612

19 Rimmelzwaan GF, Baars MM, de Lijster P, Fouchier RA, Osterhaus AD (1999) Inhibition of influenza virus replication by nitric oxide. *J Virol* 73: 8880–8883

20 Hirasawa K, Jun HS, Han HS, Zhang ML, Hollenberg MD, Yoon JW (1999) Prevention of encephalomyocarditis virus-induced diabetes in mice by inhibition of the tyrosine kinase signalling pathway and subsequent suppression of nitric oxide production in macrophages. *J Virol* 73: 8541–8548

21 Lane TE, Fox HS, Buchmeier MJ (1999) Inhibition of nitric oxide synthase-2 reduces the severity of mouse hepatitis virus-induced demyelination: implications for NOS2/NO regulation of chemokine expression and inflammation. *J Neurovirol* 5: 48–54

22 Kodukula P, Liu T, Rooijen NV, Jager MJ, Hendricks RL (1999) Macrophage control of herpes simplex virus type 1 replication in the peripheral nervous system. *J Immunol* 162: 2895–2905

23 Saura M, Zaragoza C, McMillan A, Quick RA, Hohenadl C, Lowenstein JM, Lowenstein CJ (1999) An antiviral mechanism of nitric oxide: inhibition of a viral protease. *Immunity* 10: 21–28

24 Fujioka N, Akazawa R, Ohashi K, Fujii M, Ikeda M, Kurimoto M (1999) Interleukin-

18 protects mice against acute herpes simplex virus type 1 infection. *J Virol* 73: 2401–2409

25 Pope M, Marsden PA, Cole E, Sloan S, Fung LS, Ning Q, Ding JW, Leibowitz JL, Phillips MJ, Levy GA (1998) Resistance to murine hepatitis virus strain 3 is dependent on production of nitric oxide. *J Virol* 72: 7084–7090

26 MacLean A, Wei XQ, Huang FP, Al-Alem UA, Chan WL, Liew FY (1998) Mice lacking inducible nitric-oxide synthase are more susceptible to herpes simplex virus infection despite enhanced Th1 cell responses. *J Gen Virol* 79: 825–830

27 Zaragoza C, Ocampo CJ, Saura M, McMillan A, Lowenstein CJ (1997) Nitric oxide inhibition of coxsackievirus replication *in vitro*. *J Clin Invest* 100: 1760–1767

28 Lin YL, Huang YL, Ma SH, Yeh CT, Chiou SY, Chen LK, Liao CL (1997) Inhibition of Japanese encephalitis virus infection by nitric oxide: antiviral effect of nitric oxide on RNA virus replication. *J Virol* 71: 5227–5235

29 Adler H, Beland JL, Del-Pan NC, Kobzik L, Brewer JP, Martin TR, Rimm IJ (1997) Suppression of herpes simplex virus type 1 (HSV-1)-induced pneumonia in mice by inhibition of inducible nitric oxide synthase (iNOS, NOS2). *J Exp Med* 185: 1533–1540

30 Hiraoka Y, Kishimoto C, Takada H, Nakamura M, Kurokawa M, Ochiai H, Shiraki K (1996) Nitric oxide and murine coxsackievirus B3 myocarditis: aggravation of myocarditis by inhibition of nitric oxide synthase. *J Am Coll Cardiol* 28: 1610–1615

31 Tucker PC, Griffin DE, Choi S, Bui N, Wesselingh S (1996) Inhibition of nitric oxide synthesis increases mortality in Sindbis virus encephalitis. *J Virol* 70: 3972–3927

32 Pertile TL, Karaca K, Sharma JM, Walser MM (1996) An antiviral effect of nitric oxide: inhibition of reovirus replication. *Avian Dis* 40: 342–348

33 Melkova Z, Esteban M (1995) Inhibition of vaccinia virus DNA replication by inducible expression of nitric oxide synthase. *J Immunol* 155: 5711–5718

34 Akarid K, Sinet M, Desforges B, Gougerot-Pocidalo MA (1995) Inhibitory effect of nitric oxide on the replication of a murine retrovirus *in vitro* and *in vivo*. *J Virol* 69: 7001–7005

35 Karupiah G, Harris N. Inhibition of viral replication by nitric oxide and its reversal by ferrous sulfate and tricarboxylic acid cycle metabolites. *J Exp Med* 1995 181: 2171–2179

36 Bi Z, Reiss CS (1995) Inhibition of vesicular stomatitis virus infection by nitric oxide. *J Virol* 69: 2208–2213

37 Harris N, Buller RM, Karupiah G (1995) Gamma interferon-induced, nitric oxide-mediated inhibition of vaccinia virus replication. *J Virol* 69: 910–915

38 Mannick JB, Stamler JS, Teng E, Simpson N, Lawrence J, Jordan J, Finberg RW (1999) Nitric oxide modulates HIV-1 replication. *J Acquir Immune Defic Syndr* 22: 1–9

39 Mannick JB, Asano K, Izumi K, Kieff E, Stamler JS (1994) Nitric oxide produced by human B lymphocytes inhibits apoptosis and Epstein-Barr virus reactivation. *Cell* 79: 1137–1146

40 Karupiah G, Chen JH, Mahalingam S, Nathan CF, MacMicking JD (1998) Rapid inter-

feron gamma-dependent clearance of influenza A virus and protection from consolidating pneumonitis in nitric oxide synthase 2-deficient mice. *J Exp Med* 188: 1541–1546

41 Herskowitz A, Wolfgram LJ, Rose NR, Beisel KW (1987) Coxsackievirus B3 murine myocarditis: a pathologic spectrum of myocarditis in genetically defined inbred strains. *J Am Coll Cardiol* 9: 1311–1319

42 Gauntt CJ, Godeny EK, Lutton CW, Fernandes G (1989) Role of natural killer cells in experimental murine myocarditis. *Springer Semin Immunopathol* 11: 51–59

43 Godeny EK, Gauntt CJ (1987) Murine natural killer cells limit coxsackievirus B3 replication. *J Immunol* 139: 913–918

44 Godeny EK, Gauntt CJ (1986) Involvement of natural killer cells in coxsackievirus B3-induced murine myocarditis. *J Immunol* 137: 1695–1702

45 Liu P, Penninger J, Aitken K, Sole M, Mak T (1995) The role of transgenic knockout models in defining the pathogenesis of viral heart disease. *Eur Heart J* 16 (Suppl O): 25–27

46 Lowenstein CJ, Hill SL, Lafond-Walker A, Wu J, Allen G, Landavere M, Rose NR, Herskowitz A (1996) Nitric oxide inhibits viral replication in murine myocarditis. *J Clin Invest* 97: 1837–1843

47 Mikami S, Kawashima S, Kanazawa K, Hirata K, Katayama Y, Hotta H, Hayashi Y, Ito H, Yokoyama M (1996) Expression of nitric oxide synthase in a murine model of viral myocarditis induced by coxsackievirus B3. *Biochem Biophys Res Commun* 220: 983–989

48 Zhang H, Bevan A, Inniss H, Archard LC, Robinson NM, Debelder A, Martin JF, Charles IG, Moncada S (1997) Differential expression of inducible nitric oxide synthase in murine myocardium infected with wildtype or attenuated Coxsackievirus B3. *Biochem Soc Trans* 25: 415S

49 Colston JT, Chandrasekar B, Freeman GL (1998) Expression of apoptosis-related proteins in experimental coxsackievirus myocarditis. *Cardiovasc Res* 38: 158–168

50 Zaragoza C, Ocampo C, Saura M, Leppo M, Wei XQ, Quick R, Moncada S, Liew FY, Lowenstein CJ (1998) The role of inducible nitric oxide synthase in the host response to Coxsackievirus myocarditis. *Proc Natl Acad Sci USA* 95: 2469–2474

51 Barbaro G, Di Lorenzo G, Soldini M, Giancaspro G, Grisorio B, Pellicelli A, Barbarini G (1999) Intensity of myocardial expression of inducible nitric oxide synthase influences the clinical course of human immunodeficiency virus-associated cardiomyopathy. Gruppo Italiano per lo Studio Cardiologico dei pazienti affetti da AIDS (GISCA). *Circulation* 100: 933–939

52 Horwitz MS, Krahl T, Fine C, Lee J, Sarvetnick N (1999) Protection from lethal coxsackievirus-induced pancreatitis by expression of gamma interferon. *J Virol* 73: 1756–1766

53 Robinson NM, Zhang HY, Bevan AL, De Belder AJ, Moncada S, Martin JF, Archard LC (1999) Induction of myocardial nitric oxide synthase by Coxsackie B3 virus in mice. *Eur J Clin Invest* 29: 700–7

54 Zaragoza C, Ocampo CJ, Saura M, Bao C, Leppo M, Lafond-Walker A, Thiemann DR,

Hruban R, Lowenstein CJ (1999) Inducible nitric oxide synthase protection against cox-sackievirus pancreatitis. *J Immunol* 163: 5497–5504

55   Gluck B, Merkle I, Dornberger G, Stelzner A (2000) Expression of inducible nitric oxide synthase in experimental viral myocarditis. *Herz* 25: 255–260

56   Roivainen M, Rasilainen S, Ylipaasto P, Nissinen R, Ustinov J, Bouwens L, Eizirik DL, Hovi T, Otonkoski T (2000) Mechanisms of coxsackievirus-induced damage to human pancreatic beta-cells. *J Clin Endocrinol Metab* 85: 432–440

57   De Groote MA, Granger D, Xu Y, Campbell G, Prince R, Fang FC (1995) Genetic and redox determinants of nitric oxide cytotoxicity in a *Salmonella typhimurium* model. *Proc Natl Acad Sci USA* 92: 6399–6403

58   MacMicking JD, North RJ, LaCourse R, Mudgett JS, Shah SK, Nathan CF (1997) Iden-tification of nitric oxide synthase as a protective locus against tuberculosis. *Proc Natl Acad Sci USA* 94: 5243–5248

59   Chan J, Xing Y, Magliozzo RS, Bloom BR (1992) Killing of virulent *Mycobacterium tuberculosis* by reactive nitrogen intermediates produced by activated murine macro-phages. *J Exp Med* 175: 1111–1122

60   Jang D, Williams RJ, Wang MX, Wei AQ, Murrell GA (1999) *Staphylococcus aureus* stimulates inducible nitric oxide synthase in articular cartilage. *Arthritis Rheum* 42: 2410–2417

61   McInnes IB, Leung B, Wei XQ, Gemmell CC, Liew FY (1998) Septic arthritis following *Staphylococcus aureus* infection in mice lacking inducible nitric oxide synthase. *J Immunol* 160: 308–315

62   Sasaki S, Miura T, Nishikawa S, Yamada K, Hirasue M, Nakane A (1998) Protective role of nitric oxide in *Staphylococcus aureus* infection in mice. *Infect Immun* 66: 1017–1022

63   Sakiniene E, Bremell T, Tarkowski A (1997) Inhibition of nitric oxide synthase (NOS) aggravates *Staphylococcus aureus* septicaemia and septic arthritis. *Clin Exp Immunol* 110: 370–377

64   Auguet M, Lonchampt MO, Delaflotte S, Goulin-Schulz J, Chabrier PE, Braquet P (1992) Induction of nitric oxide synthase by lipoteichoic acid from Staphylococcus aureus in vascular smooth muscle cells. *FEBS Lett* 297: 183–185

65   Kirchhoff LV (1994) Chagas' disease. In: KJ Isselbacher, E Braunwald, JD Wilson, JB Martin, AS Fauci, DL Kasper (eds): *Harrison's principles of internal medicine*. 13 ed. McGraw-Hill, New York, 176–177

66   Petray P, Rottenberg ME, Grinstein S, Orn A (1994) Release of nitric oxide during the experimental infection with *Trypanosoma cruzi*. *Parasite Immunol* 16: 193–199

67   Pakianathan DR, Kuhn RE (1994) *Trypanosoma cruzi* affects nitric oxide production by murine peritoneal macrophages. *J Parasitol* 80: 432–437

68   Rottenberg ME, Castanos-Velez E, de Mesquita R, Laguardia OG, Biberfeld P, Orn A (1996) Intracellular co-localization of *Trypanosoma cruzi* and inducible nitric oxide synthase (iNOS): evidence for dual pathway of iNOS induction. *Eur J Immunol* 26: 3203–3213

69 Abrahamsohn IA, Coffman RL (1996) *Trypanosoma cruzi*: IL-10, TNF, IFN-gamma, and IL-12 regulate innate and acquired immunity to infection. *Exp Parasitol* 84: 231–244

70 Silva JS, Vespa GN, Cardoso MA, Aliberti JC, Cunha FQ (1995) Tumor necrosis factor alpha mediates resistance to *Trypanosoma cruzi* infection in mice by inducing nitric oxide production in infected gamma interferon-activated macrophages. *Infect Immun* 63: 4862–4867

71 Munoz-Fernandez MA, Fernandez MA, Fresno M (1992) Synergism between tumor necrosis factor-alpha and interferon-gamma on macrophage activation for the killing of intracellular *Trypanosoma cruzi* through a nitric oxide-dependent mechanism. *Eur J Immunol* 22: 301–307

72 Vespa GN, Cunha FQ, Silva JS (1994) Nitric oxide is involved in control of *Trypanosoma cruzi*-induced parasitemia and directly kills the parasite *in vitro*. *Infect Immun* 62: 5177–5182

73 Petray P, Castanos-Velez E, Grinstein S, Orn A, Rottenberg ME (1995) Role of nitric oxide in resistance and histopathology during experimental infection with *Trypanosoma cruzi*. *Immunol Lett* 47: 121–126

74 Chandrasekar B, Melby PC, Troyer DA, Freeman GL (2000) Differential regulation of nitric oxide synthase isoforms in experimental acute chagasic cardiomyopathy. *Clin Exp Immunol* 121: 112–119

75 Huang H, Chan J, Wittner M, Jelicks LA, Morris SA, Factor SM, Weiss LM, Braunstein VL, Bacchi CJ, Yarlett N et al (1999) Expression of cardiac cytokines and inducible form of nitric oxide synthase (NOS2) in *Trypanosoma cruzi*-infected mice. *J Mol Cell Cardiol* 31: 75–88

76 Holscher C, Kohler G, Muller U, Mossmann H, Schaub GA, Brombacher F (1998) Defective nitric oxide effector functions lead to extreme susceptibility of *Trypanosoma cruzi*-infected mice deficient in gamma interferon receptor or inducible nitric oxide synthase. *Infect Immun* 66: 1208–1215

77 Perez-Fuentes R, Sanchez-Guillen MC, Gonzalez-Alvarez C, Monteon VM, Reyes PA, Rosales-Encina JL (1998) Humoral nitric oxide levels and antibody immune response of symptomatic and indeterminate Chagas' disease patients to commercial and autochthonous Trypanosoma cruzi antigen. *Am J Trop Med Hyg* 58: 715–720

78 Schluter D, Deckert-Schluter M, Lorenz E, Meyer T, Rollinghoff M, Bogdan C (1999) Inhibition of inducible nitric oxide synthase exacerbates chronic cerebral toxoplasmosis in *Toxoplasma gondii*-susceptible C57BL/6 mice but does not reactivate the latent disease in *T. gondii*-resistant BALB/c mice. *J Immunol* 162: 3512–3518

79 Hayashi S, Chan CC, Gazzinelli RT, Pham NT, Cheung MK, Roberge FG (1996) Protective role of nitric oxide in ocular toxoplasmosis. *Br J Ophthalmol* 80: 644–648

80 Hayashi S, Chan CC, Gazzinelli R, Roberge FG (1996) Contribution of nitric oxide to the host parasite equilibrium in toxoplasmosis. *J Immunol* 156: 1476–1481

81 Candolfi E, Villard O, Thouvenin M, Kien TT (1996) Role of nitric oxide-induced

immune suppression in toxoplasmosis during pregnancy and in infection by a virulent strain of *Toxoplasma gondii*. *Curr Top Microbiol Immunol* 219: 141–154

82   Kooy NW, Lewis SJ, Royall JA, Ye YZ, Kelly DR, Beckman JS (1997) Extensive tyrosine nitration in human myocardial inflammation: evidence for the presence of peroxynitrite. *Crit Care Med* 25: 812–819

83   de Belder AJ, Radomski MW, Why HJ, Richardson PJ, Martin JF (1995) Myocardial calcium-independent nitric oxide synthase activity is present in dilated cardiomyopathy, myocarditis, and postpartum cardiomyopathy but not in ischaemic or valvar heart disease. *Br Heart J* 74: 426–430

84   Haywood GA, Tsao PS, von der Leyen HE, Mann MJ, Keeling PJ, Trindade PT, Lewis NP, Byrne CD, Rickenbacher PR, Bishopric NH et al (1996) Expression of inducible nitric oxide synthase in human heart failure. *Circulation* 93: 1087–1094

85   Thoenes M, Forstermann U, Tracey WR, Bleese NM, Nussler AK, Scholz H, Stein B (1996) Expression of inducible nitric oxide synthase in failing and non-failing human heart. *J Mol Cell Cardiol* 28: 165–169

86   Winlaw DS, Smythe GA, Keogh AM, Schyvens CG, Spratt PM, Macdonald PS (1994) Increased nitric oxide production in heart failure. *Lancet* 344: 373–374

87   de Belder AJ, Radomski MW, Why HJ, Richardson PJ, Bucknall CA, Salas E, Martin JF, Moncada S (1993) Nitric oxide synthase activities in human myocardium. *Lancet* 341: 84–85

88   Fukuchi M, Hussain SN, Giaid A (1998) Heterogeneous expression and activity of endothelial and inducible nitric oxide synthases in end-stage human heart failure: their relation to lesion site and beta-adrenergic receptor therapy. *Circulation* 98: 132–139

89   Ishiyama S, Hiroe M, Nishikawa T, Shimojo T, Hosokawa T, Ikeda I, Toyozaki T, Kasajima T, Marumo F (1999) Inhibitory effects of vesnarinone in the progression of myocardial damage in experimental autoimmune myocarditis in rats. *Cardiovasc Res* 43: 389–397

90   Goren N, Leiros CP, Sterin-Borda L, Borda E (1998) Nitric oxide synthase in experimental autoimmune myocarditis dysfunction. *J Mol Cell Cardiol* 30: 2467–2474

91   Shin T, Tanuma N, Kim S, Jin J, Moon C, Kim K, Kohyama K, Matsumoto Y, Hyun B (1998) An inhibitor of inducible nitric oxide synthase ameliorates experimental autoimmune myocarditis in Lewis rats. *J Neuroimmunol* 92: 133–138

92   Ishiyama S, Hiroe M, Nishikawa T, Abe S, Shimojo T, Ito H, Ozasa S, Yamakawa K, Matsuzaki M, Mohammed MU et al (1997) Nitric oxide contributes to the progression of myocardial damage in experimental autoimmune myocarditis in rats. *Circulation* 95: 489–496

93   Hirono S, Islam MO, Nakazawa M, Yoshida Y, Kodama M, Shibata A, Izumi T, Imai S (1997) Expression of inducible nitric oxide synthase in rat experimental autoimmune myocarditis with special reference to changes in cardiac hemodynamics. *Circ Res* 80: 11–20

94   Bachmaier K, Neu N, Pummerer C, Duncan GS, Mak TW, Matsuyama T, Penninger JM (1997) iNOS expression and nitrotyrosine formation in the myocardium in response to

inflammation is controlled by the interferon regulatory transcription factor 1. *Circulation* 96: 585–591

95 Cooper LT Jr (2000) Giant cell myocarditis: diagnosis and treatment. *Herz* 25: 291–298

96 Cooper LT Jr, Berry GJ, Shabetai R (1997) Idiopathic giant-cell myocarditis – natural history and treatment. Multicenter Giant Cell Myocarditis Study Group Investigators. *N Engl J Med* 336: 1860–1866

97 Feron O, Belhassen L, Kobzik L, Smith TW, Kelly RA, Michel T (1996) Endothelial nitric oxide synthase targeting to caveolae. Specific interactions with caveolin isoforms in cardiac myocytes and endothelial cells. *J Biol Chem* 271: 22810–22814

98 Xu KY, Huso DL, Dawson TM, Bredt DS, Becker LC (1999) Nitric oxide synthase in cardiac sarcoplasmic reticulum. *Proc Natl Acad Sci USA* 96: 657–662

99 Skarsgard PL, Wang X, McDonald P, Lui AH, Lam EK, McManus BM, van Breemen C, Laher I (2000) Profound inhibition of myogenic tone in rat cardiac allografts is due to eNOS- and iNOS-based nitric oxide and an intrinsic defect in vascular smooth muscle contraction. *Circulation* 101: 1303–1310

100 Finkel MS, Oddis CV, Jacob TD, Watkins SC, Hattler BG, Simmons RL (1992) Negative inotropic effects of cytokines on the heart mediated by nitric oxide. *Science* 257: 387–389

101 Vila-Petroff MG, Younes A, Egan J, Lakatta EG, Sollott SJ (1999) Activation of distinct cAMP-dependent and cGMP-dependent pathways by nitric oxide in cardiac myocytes. *Circ Res* 84: 1020–1031

102 Campbell DL, Stamler JS, Strauss HC (1996) Redox modulation of L-type calcium channels in ferret ventricular myocytes. Dual mechanism regulation by nitric oxide and S-nitrosothiols. *J Gen Physiol* 108: 277–293

103 Xu L, Eu JP, Meissner G, Stamler JS (1998) Activation of the cardiac calcium release channel (ryanodine receptor) by poly-S-nitrosylation. *Science* 279: 234–237

104 Forfia PR, Hintze TH, Wolin MS, Kaley G (1999) Role of nitric oxide in the control of mitochondrial function. *Adv Exp Med Biol* 471: 381–388

105 Loke KE, Laycock SK, Mital S, Wolin MS, Bernstein R, Oz M, Addonizio L, Kaley G, Hintze TH (1999) Nitric oxide modulates mitochondrial respiration in failing human heart. *Circulation* 100: 1291–1297

106 Zhao G, Bernstein RD, Hintze TH (1999) Nitric oxide and oxygen utilization: exercise, heart failure and diabetes. *Coron Artery Dis* 10: 315–320

107 Wolin MS, Xie YW, Hintze TH (1999) Nitric oxide as a regulator of tissue oxygen consumption. *Curr Opin Nephrol Hypertens* 8: 97–103

108 Xie YW, Shen W, Zhao G, Xu X, Wolin MS, Hintze TH (1996) Role of endothelium-derived nitric oxide in the modulation of canine myocardial mitochondrial respiration *in vitro*. Implications for the development of heart failure. *Circ Res* 79: 381–387

109 Shen W, Hintze TH, Wolin MS (1995) Nitric oxide. An important signaling mechanism between vascular endothelium and parenchymal cells in the regulation of oxygen consumption. *Circulation* 92: 3505–3512

110 Dimmeler S, Haendeler J, Nehls M, Zeiher AM (1997) Suppression of apoptosis by

nitric oxide *via* inhibition of interleukin-1beta-converting enzyme (ICE)-like and cysteine protease protein (CPP)-32-like proteases. *J Exp Med* 185: 601–607

111 Li J, Billiar TR, Talanian RV, Kim YM (1997) Nitric oxide reversibly inhibits seven members of the caspase family *via* S-nitrosylation. *Biochem Biophys Res Commun* 240: 419–424

112 Mohr S, Zech B, Lapetina EG, Brune B (1997) Inhibition of caspase-3 by S-nitrosation and oxidation caused by nitric oxide. *Biochem Biophys Res Commun* 238: 387–391

113 Gow A, Foust R, Malcolm S, Gole M, Ischiropoulos H (1999) Biochemical regulation of nitric oxide cytotoxicity. In: FC Fang (ed): *Nitric oxide and infection*. Plenum Publishers, New York 180–183

Nitric oxide in shock: sepsis and hemorrhage

Carol A. McCloskey and Timothy R. Billiar

Department of Surgery, University of Pittsburgh, 676 Scaife Hall, 3550 Terrace Street, Pittsburgh, PA 15213, USA

Introduction

The past decade of nitric oxide (NO) research was highlighted by the awarding of the 1998 Nobel Prize in Physiology and Medicine to Drs. Robert Furchgott, Louis Ignarro, and Ferid Murad for their discoveries that endothelial cells synthesize nitric oxide (NO), and that endothelial derived NO regulates vascular smooth muscle relaxation. Although NO is one of the smallest synthetic products of mammalian cells, its contributions are large. Continued research in the field of NO has not only emphasized the important physiologic functions of NO, but has revealed its paradoxical role in pathophysiologic states as well.

Shock is defined as a clinical syndrome characterized by tissue perfusion that is inadequate to maintain normal metabolic functions. Two major types of shock, septic and hemorrhagic, often culminate in the final common pathway of a systemic inflammatory response (SIRS) and multiple organ failure (MOF). However, growing understanding has made it apparent that each situation involves its own specific sets of programmed responses that distinguish it from the other. Although nitric oxide is a common integral mediator in both types of shock, its overall pathophysiological role in each cannot be generalized and comparison between them has been avoided. The current knowledge of nitric oxide as it relates to both hemorrhage and sepsis will therefore be individually addressed below.

Biochemistry of nitric oxide

Nitric oxide is involved in diverse physiologic processes, including maintenance of vascular tone, neurotransmission, inhibition of platelet aggregation, and microbial killing. It is a small, uncharged, unstable free radical which readily diffuses across cell membranes. The half-life of NO is only seconds, and therefore its effect depends on the magnitude and duration of its production. Its targets include heavy metals, other radicals, and protein thiol groups. NO rapidly oxidizes in the presence of oxygen or hemoglobin to form stable, measurable end products, nitrite and nitrate. This rapid inactivation of NO by hemoglobin limits the effects of NO to the local level,

Nitric Oxide and Inflammation, edited by Daniela Salvemini, Timothy R. Billiar and Yoram Vodovotz
© 2001 Birkhäuser Verlag Basel/Switzerland

with systemic effects being the cumulative result of local action [1]. A family of enzymes known as nitric oxide synthases (NOS) stereospecifically oxidize the terminal guanidino group of the amino acid L-arginine to produce NO and citrulline. There are three known forms of synthases, each encoded by a distinct gene [2]: neuronal NOS (nNOS, NOS1), inducible NOS (iNOS, NOS2), and endothelial NOS (eNOS, NOS 3). All of the synthases are homodimers, which require the presence of the cofactors nicotinamide adenine dinucleotide phosphate (NADPH), flavin adenine dinucleotide (FAD), flavin mononucleotide (FMN), and tetrahydrobiopterin (H4B). However, they have important differences in regards to the regulation of their expression (Tab. 1). The nNOS and eNOS families are collectively named constitutive NOS (cNOS), because of their constant low level of NO production (picomolar). Their activity is tightly controlled, regulated by intracellular calcium levels. In the case of eNOS, vasoactive substances such as acetylcholine, bradykinin, and histamine bind to endothelial cells, resulting in calcium influx. Calcium binds to calmodulin, which then transiently binds to eNOS, leading to the production of NO. NO then diffuses across the cell membrane of adjacent smooth muscle cells, where it activates guanylate cyclase by binding to its heme moiety, resulting in increased cyclic GMP levels, decreased intracellular calcium levels, and ultimately leading to vasorelaxation. The constitutive production of NO by eNOS serves to regulate normal blood pressure by balancing sympathetic mediated vasoconstriction. Basal release of NO is greater in arteries than veins, and also greater in small vessels than conductance vessels. In addition, the ability of endothelial cells to convert changes in physical forces into biochemical signals allows NO production to be influenced by viscosity and flow. In the case of nNOS, excitatory amino acids stimulate neuronal production of NO, also resulting in increased levels of cyclic GMP. NO therefore has a role as a neurotransmitter in both the peripheral and central nervous systems. In contrast, iNOS is not present in unstimulated cells, and instead is synthesized *de novo* in response to immunologic and inflammatory stimuli, including TNFα, endotoxin, interferon γ (IFNγ), IL-2 and IL-1β [3]. Its regulation is calcium independent, and it is produced in much higher levels (micromolar). Virtually every cell type is able to produce it. Once stimulated, the production is sustained by calmodulin, which permanently binds to each subunit of the homodimers. The production is then limited only by the concentration of the enzyme and the substrate and cofactor availability. This can result in high levels of potentially toxic NO over sustained periods of time.

NO and sepsis

Sepsis, a systemic inflammatory response to infection, remains the leading cause of death in the ICU, with mortality ranging from 40 to 70% despite treatment [4]. The incidence is increasing, partially due to rising numbers of patients with depressed

Table 1 - Isoforms of NOS

NOS isoform	Chromosome (human)	Protein size	NO production	Subcellular localization	Tissue localization	Activated by	Function/actions
Type I (neuronal)	12	160–161 kDa (1433 aa)	Constitutive short-acting, picomolar quantities	Cytosolic, binds to specific proteins. Also particulate	Neuronal cells, Neuronal cells, adrenal medulla	Acetylcholine, bradykinin, glutamate, histamine	Cell signalling, neurotransmission
Type II (inducible)	17	130–135kDa (1144 aa)	Inducible, long lasting, micromolar quantities	Cytosolic, "nitroxysomal", peroxisomal	Macrophages, liver, lung, aorta, PMNs and others	Endotoxins, cytokines	Cytotoxicity, immuno-regulation
Type III (endothelial)	7	133–134 kDa (1200 aa)	Constitutive, short-acting, picomolar quantities	Cytosolic, membrane bound (caveolae)	Epithelial cells, endothelial cells, platelets, cardiac myocytes	Acetylcholine, bradykinin, glutamate, histamine	Cell signaling, vasomotor tone regulation

Collins J et al (2001) Biology of NO: measurement, modulation, and models. In: WW Souba, DW Wilmore (eds): *Surgical research*, Academic Press, San Diego, CA, 949–969 immune systems, including the elderly, organ transplant recipients, and AIDS patients. Clinically, patients exhibit a hyperdynamic state with tachycardia, increased cardiac output, decreased systemic vascular resistance, oliguria, and lactic acidosis [5]. This is subsequently accompanied by an overproduction of inflammatory mediators that results in hypotension refractory to vasopressors. Later, cardiac failure develops, with a corresponding fall in cardiac output, maldistribution of blood flow, tissue injury, multi-organ dysfunction, and ultimately death. The most common etiologic agent in sepsis is endotoxin secondary to gram negative organisms. However, gram positive organisms account for an increasing number of cases, in which peptidoglycan and lipoteichoic acids of the cell wall are the important mediators [6].

Serum levels of TNFα, IL-1β, IFNγ, and IL-6 have been demonstrated in patients with septic shock [7]. Administration of TNFα and IL-1β reproduces the pathologic effects of septic shock in both animals and man [8, 9]. Animals pretreated with anti-TNFα antibodies or IL-1β receptor antagonists are protected against the development of shock, but are without benefit if the same agents are given after shock has already been initiated [7, 10]. This suggests that these cytokines act by further stimulating other important mediators. There is now a substantial amount of publications regarding the role of NO in septic shock as one such mediator. It is known that the only endogenous source of nitrite/nitrate is *via* the degradation of NO [11], and elevated levels of nitrates and nitrites have been detected in the plasma of clinically septic patients with normal renal function [12]. These levels inversely correlated with systemic vascular resistance, suggesting that the overproduction of NO is at least partially responsible for the hypotension that occurs during septic shock. Another study demonstrated that plasma levels of nitrite/nitrate in critically ill trauma patients correlated with worsening sepsis, decreased vascular tone, and death [13]. Similarly, increased urinary nitrite/nitrate concentrations have also been found in septic patients [14]. Formation of a hemoglobin/NO adduct in the blood of endotoxemic rats has been detected by electron spin resonance [15]. The excess NO that is produced during septic shock is believed to be due to an initial activation of eNOS [16] followed by induction of iNOS, secondary to endotoxin, lipoteichoic acid, or proinflammatory cytokines. The specific requirement of the above factors in iNOS induction is tissue dependent, and there appears to be synergy between them. During the late phase of shock, the synthesis of NO by eNOS is impaired [17], while iNOS expression predominates [7]. IL-1β, IL-2, TNFα, IFNγ, and endotoxin have all been shown to induce NO *in vitro* [2]. Pretreatment of animals with IL-1β receptor antagonist attenuates the induction of iNOS in rats, and ameliorates the delayed hypotension and tachycardia in response to endotoxin [18]. Similarly, anti-TNFα antibodies, soluble TNFα receptor antagonist, and anti-IFNγ antibodies all demonstrate the ability to partially block LPS induced iNOS expression [19]. Initial studies demonstrated that macrophages synthesize NO in response to bacterial LPS [20]. However, increases in iNOS mRNA and protein have since been observed in a wide variety of cell types during endotoxemia, including endothelial cells, Kupffer cells, hepatocytes, vascular smooth muscle cells, kidney cells, chondrocytes, cardiac myocytes, pancreatic islets, and fibroblasts [11, 21–23]. Gram positive models of sepsis using lipoteichoic acid (LTA) alone or in combination with peptidoglycan also induce iNOS, in vascular smooth muscle cells and macrophages *in vitro*, and lung, aorta, heart, liver, pancreas, and kidney *in vivo* [24–26].

Sepsis, NO, and the cardiovascular system

Taking into account the physiologic role of NO in the maintenance of vascular tone, it is easily conceivable that overproduction of NO can contribute to the loss of systemic vascular resistance, persistent hypotension, and impaired tissue perfusion that is characteristic of sepsis. Although iNOS induction occurs in endothelial cells, the NO produced by vascular smooth muscle cell iNOS is probably the most important determinant of vasodilation and vasoplegia seen in shock. NOS inhibition in both septic patients and experimental models have demonstrated reversal of hypotension. Kilbourn et al. [27] have shown that both endotoxin and TNF induced hypotension in dogs can be reversed by the administration of the nonselective NOS inhibitor L-NMA (N^6-methyl-L-arginine). Administration of L-arginine restored the hypotension. They therefore concluded that NO mediates the hypotensive effect of TNFα. The degree of hypotension following LPS administration is also significantly less in iNOS knockout mice compared to their wildtype counterparts [28]. In a human study, Petros et al. demonstrated increased blood pressure and systemic vascular resistance in septic patients treated with N(G)-monomethyl-L-arginine (L-NMMA) or N^ω-nitro-L-arginine-methyl-ester (L-NAME) [29].

Classically, the peripheral vasodilation in septic shock is also accompanied by vascular hyporeactivity to vasopressors. *In vivo*, methylene blue, an inhibitor of NO mediated activation of guanylyl cyclase, restores vasoreactivity to norepinephrine in endotoxemic rats, suggesting a cyclic GMP dependent mechanism [30]. In addition, NO or peroxynitrite can exhibit direct, cGMP-independent effects on vascular smooth muscle, resulting in decreased contractility secondary to energy depletion, and activation of calcium dependent potassium channels and ATP-sensitive potassium channels [27]. Landin et al has shown that vascular hyporeactivity in sheep given endotoxin was restored by the administration of LNNA (N^ω-nitro-L-arginine) [31]. This was also demonstrated at the level of resistance arterioles in a rat sepsis model utilizing a nonspecific NOS inhibitor [32].

Increases in vascular permeability and edema formation have also been linked to NO. Endothelial toxicity secondary to iNOS production of NO has been demonstrated, possibly due to peroxynitrite or other free radical production [33]. NOS inhibition in a rodent model attenuates changes in vascular permeability and edema formation induced by endotoxin and proinflammatory cytokines in a variety of tissues [33].

It is now well recognized that intrinsic myocardial dysfunction also occurs during septic shock, although this is sometimes masked by the overall increased cardiac index that occurs in the hyperdynamic state. NO is among a group of other candidates, including LPS, TNFα, PAF, C5a, and COX2, which have all been implicated in contributing to the myocardial depression seen during sepsis. Under physiologic conditions, NO is thought to have a role in modulating systolic and diastolic cardiac function. It acts in the heart *via* 3 different mechanisms: altering protein kinase activity and thus L-type calcium channels, decreasing myofibril response to calcium, and decreasing cAMP *via* phosphodiesterase [34]. These are potential mechanisms by which NO may also modulate the myocardial dysfunction seen during sepsis. NO production in the heart includes iNOS expression in vascular and endocardial endothelium, cardiac myocytes, as well as eNOS in the coronary endothelium and endocardium [7]. Upon exposure to NO or cytokines which induce NO, cardiac myocytes, isolated papillary muscle, and heart preparations all show decreased contractility [35–37]. Inhibition of iNOS reverses the impaired contractility of cardiac myocytes isolated from endotoxic rats [38]. Similarly, the negative inotropic effects of cytokines on myocardial contractility were blocked with N^G-monomethyl-L-arginine (L-NMMA) which could subsequently be reversed by L-arginine administration [37]. It has also been suggested that the eventual impairment of eNOS function in cardiac microvasculature may result in vasoconstriction and platelet aggregation, leading to myocardial ischemia [7]. As cardiovascular dysfunction in sepsis is an important determinant of outcome, continued research is important in clarifying the underlying basis.

Sepsis, NO and the liver

An important component of MODS is hepatocellular damage. Elevated levels of aspartate aminotransferase, bilirubin, ornithine carbamoyltransferase, and lactate dehydrogenase appear in the bloodstream. While Kupffer cells have been shown *in vitro* to synthesize NO in response to LPS alone, hepatocyte NO production requires a combination of LPS and cytokines, including TNFα, IL-1, and IFNγ [39, 40]. In response to endotoxin, Kupffer cells release a variety of cytokines and eicosanoids in addition to nitric oxide. These products interact with adjacent hepatocytes to alter parenchymal cell function, including profoundly decreasing total protein synthesis and inhibition of mitochondrial enzymes. Although eNOS is eventually downregulated in vascular endothelium during sepsis, there is evidence for increased eNOS expression in addition to the iNOS induction in the liver following endotoxin [26]. The significance of this remains to be determined. Satoi et al. [41] report increased plasma nitrite/nitrate levels in nonsurviving septic patients compared to survivors, which correlated with decreased arterial ketone body ratios, indicative of hepatocyte mitochondrial dysfunction.

NO is speculated to play a role in the inhibition of gluconeogenesis and resulting hypoglycemia that occurs during advanced sepsis. Ruetten et al. [42] demonstrated that prevention of IκB degradation with administration of a calpain I inhibitor in a rat endotoxemic model prevents lung and liver iNOS induction as well as development of hypoglycemia. Similarly, Stadler et al. [43] observed that the inhibition of glucose output following cytokine stimulation of hepatocytes can be reversed by L-NMMA. However, others studies have failed to show an effect following NOS inhibitor administration [44] and the overall effect of NO on glucose levels is likely dependent on the specific hormonal milieu at any given time [45].

Experiments assessing the role of NO in liver injury have produced conflicting results secondary to the use of nonselective NOS inhibitors. In a *C. parvum* plus LPS murine model of endotoxic shock, a bolused dose of L-NMMA prevented NO formation, but exacerbated the endotoxin induced liver injury. Histologically, this manifested as hepatic necrosis, microinfarcts and platelet thrombi within small vessels. This suggested that vasoconstriction and clotting of microvasculature might result in local ischemia and subsequent parenchymal damage. This effect was exacerbated by aspirin, suggesting that eNOS and prostacyclins act together to maintain hepatic blood flow during sepsis [46]. A subsequent study comparing nonselective *versus* iNOS selective inhibitors administrated simultaneously with LPS has shown increased LPS induced necrosis, increased ICAM-1 expression, and increased neutrophil migration into the liver in the animals treated with the nonselective inhibitors. Delivery of exogenous NO *via* V-PYRRO/NO (O^2-vinyl-1-(pyrrolidin-1-yl)diazen-1-ium-1,2-diolate) directly to the liver prevented the adverse effects of nonselective NOS inhibitors. In the same study, specific iNOS inhibition did not affect liver necrosis, ICAM-1 expression, or neutrophil infiltration [47]. Another study in which a bolus of a selective iNOS inhibitor was administered under the conditions where NMMA exacerbated hepatic damage showed attenuation of liver injury, suggesting that iNOS, in contrast to eNOS, plays a role in the induction of hepatic damage [5]. In iNOS deficient mice, however, some liver injury does occur [28], illustrating that factors independent of iNOS may also contribute to injury. Overall, it appears that at the microcirculatory level of the liver, eNOS has a protective role in response to inflammatory stimuli, including preservation of blood flow and prevention of platelet adhesion, while excessive production of iNOS within the parenchyma is injurious.

Sepsis, NO, and the gastrointestinal system

The gastrointestinal tract is a major site of injury during septic shock [48]. Experimental LPS administration has been shown to decrease motility [49], increase both endothelial and epithelial permeability [50], and promote bacterial translocation [51]. A variety of factors have been implicated, including diminished perfusion, oxidant stress, and tissue acidosis. Recently, the contribution of NO overproduction has been examined. LPS induced iNOS expression is differentially regulated both along the crypt villus axis as well as the intestinal mucosa, being most prominent in the villus cells of the ileum [52]. Experiments assessing the effect of both specific and nonspecific NOS inhibitors on the GI tract during septic shock has revealed results that parallel those found in the liver. An increase in iNOS following *in vivo* endotoxin challenge is associated with decreased cell viability, mitochondrial dysfunction, and vasocongestion in rat small intestine. Inhibition of iNOS induction with dexamethasone or iNOS specific inhibitors attenuates the damage [53, 54]. Administration of the relatively selective iNOS inhibitor aminoguanidine significantly reduced bacterial translocation in animals following LPS administration [55]. However, pretreatment with the nonspecific inhibitor L-NMMA prevents NO formation but enhances endotoxin induced intestinal damage and plasma leakage. Co-administration of a bioactive NO adduct attenuates this damage [56]. Pretreatment with the drug NOX selectively scavenges "excess" NO while preserving essential low levels of NO, and has been shown to maintain enterocyte viability and reduce bacterial translocation in rats following endotoxin challenge [57]. It has therefore been suggested that eNOS is important in the maintenance of microvascular flow and epithelial cell integrity while excessive production of iNOS contributes to cell damage.

Sepsis, NO, and apoptosis

The comprehensive role of NO in apoptosis, or programmed cell death, is beyond the scope of this chapter. However, it is important to note that apoptosis has been demonstrated in a variety of tissues in rodent models of endotoxemia, including liver, lung, kidneys, thymus, and intestines [58, 59]. NO has been shown to prevent apoptosis in various cell types, including hepatocytes, endothelial cells, and lymphocytes, while inducing it in macrophages, B cells, and thymocytes [60]. Whether NO prevents or promotes apoptosis appears to depend not only on cell type, but also the conditions involved, and the level of NO present. Multiple mechanisms of inhibition of apoptosis by NO exist, including the ability of NO to interfere with caspase-3 activation and activity. NO can directly inhibit caspase 3 activity by S-nitrosylation, as well as indirectly *via* a cGMP-dependent mechanism [61]. Both gene transfer and induction of iNOS are effective at blocking hepatic apoptosis *in vitro* [61]. *In vivo*, the liver specific NO donor V-PYRRO/NO administered continuously following TNF/Gal N (TNFα plus galactosamine) in rats inhibited hepatic apoptosis and reduced transaminase levels by greater than 90% [62]. In the liver, iNOS specific inhibitors and nonspecific inhibitors are equally potent in inducing apoptosis, suggesting that inhibition of apoptosis is a result of either iNOS alone or a combination of both iNOS and eNOS activation [47].

Sepsis, NO and energy metabolism

Severe sepsis is accompanied by a marked decrease in tissue oxygen extraction, resulting in tissue hypoxia and increased venous oxygen concentration in both septic patients and animal models of sepsis [63]. Although this may be caused by tissue hypoperfusion, it also suggests an impairment of oxygen utilization. Inhibition of mitochondrial respiratory chain activity secondary to LPS or cytokine induction of iNOS has been shown in a variety of cell types, including macrophages, hepatocytes, astrocytes, and cardiac myocytes [64]. In experiments utilizing both intact cells and isolated mitochondria, NO competes with oxygen at cytochrome oxidase complex IV, resulting in a reversible inhibition of oxygen consumption. Therefore, during shock, where less oxygen is available to compete with NO, the inhibition of cytochrome oxidase is enhanced. Elevated levels of peroxynitrite, the product of NO and superoxide, have also been well documented in septic shock [65, 66]. Peroxynitrite irreversibly inhibits complexes I and II, possibly III, the ATPase, and mitochondrial aconitase, further contributing to the impairment of oxygen utilization. Another known toxicity of peroxynitrite is its single strand breakage of DNA. This breakage stimulates the activation of the nuclear repair enzyme PARS (poly-ADP-ribosyl-transferase). The activation of PARS results in intracellular NAD^+ depletion, potentially decreasing ATP levels and resulting in cell death.

NOS inhibition and therapeutic trials

Persistent hypotension (MAP < 85mm Hg after 24 h of treatment) is a major risk factor for mortality in patients with septic shock [67], and therefore its prevention is an important therapeutic target. Because NO appears to play an integral role in the pathophysiology of septic shock, several strategies directed at antagonism of NO production have been attempted. However, the results have been conflicting. There are numerous approaches to decreasing NO levels. Corticosteroids are the only known agents with the capability of blocking iNOS induction [68]. However, their use in sepsis is controversial secondary to other biological effects [69]. The most commonly utilized inhibitors have been analogues of L-arginine, which reduce substrate availability by competitive, nonselective inhibition. These include N^G-methyl-L-arginine (L-NMA), N^w-nitro-L-arginine (LNNA), and N^w-nitro-L-arginine-methyl-ester (L-NAME). L-NMA has a short half-life, making it an easily reversible, continuous infusion in clinical trials. L-NAME is a pro-drug that is converted to L-NNA by serum esterases. This may provide a prolonged effect, but also may potentiate toxicity. However, the use of nonspecific inhibitors as a therapy assumes that negation of the physiologic function of eNOS has no deleterious consequences.

Nonselective NOS inhibitors have been tested in a variety of large animal models with both positive and negative results. The proper dosing and timing of the inhibitor remains controversial. For example, Nava et al. [36] have shown in animal models of sepsis that higher doses of the nonselective inhibitor L-NMMA are associated with a substantial increase in mortality, suggesting a narrow therapeutic window for the drug. Bacteremic sheep, pigs, and baboons treated with NMA after established vasodilation showed reversal of cardiovascular abnormalities and increased survival [70–72]. However, a study of septic canines treated with N^w-amino-L-arginine increased vascular resistance but also increased mortality rates [73].

Petros et al. [29] were the first to administer a NOS inhibitor to septic humans. They observed the reversal of refractory hypotension and vascular dilation following the administration of L-NMMA and L-NAME in two patients with septic shock, one of whom survived. They followed this study with a randomized trial investigating the effect of L-NMMA administered by an initial bolus followed by a continuous infusion in 12 patients with septic shock. They demonstrated dose-dependent increases in systemic vascular resistance, MAP and pulmonary artery pressure. There was also an observed decrease in cardiac output, although no serious side-effects were observed [74].

A subsequent human clinical trial utilizing a continuous infusion of the nonselective inhibitor L-NMA in vasopressor dependent shock decreased plasma nitrite/nitrate levels, restored systemic vascular resistance, and reduced the need for concurrent pressors [75]. Also reported in this study, however, was a significant fall in cardiac index, a small but significant worsening of pulmonary hypertension, and EKG changes consistent with ischemia in a few patients treated at the highest dosage. A subsequent randomized multicenter phase III trial based on the positive findings of this study was recently closed after an interim safety analysis revealed worse survival in the L-NMA treated group.

There is no debate that NOS inhibition increases MAP and SVR, however the majority of studies involving NOS inhibitors also report an accompanying decrease in cardiac output. Albert et al. [76] examined the effects of a 60-min infusion of L-NMMA in healthy volunteers. They found a 12% increase in MAP, and reduction of cardiac output by 23%, due to a decrease in stroke volume, as the heart rate remained constant. Forearm vascular resistance actually decreased, with increased forearm bloodflow. They therefore concluded that the overall increase in systemic vascular resistance is due to vasoconstriction in regions other than skeletal muscle and skin, indicating that there may be a considerable reduction in visceral flow, which could potentially aggravate end organ failure.

Experience from the above studies utilizing nonspecific NOS inhibitors has caused investigators to proceed with caution, considering the possibility that serious side-effects may result from blocking the protective effects of eNOS, which include maintenance of microvascular flow, inhibition of platelet aggregation and leukocyte adhesion, nonspecific immunity, and inhibition of stress induced apoptosis. There is now growing interest in studying selective iNOS inhibitors, which can potentially preserve the physiologic functions of eNOS while preventing deleterious overproduction of iNOS. Animal studies utilizing the relatively selective iNOS inhibitor aminoguanidine showed significantly decreased bacterial translocation following high dose endotoxin, suggesting decreased damage to the gut mucosal barrier [55]. Other studies utilizing aminoguanidine demonstrated attenuation of circulatory failure in rats and decreased mortality in murine endotoxic models [77]. At present there is no human data on the effects of selective iNOS inhibition, as currently developed compounds have had unwanted side-effects apparently unrelated to their action on NOS. Efforts continue in the pharmaceutical industry to develop specific iNOS inhibitors, which may be a powerful tool. In the meantime, further animal studies utilizing alternative regimens also continue. This includes the use of nonspecific inhibitors with adjuncts such as inhaled NO, which can prevent the development of pulmonary hypertension without systemic effects. In a porcine endotoxemia model utilizing inhaled NO in combination with nonspecific inhibition of NOS, Klemm et al. [78] demonstrated improved MAP and CO, but also prevented pulmonary hypertension and a decrease in paO_2 during infusion of L-NMMA. This was accompanied by a substantial reduction in mortality compared to L-NMMA alone. Because the levels and importance of NO in different tissues may vary, site-specific NO delivery may be beneficial in combination with systemic nonspecific NO inhibition. Another class of drugs undergoing investigation include NO scavengers which are designed to remove "excess" NO. Because NO diffuses rapidly, the drug is unlikely to scavenge all nitric oxide, theoretically maintaining essential levels of NO while limiting the toxic effects of NO overproduction. The ruthenium-based NO scavenger AMD-6245 demonstrated reversal of hypotension and vasoplegia in a rat endotoxemic model [79]. Hydroxycobalamin (vitamin B_{12}) is another NO scavenger which has been shown to improve survival in a murine endotoxemic model [80]. Inhibition of cGMP is yet another mode of experimentation, given that NO mediates its vasodilatory effect *via* cGMP. Endotoxemic mice treated with cGMP inhibitor ODQ (4H-8-bromo-1,2,4oxadiazolo(3,4-d)benz(b) (1,4)oxazin-1-one) demonstrated improved survival [81]. However, given the deleterious effects attributed to eNOS inhibition in experiments using nonspecific inhibitors, the use of such agents would theoretically be expected to eradicate the benefit of eNOS while failing to prevent the deleterious effects of the cGMP-independent iNOS.

Overall, the ubiquitous nature of NO makes extensive preclinical knowledge of various inhibitors mandatory prior to human trials. Currently available inhibitors may be too nonspecific, and therefore intensivists await the development of selective inhibitors which may prove to be a powerful tool.

INOS deficient mice

An important adjunct in studying isoform specific contributions is the utilization of iNOS knockout mice. These mice undergo normal development, but do not produce nitrite/nitrate in response to LPS challenge. Survival studies following endotoxemia in these mice have produced conflicting results. Laubach et al. [82] found no difference in survival between iNOS knockout mice and their wildtype counterpart following high dose endotoxin administration, while Wei et al. [83] found that iNOS deficient mice were completely protected from death. MacMicking et al. [28] observed that anesthetized knockout mice were significantly protected from hypotension and death following a moderate dose of endotoxin. However, unanesthetized mice were protected only at high doses of LPS. The explanations for the discrepancies between these studies have been unclear. A potential reason for a lack of benefit in iNOS deficient mice is that iNOS independent mechanisms may also play an important role in shock. Also, it must be considered that these mice may have developed compensatory mechanisms that could also alter the pathophysiology seen in shock. Therefore it is important to interpret data from these mice in parallel with pharmacological inhibition studies.

NO and hemorrhagic shock

Trauma remains the leading cause of mortality during the first three decades of life in the United States. Severe hemorrhagic shock, a frequent consequence of accidental trauma, is characterized by an initial decrease in blood pressure and cardiac output, followed by a compensatory phase during which the release of endogenous vasoconstrictors attempt to restore blood pressure. There is subsequently a phase of decompensation during which there is a progressive vasodilatation despite the augmented sympathetic activity. During this time there is hyporeactivity to norepinephrine, epinephrine, and angiotensin. Mortality following trauma occurs in three distinct phases. The first is immediate death, which often occurs during the first hour following injury as a result of either major vessel injury/exsanguination or massive CNS injury [63]. Second is early death that occurs following arrival to the trauma center, often secondary to missed injuries. Lastly is late death, which is secondary to multiple organ failure and septic complications. Understanding the pathophysiology of late death is the subject of intense research. In patients who survive the initial resuscitation from hemorrhagic shock, a systemic inflammatory response is already in evolution. Hypovolemic shock followed by resuscitation can activate many mediator systems, including free radicals, arachidonic acid metabolites, and upregulation of inflammatory cytokine expression and accumulation of neutrophils in a variety of tissues. Ultimately, the combined oxidative and inflammatory insult to tissues can progress along a continuum into multiple organ dysfunction, multiple organ failure, and possibly death. Hemorrhage and resuscitation results in myocardial [84], pulmonary [85], hepatocellular [86], renal [84], and splenic [87] dysfunction. In addition, this early hyperinflammatory response triggers a later counteracting anti-inflammatory response, which leaves the patient vulnerable to infection and

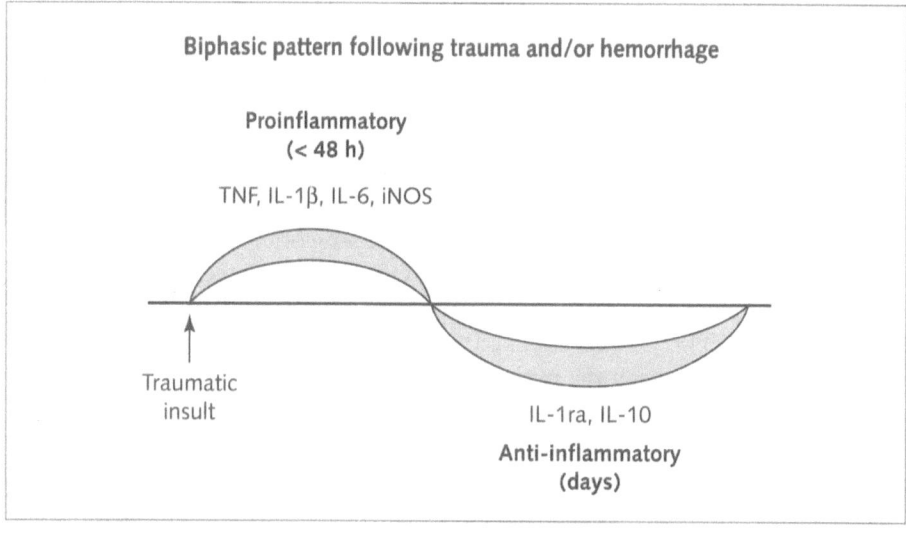

Figure 1

The early proinflammatory response following trauma and/or hemorrhage is followed by a late compensatory anti-inflammatory response, which can be complicated by infection and sepsis.

sepsis (Fig. 1). However, the early signaling pathways initiating the proinflammatory response remain unclear. Understanding such pathways may one day be pivotal in future prevention of the patients' progression to organ failure. There is now emerging interest in examining the role of nitric oxide in the pathophysiology of hemorrhagic shock, not only in terms of the directly toxic effect of nitric oxide and its products on tissues, but also through the unique role of nitric oxide in proinflammatory signaling.

Thiemermann et al. [88] demonstrated iNOS induction in various tissues, including the liver, during the period of vascular decompensation in an animal model of hemorrhagic shock. Szabo et al. [65] has confirmed that NO or peroxynitrite activation of poly(ADP-ribose)synthetase contributes to the vascular failure in irreversible shock. INOS mRNA was detectable by reverse transcriptase PCR in liver biopsies of hypotensive trauma patients who underwent laparotomies for control of hemorrhage and abdominal injuries within 2 h of presentation to the emergency room [89]. In addition, macrophages obtained from mice subjected to hemorrhagic shock have increased iNOS mRNA expression [90]. INOS mRNA can be detected in the livers of rats subjected to hemorrhagic shock at timepoints as early as 1 h [91]. INOS mRNA levels increase in parallel with the duration of shock, and remain elevated even after resuscitation [89]. INOS protein is detectable in rat liver by immunohistochemistry within 2.5 h of hemorrhage, assuming a centrilobular distribution [91]. Although the levels of NO observed in hemorrhagic shock are not increased to the large magnitudes seen in septic shock, the high activity of even low levels of iNOS, as well as the potency of nitric oxide at the local level appear to have a profound effect.

Unlike sepsis, where a specific agent (endotoxin) is held accountable for activation of the inflammatory cascade, the factors responsible in the setting of hemorrhagic shock remain unelucidated. However, several theories regarding the upregulation of NO during hemorrhagic shock exist. One such theory is that the induction of iNOS is secondary to increased circulating levels of inflammatory cytokines such as TNFα and IL-1β [92]. Ayala A et al. [93] has reported elevated plasma TNF levels within 45 min following the initiation of hypotension, and this was not associated with the presence of endotoxin. However, other studies have not found a significant elevation of TNF following hemorrhage when compared to controls [94]. A second theory is that NO induction is the result of endotoxin stimulation, secondary to bacterial translocation across an impaired gut mucosal barrier [95]. Although elevated systemic plasma endotoxin levels have been reported both during the hypotensive phase and following resuscitation in animal models of hemorrhagic shock [96, 97], other studies report that endotoxin was undetectable [88, 93]. However, detection limits of the assays that were utilized, as well as differing severity of the hemorrhage models must be considered when interpreting this type of data. A third theory attributes the upregulation of iNOS to the activation of hypoxia-sensitive transcription factors such as hypoxia inducible factor-1 [98]. In addition, Angele et al. [99] has demonstrated that hypoxemia in the absence of blood loss upregulates iNOS expression and activity in macrophages. Overall, the stimulus for iNOS upregulation during hemorrhagic shock remains controversial, and remains the subject of active research.

Studies utilizing NOS inhibitors have shed light on the consequences of NO in hemorrhagic shock. In rats subjected to hemorrhagic shock and resuscitation, infusion of the nonselective inhibitor L-NAME worsened organ injury [100– 102]. In contrast, selective iNOS inhibitors appear to have both an organ protective effect as well as improved survival in hemorrhagic shock [5, 103–105]. Aminoguanidine, an inhibitor with low potency but high selectivity for iNOS, improved survival in rodent models of hemorrhagic shock [106]. Mercaptoethylguanidine (MEG), another class of relatively selective iNOS inhibitors, also exhibits an additional independent effect of inhibition of peroxynitrite-induced oxidations [105]. MEG decreases nitrate/nitrite production, prevents vascular decompensation *in vivo*, and improves *ex vivo* cellular metabolic alterations in a rat model of hemorrhagic shock when administered just prior to resuscitation [107]. In pigs, MEG treatment significantly reduced the fall in blood pressure and cardiac output during resuscitation and dramatically increased survival [108]. Similarly, rats treated with an infusion of NOX, a scavenger of "excess" NO, during hemorrhagic shock had reduced liver injury, hepatic neutrophil infiltration, and improved survival compared to saline treated animals [109]. Overall, it appears that physiologic levels of NO provided by eNOS are beneficial, while the overproduction of NO by iNOS is detrimental.

NO, peroxynitrite, and direct toxicity

Overproduction of oxygen radicals is characteristic of hemorrhagic shock and resuscitation. In addition to the increase in NO described above, there is also generation of superoxide at the time or resuscitation by sources such as xanthine oxidase and NADPH. In this setting, the reaction of NO with superoxide results in a directly toxic product, peroxynitrite. This reaction outcompetes the reaction of superoxide with superoxide dismutase [66]. Under physiologic conditions, the cell is easily protected from the low levels of peroxynitrite by endogenous antioxidant systems. However, when the antioxidant system becomes overwhelmed, peroxynitrite accumulation can have several toxic effects. One such mechanism of direct toxicity is the ability of peroxynitrite to interact with enzymes by oxidation of sulfhydryl groups and thioethers, and the nitration and hydroxylation of aromatic compounds. These reactions can modify enzymatic activity. Peroxynitrite can also interact with nucleic acids by both DNA single strand breakage and DNA base modifications [110]. Subsequent triggering of the nuclear enzyme poly(ADP-ribose)synthetase (PARS) by this DNA single strand breakage is an indirect action of peroxynitrite. PARS catalyzes the cleavage of NAD into nicotinamide and ADP ribose, covalently attaching ADP-ribose to various nuclear proteins, and depleting NAD pools. This results in slowing of glycolysis, electron transport, and ATP formation, ultimately causing cell dysfunction and death *via* a necrotic pathway. Evidence for the role of peroxynitrite, however, is indirect, as specific peroxynitrite scavengers are not available. Nitrotyrosine formation detected by immunostaining was initially deemed as a relatively specific "footprint" of peroxynitrite [111]. However, recent evidence indicates that other reactions can also induce tyrosine nitration [112]. Therefore, recent reviews now refer to nitrotyrosine formation as an indicator of nitrosative stress in general [113].

NO and proinflammatory signaling in hemorrhagic shock

In addition to the directly toxic effects described above, NO appears to have a second, indirect contribution to the pathophysiology of hemorrhagic shock *via* its role in proinflammatory signaling (Fig. 2). A double approach was undertaken to examine the potential participation of NO in the signaling cascade that follows resuscitation from hemorrhagic shock. Rats subjected to hemorrhagic shock

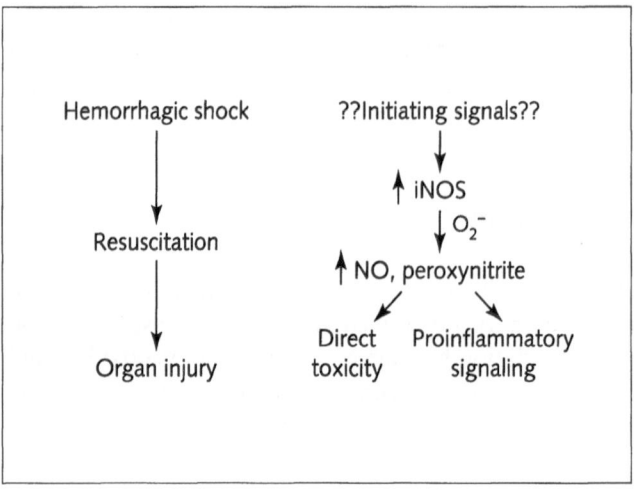

Figure 2
The figure summarizes the role of NO in parallel with the course of events which occur in hemorrhagic shock.

received infusion of the selective iNOS inhibitor N^6(iminoethyl)-L-lysine (L-NIL) prior to resuscitation. In parallel, iNOS knockout mice were also subjected to hemorrhagic shock. Both the iNOS knockout and L-NIL treated groups demonstrated a significant attenuation in the upregulation of the proinflammatory cytokines IL-6 and G-CSF as well as diminished activation of the proinflammatory transcription factors NF-κB (nuclear factor kappa B) and Stat3 (signal transducer and activator of transcription) in lungs and liver 4–6 h following resuscitation [114], as compared to respective controls. These findings correlated with a decrease in lung and liver injury, as assessed by decreased PMN accumulation and edema formation in the lungs following hemorrhagic shock and resuscitation, as well as an attenuation of the level of plasma liver enzymes. These data indicate that NO has an important role in upregulation of the inflammatory cascade in resuscitated hemorrhagic shock. Under conditions of reduced antioxidant capacity such as hemorrhagic shock, redox-sensitive signaling pathways are a potential mechanism. Landers et al. demonstrated that NO can S-nitrosylate p21(ras), thereby activating it and subsequently resulting in NF-κB activation [115]. This provides an interesting forum for continued research in further elucidating the role of NO in the amplification of the inflammatory response of hemorrhagic shock, as the point of resuscitation of trauma patients may one day provide a unique therapeutic window of opportunity to remove excess nitric oxide and attenuate the downstream inflammatory response.

Conclusions

Nitric oxide is clearly a common mediator in both septic and hemorrhagic shock. However, it is apparent that each type of shock has distinguishing features from the other despite their common endpoints, precluding generalizations regarding the role of NO. There is still a great deal to learn about both. While previous clinical trial failures of NO inhibition in sepsis have pointed us in the direction of modifying our approach to more specific inhibitors, knowledge of the role of NO in hemorrhagic shock remains in its infancy. Actively growing research in both fields will continue to identify potential points of future therapeutic intervention.

References

1   Palmer RM, Ferrige AG, Moncada S (1987) Nitric oxide release accounts for the biological activity of endothelium-derived relaxing factor. *Nature* 327: 524–526
2   Nathan C, Xie QW (1994) Nitric oxide synthases: roles, tolls, and controls. *Cell* 78: 915–918
3   Forstermann U, Schmidt HH, Pollock JS, Sheng H, Mitchell JA, Warner TD et al (1991) Isoforms of nitric oxide synthase. Characterization and purification from different cell types. *Biochem Pharmacol* 42: 1849–1857
4   Rackow EC, Astiz ME (1991) Pathophysiology and treatment of septic shock. *JAMA* 266: 548–554
5   Thiemermann C (1997) Nitric oxide and septic shock. *Gen Pharmacol* 29: 159–166
6   Bone RC (1994) Gram-positive organisms and sepsis. *Arch Intern Med* 154: 26–34
7   Kilbourn RG, Traber DL, Szabo C (1997) Nitric oxide and shock. *Dis Mon* 43: 277–348
8   Rees DD, Cellek S, Palmer RM, Moncada S (1990) Dexamethasone prevents the induction by endotoxin of a nitric oxide synthase and the associated effects on vascular tone: an insight into endotoxin shock. *Biochem Biophys Res Commun* 173: 541–547
9   Natanson C, Eichenholz PW, Danner RL, Eichacker PQ, Hoffman WD, Kuo GC et al (1989) Endotoxin and tumor necrosis factor challenges in dogs simulate the cardiovascular profile of human septic shock. *J Exp Med* 169: 823–832
10 Novogrodsky A, Vanichkin A, Patya M, Gazit A, Osherov N, Levitzki A (1994) Prevention of lipopolysaccharide-induced lethal toxicity by tyrosine kinase inhibitors. *Science* 264: 1319–1322
11 Moncada S, Palmer RM, Higgs EA (1991) Nitric oxide: physiology, pathophysiology, and pharmacology. *Pharmacol Rev* 43: 109–142
12 Ochoa JB, Udekwu AO, Billiar TR, Curran RD, Cerra FB, Simmons RL et al (1991) Nitrogen oxide levels in patients after trauma and during sepsis. *Ann Surg* 214: 621–626
13 Rixen D, Siegel JH, Espina N, Bertolini M (1997) Plasma nitric oxide in posttrauma critical illness: a function of "sepsis" and the physiologic state severity classification quan-

tifying the probability of death [published erratum appears in *Shock* 1997 Feb 7(2): 156]. *Shock* 7: 17–28

14 Gomez-Jimenez J, Salgado A, Mourelle M, Martin MC, Segura RM, Peracaula R et al (1995) L-arginine: nitric oxide pathway in endotoxemia and human septic shock. *Crit Care Med* 23: 253–258

15 Westenberger U, Thanner S, Ruf HH, Gersonde K, Sutter G, Trentz O (1990) Formation of free radicals and nitric oxide derivative of hemoglobin in rats during shock syndrome. *Free Radic Res Commun* 11: 167–178

16 Salvemini D, Korbut R, Anggard E, Vane J (1990) Immediate release of a nitric oxide-like factor from bovine aortic endothelial cells by *Escherichia coli* lipopolysaccharide [published erratum appears in *Proc Natl Acad Sci USA* (1990) Aug 87 (15): 6007]. *Proc Natl Acad Sci USA* 87: 2593–2597

17 MacNaul KL, Hutchinson NI Differential expression of iNOS and cNOS mRNA in human vascular smooth muscle cells and endothelial cells under normal and inflammatory conditions. *Biochem Biophys Res Commun* 1993 196: 1330–1334

18 Szabo C, Wu CC, Gross SS, Thiemermann C, Vane JR (1993) Interleukin-1 contributes to the induction of nitric oxide synthase by endotoxin *in vivo*. *Eur J Pharmacol* 250: 157–160

19 Salkowski CA, Detore G, McNally R, van Rooijen N, Vogel SN (1997) Regulation of inducible nitric oxide synthase messenger RNA expression and nitric oxide production by lipopolysaccharide *in vivo*: the roles of macrophages, endogenous IFN-gamma, and TNF receptor-1-mediated signaling. *J Immunol* 158: 905–912

20 Stuehr DJ, Marletta MA (1985) Mammalian nitrate biosynthesis: mouse macrophages produce nitrite and nitrate in response to *Escherichia coli* lipopolysaccharide. *Proc Natl Acad Sci USA* 82: 7738–7742

21 Morris SM Jr, Billiar TR (1994) New insights into the regulation of inducible nitric oxide synthesis. *Am J Physiol* 266: E829–E839

22 Nathan C (1992) Nitric oxide as a secretory product of mammalian cells. *FASEB J* 6: 3051–3064

23 Salter M, Knowles RG, Moncada S (1991) Widespread tissue distribution, species distribution and changes in activity of Ca(2+)-dependent and Ca(2+)-independent nitric oxide synthases. *FEBS Lett* 291: 145–149

24 De Kimpe SJ, Kengatharan M, Thiemermann C, Vane JR (1995) The cell wall components peptidoglycan and lipoteichoic acid from *Staphylococcus aureus* act in synergy to cause shock and multiple organ failure. *Proc Natl Acad Sci USA* 92: 10359–10363

25 Kengatharan M, De Kimpe SJ, Thiemermann C (1996) Analysis of the signal transduction in the induction of nitric oxide synthase by lipoteichoic acid in macrophages. *Br J Pharmacol* 117: 1163–1170

26 Bucher M, Ittner KP, Zimmermann M, Wolf K, Hobbhahn J, Kurtz A (1997) Nitric oxide synthase isoform III gene expression in rat liver is up-regulated by lipopolysaccharide and lipoteichoic acid. *FEBS Lett* 412: 511–514

27 Kilbourn RG, Gross SS, Jubran A, Adams J, Griffith OW, Levi R et al (1990) N^G-

methyl-L-arginine inhibits tumor necrosis factor-induced hypotension: implications for the involvement of nitric oxide. *Proc Natl Acad Sci USA* 87: 3629–3632

28 MacMicking JD, Nathan C, Hom G, Chartrain N, Fletcher DS, Trumbauer M et al (1995) Altered responses to bacterial infection and endotoxic shock in mice lacking inducible nitric oxide synthase [published erratum appears in *Cell* (1995) Jun 30 81(7): following 1170] *Cell* 81: 641–650

29 Petros A, Bennett D, Vallance P (1991) Effect of nitric oxide synthase inhibitors on hypotension in patients with septic shock. *Lancet* 338: 1557–1558

30 Paya D, Gray GA, Stoclet JC (1993) Effects of methylene blue on blood pressure and reactivity to norepinephrine in endotoxemic rats. *J Cardiovasc Pharmacol* 21: 926–930

31 Landin L, Lorente JA, Renes E, Canas P, Jorge P, Liste D (1994) Inhibition of nitric oxide synthesis improves the vasoconstrictive effect of noradrenaline in sepsis. *Chest* 106: 250–256

32 Hollenberg SM, Cunnion RE, Zimmerberg J (1993) Nitric oxide synthase inhibition reverses arteriolar hyporesponsiveness to catecholamines in septic rats. *Am J Physiol* 264: H660–H663

33 Whittle BJ (1995) Nitric oxide in physiology and pathology. *Histochem J* 27: 727–737

34 Price S, Anning PB, Mitchell JA, Evans TW (1999) Myocardial dysfunction in sepsis: mechanisms and therapeutic implications. *Eur Heart J* 20: 715–24

35 Brady AJ, Warren JB, Poole-Wilson PA, Williams TJ, Harding SE (1993) Nitric oxide attenuates cardiac myocyte contraction. *Am J Physiol* 265: H176–H182

36 Schulz R, Nava E, Moncada S (1992) Induction and potential biological relevance of a Ca(2+)-independent nitric oxide synthase in the myocardium. *Br J Pharmacol* 105: 575–580

37 Finkel MS, Oddis CV, Jacob TD, Watkins SC, Hattler BG, Simmons RL (1992) Negative inotropic effects of cytokines on the heart mediated by nitric oxide. *Science* 257: 387–389

38 Brady AJ, Poole-Wilson PA, Harding SE, Warren JB (1992) Nitric oxide production within cardiac myocytes reduces their contractility in endotoxemia. *Am J Physiol* 263: H1963–H1966

39 Billiar TR, Curran RD, Stuehr DJ, West MA, Bentz BG, Simmons RL (1989) An L-arginine-dependent mechanism mediates Kupffer cell inhibition of hepatocyte protein synthesis *in vitro*. *J Exp Med* 169: 1467–1472

40 Curran RD, Billiar TR, Stuehr DJ, Ochoa JB, Harbrecht BG, Flint SG et al (1990) Multiple cytokines are required to induce hepatocyte nitric oxide production and inhibit total protein synthesis. *Ann Surg* 212: 462–469

41 Satoi S, Kamiyama Y, Kitade H, Kwon AH, Takahashi K, Wei T et al (2000) Nitric oxide production and hepatic dysfunction in patients with postoperative sepsis. *Clin Exp Pharmacol Physiol* 27: 197–201

42 Ruetten H, Thiemermann C (1997) Effect of calpain inhibitor I, an inhibitor of the proteolysis of I kappa B, on the circulatory failure and multiple organ dysfunction caused by endotoxin in the rat. *Br J Pharmacol* 121: 695–704

43 Stadler J, Barton D, Beil-Moeller H, Diekmann S, Hierholzer C, Erhard W et al (1995) Hepatocyte nitric oxide biosynthesis inhibits glucose output and competes with urea synthesis for L-arginine. *Am J Physiol* 268: G183–G188

44 Ceppi ED, Smith FS, Titheradge MA (1996) Effect of multiple cytokines plus bacterial endotoxin on glucose and nitric oxide production by cultured hepatocytes. *Biochem J* 317 (Pt 2): 503–507

45 Titheradge MA (1999) Nitric oxide in septic shock. *Biochim Biophys Acta* 1411: 437–455

46 Harbrecht BG, Billiar TR, Stadler J, Demetris AJ, Ochoa J, Curran RD et al (1992) Inhibition of nitric oxide synthesis during endotoxemia promotes intrahepatic thrombosis and an oxygen radical-mediated hepatic injury. *J Leukoc Biol* 52: 390–394

47 Ou J, Carlos TM, Watkins SC, Saavedra JE, Keefer LK, Kim YM et al (1997) Differential effects of nonselective nitric oxide synthase (NOS) and selective inducible NOS inhibition on hepatic necrosis, apoptosis, ICAM-1 expression, and neutrophil accumulation during endotoxemia. *Nitric Oxide* 1: 404–416

48 Fink MP (1991) Gastrointestinal mucosal injury in experimental models of shock, trauma, and sepsis. *Crit Care Med* 19: 627–641

49 Pons L, Droy-Lefaix MT, Braquet P, Bueno L (1991) Role of free radicals and platelet-activating factor in the genesis of intestinal motor disturbances induced by *Escherichia coli* endotoxins in rats. *Gastroenterology* 100: 946–953

50 Laszlo F, Whittle BJ, Moncada S (1994) Interactions of constitutive nitric oxide with PAF and thromboxane on rat intestinal vascular integrity in acute endotoxaemia. *Br J Pharmacol* 113: 1131–1136

51 Deitch EA, Specian RD, Berg RD (1991) Endotoxin-induced bacterial translocation and mucosal permeability: role of xanthine oxidase, complement activation, and macrophage products. *Crit Care Med* 19: 785–791

52 Morin MJ, Unno N, Hodin RA, Fink MP (1998) Differential expression of inducible nitric oxide synthase messenger RNA along the longitudinal and crypt-villus axes of the intestine in endotoxemic rats. *Crit Care Med* 26: 1258–1264

53 Tepperman BL, Brown JF, Whittle BJ (1993) Nitric oxide synthase induction and intestinal epithelial cell viability in rats. *Am J Physiol* 265: G214–G218

54 Unno N, Wang H, Menconi MJ, Tytgat SH, Larkin V, Smith M et al (1997) Inhibition of inducible nitric oxide synthase ameliorates endotoxin-induced gut mucosal barrier dysfunction in rats. *Gastroenterology* 113: 1246–1257

55 Sorrells DL, Friend C, Koltuksuz U, Courcoulas A, Boyle P, Garrett M et al (1996) Inhibition of nitric oxide with aminoguanidine reduces bacterial translocation after endotoxin challenge *in vivo*. *Arch Surg* 131: 1155–1163

56 Hutcheson IR, Whittle BJ, Boughton-Smith NK (1990) Role of nitric oxide in maintaining vascular integrity in endotoxin-induced acute intestinal damage in the rat. *Br J Pharmacol* 101: 815–20

57 Dickinson E, Tuncer R, Nadler E, Boyle P, Alber S, Watkins S et al (1999) NOX, a novel

nitric oxide scavenger, reduces bacterial translocation in rats after endotoxin challenge. *Am J Physiol* 277: G1281–G1287

58   Bohlinger I, Leist M, Gantner F, Angermuller S, Tiegs G, Wendel A (1996) DNA fragmentation in mouse organs during endotoxic shock. *Am J Pathol* 149: 1381–1393

59   Fehsel K, Kroncke KD, Meyer KL, Huber H, Wahn V, Kolb-Bachofen V (1995) Nitric oxide induces apoptosis in mouse thymocytes. *J Immunol* 155: 2858–2865

60   Dimmeler S, Zeiher AM (1997) Nitric oxide and apoptosis: another paradigm for the double-edged role of nitric oxide. *Nitric Oxide* 1: 275–281

61   Kim YM, Talanian RV, Billiar TR (1997) Nitric oxide inhibits apoptosis by preventing increases in caspase-3-like activity *via* two distinct mechanisms. *J Biol Chem* 272: 31138–31148

62   Saavedra JE, Billiar TR, Williams DL, Kim YM, Watkins SC, Keefer LK (1997) Targeting nitric oxide (NO) delivery *in vivo* Design of a liver-selective NO donor prodrug that blocks tumor necrosis factor-alpha-induced apoptosis and toxicity in the liver. *J Med Chem* 40: 1947–1954

63   Chaudry IH, Ayala A, Ertel W, Stephan RN (1990) Hemorrhage and resuscitation: immunological aspects [editorial]. *Am J Physiol* 259: R663–R678

64   Brown GC, McBride AG, Fox EJ, McNaught KS, Borutaite V (1997) Nitric oxide and oxygen metabolism. *Biochem Soc Trans* 25: 901–904

65   Szabo C (1997) Role of poly(ADP-ribose) synthetase activation in the suppression of cellular energetics in response to nitric oxide and peroxynitrite. *Biochem Soc Trans* 25: 919–924

66   Beckman JS, Koppenol WH (1996) Nitric oxide, superoxide, and peroxynitrite: the good, the bad, and ugly. *Am J Physiol* 271: C1424–C1437

67   Bernardin G, Pradier C, Tiger F, Deloffre P, Mattei M (1996) Blood pressure and arterial lactate level are early indicators of short-term survival in human septic shock. *Intensive Care Med* 22: 17–25

68   Di Rosa M, Radomski M, Carnuccio R, Moncada S (1990) Glucocorticoids inhibit the induction of nitric oxide synthase in macrophages. *Biochem Biophys Res Commun* 172: 1246–1252

69   Bone RC, Fisher CJ, Jr , Clemmer TP, Slotman GJ, Metz CA, Balk RA (1987) A controlled clinical trial of high-dose methylprednisolone in the treatment of severe sepsis and septic shock. *N Engl J Med* 317: 653–658

70   Brooke M, Hinder F, McGuire R, Traber LD, Traber DL (1996) Nitric oxide synthase inhibitor *versus* norepinephrine in bovine sepsis: effects on regional blood flows. *Shock* 5: 362–370

71   Strand OA, Leone AM, Giercksky KE, Skovlund E, Kirkeboen KA (1998) N(G)-monomethyl-L-arginine improves survival in a pig model of abdominal sepsis. [published errata appear in *Crit Care Med* (1999) Jan 27 (1): 226 and 1999 Feb 27 (2): 444]. *Crit Care Med* 26: 1490–1499

72   Redl H, Schlag G, Bahrami S (1998) Animal models of sepsis and shock: a review and

lessons learned. Edwin A Deitch *Shock* 9 (1): 1–11, 1998 [letter comment]. *Shock* 10: 442–445

73 Cobb JP, Natanson C, Hoffman WD, Lodato RF, Banks S, Koev CA et al (1992) N omega-amino-L-arginine, an inhibitor of nitric oxide synthase, raises vascular resistance but increases mortality rates in awake canines challenged with endotoxin. *J Exp Med* 176: 1175–1182

74 Petros A, Lamb G, Leone A, Moncada S, Bennett D, Vallance P (1994) Effects of a nitric oxide synthase inhibitor in humans with septic shock. *Cardiovasc Res* 28: 34–39

75 Grover R, Zaccardelli D, Colice G, Guntupalli K, Watson D, Vincent JL (1999) An open-label dose escalation study of the nitric oxide synthase inhibitor, N(G)-methyl-L-arginine hydrochloride (546C88), in patients with septic shock. Glaxo Wellcome International Septic Shock Study Group [see comments]. *Crit Care Med* 27: 913–922

76 Albert J, Schedin U, Lindqvist M, Melcher A, Hjemdahl P, Frostell C (1997) Blockade of endogenous nitric oxide production results in moderate hypertension, reducing sympathetic activity and shortening bleeding time in healthy volunteers. *Acta Anaesthesiol Scand* 41: 1104–1113

77 Wu CC, Chen SJ, Szabo C, Thiemermann C, Vane JR (1995) Aminoguanidine attenuates the delayed circulatory failure and improves survival in rodent models of endotoxic shock. *Br J Pharmacol* 114: 1666–1672

78 Klemm P, Thiemermann C, Winklmaier G, Martorana PA, Henning R (1995) Effects of nitric oxide synthase inhibition combined with nitric oxide inhalation in a porcine model of endotoxin shock. *Br J Pharmacol* 114: 363–368

79 Fricker SP, Slade E, Powell NA, Vaughan OJ, Henderson GR, Murrer BA et al (1997) Ruthenium complexes as nitric oxide scavengers: a potential therapeutic approach to nitric oxide-mediated diseases. *Br J Pharmacol* 122: 1441–1449

80 Greenberg SS, Xie J, Zatarain JM, Kapusta DR, Miller MJ (1995) Hydroxocobalamin (vitamin B12a) prevents and reverses endotoxin-induced hypotension and mortality in rodents: role of nitric oxide. *J Pharmacol Exp Ther* 273: 257–265

81 Zingarelli B, Hasko G, Salzman AL, Szabo C (1999) Effects of a novel guanylyl cyclase inhibitor on the vascular actions of nitric oxide and peroxynitrite in immunostimulated smooth muscle cells and in endotoxic shock. *Crit Care Med* 27: 1701–1707

82 Laubach VE, Shesely EG, Smithies O, Sherman PA (1995) Mice lacking inducible nitric oxide synthase are not resistant to lipopolysaccharide-induced death. *Proc Natl Acad Sci USA* 92: 10688–10692

83 Wei XQ, Charles IG, Smith A, Ure J, Feng GJ, Huang FP et al (1995) Altered immune responses in mice lacking inducible nitric oxide synthase. *Nature* 375: 408–411

84 Wang P, Ba ZF, Meldrum DR, Chaudry IH (1992) Diltiazem restores cardiac output and improves renal function after hemorrhagic shock and crystalloid resuscitation. *Am J Physiol* 262: H1435–H1440

85 Anderson BO, Moore EE, Moore FA, Leff JA, Terada LS, Harken AH et al (1991) Hypovolemic shock promotes neutrophil sequestration in lungs by a xanthine oxidase-related mechanism. *J Appl Physiol* 71: 1862–1865

86 Wang P, Ba ZF, Burkhardt J, Chaudry IH (1992) Measurement of hepatic blood flow after severe hemorrhage: lack of restoration despite adequate resuscitation. *Am J Physiol* 262: G92–G98

87 Meldrum DR, Ayala A, Wang P, Ertel W, Chaudry IH (1991) Association between decreased splenic ATP levels and immunodepression: amelioration with ATP-MgCl2. *Am J Physiol* 261: R351–R357

88 Thiemermann C, Szabo C, Mitchell JA, Vane JR (1993) Vascular hyporeactivity to vasoconstrictor agents and hemodynamic decompensation in hemorrhagic shock is mediated by nitric oxide. *Proc Natl Acad Sci USA* 90: 267–271

89 Kelly E (1996) Traumatic shock induces Type II nitric oxide synthase mRNA expression in the liver (abstract). *Surgical Forum* 47: 32–33   ·

90 Zhu XL, Zellweger R, Zhu XH, Ayala A, Chaudry IH (1995) Cytokine gene expression in splenic macrophages and Kupffer cells following haemorrhage. *Cytokine* 7: 8–14

91 Villavicencio R (2000) *Unpublished work*

92 Szabo C, Thiemermann C (1994) Invited opinion: role of nitric oxide in hemorrhagic, traumatic, and anaphylactic shock and thermal injury. *Shock* 2: 145–155

93 Ayala A, Perrin MM, Meldrum DR, Ertel W, Chaudry IH (1990) Hemorrhage induces an increase in serum TNF which is not associated with elevated levels of endotoxin. *Cytokine* 2: 170–4

94 Rabinovici R, John R, Esser KM, Vernick J, Feuerstein G (1993) Serum tumor necrosis factor-alpha profile in trauma patients. *J Trauma* 35: 698–702

95 LaRocco MT, Rodriguez LF, Chen CY, Smith GS, Russell DH, Myers SI et al (1993) Reevaluation of the linkage between acute hemorrhagic shock and bacterial translocation in the rat. *Circ Shock* 40: 212–220

96 Jiang J, Bahrami S, Leichtfried G, Redl H, Ohlinger W, Schlag G (1995) Kinetics of endotoxin and tumor necrosis factor appearance in portal and systemic circulation after hemorrhagic shock in rats. *Ann Surg* 221: 100–106

97 Yao YM, Bahrami S, Leichtfried G, Redl H, Schlag G (1996) Significance of NO in hemorrhage-induced hemodynamic alterations, organ injury, and mortality in rats. *Am J Physiol* 270: H1616–H1623

98 Guillemin K, Krasnow MA (1997) The hypoxic response: huffing and HIFing. *Cell* 89: 9–12

99 Angele MK, Schwacha MG, Smail N, Catania RA, Ayala A, Cioffi WG et al (1999) Hypoxemia in the absence of blood loss upregulates iNOS expression and activity in macrophages. *Am J Physiol* 276: C285–C290

100 Harbrecht BG, Wu B, Watkins SC, Marshall HP, Jr , Peitzman AB, Billiar TR (1995) Inhibition of nitric oxide synthase during hemorrhagic shock increases hepatic injury. *Shock* 4: 332–337

101 Adachi T, Hori S, Miyazaki K, Nakagawa M, Inoue S, Ohnishi Y et al (1998) Inhibition of nitric oxide synthesis aggravates myocardial ischemia in hemorrhagic shock in constant pressure model. *Shock* 9: 204–209

102 Todorovic Z, Prostran MS, Varagic V, Zunic G, Savic J, Vujnov S (1998) The cardio-

vascular effects of the administration of L-NAME during the early posthemorrhagic period. *Gen Pharmacol* 30: 763–769

103 Hua TC, Moochhala SM (1999) Influence of L-arginine, aminoguanidine, and N^G-nitro-L-arginine methyl ester (L-name) on the survival rate in a rat model of hemorrhagic shock. *Shock* 11: 51–57

104 Southan GJ, Zingarelli B, O'Connor M, Salzman AL, Szabo C (1996) Spontaneous rearrangement of aminoalkylisothioureas into mercaptoalkylguanidines, a novel class of nitric oxide synthase inhibitors with selectivity towards the inducible isoform. *Br J Pharmacol* 117: 619–632

105 Szabo C, Ferrer-Sueta G, Zingarelli B, Southan GJ, Salzman AL, Radi R (1997) Mercaptoethylguanidine and guanidine inhibitors of nitric-oxide synthase react with peroxynitrite and protect against peroxynitrite-induced oxidative damage. *J Biol Chem* 272: 9030–9036

106 Zingarelli B, Squadrito F, Altavilla D, Calapai G, Campo GM, Calo M et al (1992) Evidence for a role of nitric oxide in hypovolemic hemorrhagic shock. *J Cardiovasc Pharmacol* 19: 982–986

107 Zingarelli B, Ischiropoulos H, Salzman AL, Szabo C (1997) Amelioration by mercaptoethylguanidine of the vascular and energetic failure in haemorrhagic shock in the anesthetised rat. *Eur J Pharmacol* 338: 55–65

108 Szabo A, Hake P, Salzman AL, Szabo C (1999) Beneficial effects of mercaptoethylguanidine, an inhibitor of the inducible isoform of nitric oxide synthase and a scavenger of peroxynitrite, in a porcine model of delayed hemorrhagic shock. *Crit Care Med* 27: 1343–1350

109 Menezes J, Hierholzer C, Watkins SC, Lyons V, Peitzman AB, Billiar TR et al (1999) A novel nitric oxide scavenger decreases liver injury and improves survival after hemorrhagic shock. *Am J Physiol* 277: G144–G151

110 Szabo C, Ohshima H (1997) DNA injury induced by peroxynitrite. *Nitric Oxide: Biological Chemistry* 1: 323–385

111 Ischiropoulos H, Zhu L, Chen J, Tsai M, Martin JC, Smith CD et al (1992) Peroxynitrite-mediated tyrosine nitration catalyzed by superoxide dismutase. *Arch Biochem Biophys* 298: 431–437

112 Eiserich JP, Hristova M, Cross CE, Jones AD, Freeman BA, Halliwell B et al (1998) Formation of nitric oxide-derived inflammatory oxidants by myeloperoxidase in neutrophils. *Nature* 391: 393–397

113 Halliwell B (1997) What nitrates tyrosine? Is nitrotyrosine specific as a biomarker of peroxynitrite formation *in vivo*? *FEBS Lett* 411: 157–160

114 Hierholzer C, Harbrecht B, Menezes JM, Kane J, MacMicking J, Nathan CF et al (1998) Essential role of induced nitric oxide in the initiation of the inflammatory response after hemorrhagic shock. *J Exp Med* 187: 917–928

115 Lander HM, Hajjar DP, Hempstead BL, Mirza UA, Chait BT, Campbell S et al (1997) A molecular redox switch on p21(ras) Structural basis for the nitric oxide-p21(ras) interaction. *J Biol Chem* 272: 4323–4326

Nitric oxide as a mediator of interleukin-2 induced cardiovascular toxicity and antitumor activity

Wolfram E. Samlowski

Huntsman Cancer Institute, University of Utah, 2000 Circle of Hope Dr., Salt Lake City, UT 84112, USA

Preclinical and clinical evaluation of IL-2 as an anticancer agent

IL-2 activation of T and NK cells

Interleukin-2 (IL-2) is a 15 kDa cytokine which is primarily synthesized by activated T lymphocytes. IL-2 activates lymphocytes *via* a well-characterized heterotrimeric receptor [1, 2], and therefore plays a central role in the development of cell-mediated immunity [3]. Low concentrations (10–100 IU/ml) of IL-2 in the presence of appropriately processed and presented antigenic peptides appear to be critical for activation of cytolytic lymphocytes, as well as in clonal expansion of these effector cells [4].

IL-2 is also involved in an additional pathway of lymphocyte activation. Exposure of murine or human lymphocytes to high concentrations of IL-2 (> 600 IU/ml) over 3–4 days either *in vitro* or *in vivo* results in the rapid activation of a population of cytotoxic lymphocytes termed lymphokine-activated killer (LAK) cells [5]. Once activated, LAK cells demonstrate cytotoxicity against a wide variety of freshly isolated cancer cells or cultured cancer cell lines derived from syngeneic, allogeneic or even xenogeneic hosts [6, 7]. Since the pattern of cytotoxicity is not tumor specific and does not require antigen presentation in the context of self-MHC on target cells for cytotoxicity, LAK cells are termed "non-specific" killer cells. A major subset of the cytolytic cells in the LAK population are CD3⁻ and express CD56 (N-CAM: or neural cell adhesion molecule), indicating NK lymphocyte derivation [8]. Almost all freshly isolated and cultured malignant cells, including multidrug-resistant tumor cells, are susceptible to LAK mediated cytolysis [9].

Preclinical models of IL-2 treatment

Since IL-2 was shown to activate cytolytic T lymphocyte as well as LAK cell killing of tumor cells *in vitro*, this agent was evaluated in preclinical studies as an anticancer agent at the Surgery Branch, NCI by Rosenberg and colleagues. When IL-2 was administered to tumor bearing mice with concomitant administration of LAK cells, regression of lung or liver metastases were seen [10, 11]. Tumor regression was associated with prolonged survival of experimental mice [12, 13]. Responses correlated with both increasing doses of cells (up to 10^8/mouse) and of IL-2 (maximizing at 10^5 units every 8 h) [11, 14, 15]. Higher doses of IL-2 proved fatal to mice due to the development of a "vascular leak syndrome" (discussed below) [16, 17].

Clinical trials with IL-2 in patients

IL-2 treatment was subsequently evaluated in the treatment of refractory human cancers. Although high-dose i.v. bolus schedules of IL-2 administration have been most widely used and appear to produce the highest frequency of complete responses, a number of other IL-2 schedules and routes of administration have also shown effectiveness. High-dose i.v. bolus IL-2 has been shown to induce objective regressions in 11–21% of patients with advanced melanoma, with 4–8.3% complete response (CR) rates [18, 19]. In renal cell carcinoma, response rates range from 13–35%, with 3–11% CRs [18, 19]. Responses have been observed in most anatomic sites, except in the CNS. Approximately two-thirds of the complete responses to IL-2/LAK have proven durable, with up to 15 years of follow-up [20–22]. This unusual property has maintained clinical interest in IL-2 as a therapeutic agent. The human IL-2 treatment experience has differed somewhat from murine models, as addition of adoptively transferred autologous LAK cells to high-dose i.v. bolus IL-2 has not increased therapeutic responses to IL-2 in patients [18]. Currently, high-dose IL-2 therapy is FDA approved for treatment of metastatic melanoma and renal cell carcinoma and is showing promise as a consolidation therapy following cytoreductive chemotherapy in acute myelogenous leukemia, non-Hodgkin's lymphoma and breast cancer. Recent studies by Legha and colleagues, using a regimen consisting of cisplatin, vinblastine, DTIC, IL-2 and IFNα (CVD-biochemotherapy) in metastatic melanoma, have shown encouraging response rates (~60%), including approximately 10% 3-year disease-free survival [23, 24]. Whether the long-term survival rates are improved over high-dose i.v. bolus IL-2 therapy in melanoma remains to be tested. IL-2 is also being evaluated as an immunostimulant to increasing T-cell number and cell-mediated immunity in HIV-induced immunodeficiency [25, 26].

Cardiovascular toxicity during IL-2 therapy

IL-2 induced hypotension

IL-2 treatment can affect the function of virtually every organ system (reviewed in [27, 28]). Most toxicity is not caused directly by IL-2, but rather *via* a plethora of secondarily released cytokines, including IFNγ, TNFα, lymphotoxin, IL-1α, IL-1β, IL-6 [29, 30]. The major dose-limiting toxicity of IL-2 is hypotension, due to a marked decrease in systemic vascular resistance, resulting in hypoperfusion of vital organs, such as heart, brain and kidneys [31]. The lowest daily blood pressure (mean ± SD) in 13 typical patients treated with high-dose IL-2 (600 000 IU/kg by i.v. bolus every 8 h on days 1–5 and 11–15) at the University of Utah is shown (Fig. 1, Panel A). Despite maximal medical therapy (described below) each of these patients developed a reproducible pattern of systolic and diastolic hypotension, peaking on days 3–5 and 13–15 of IL-2 administration.

Vascular leak syndrome

IL-2 administration also resulted in development of a "vascular leak syndrome" (VLS), with generalized and dose-dependent increases in vascular permeability and loss of intravascular fluid into interstitial tissues. VLS is associated with marked fluid retention (Fig. 1, Panel B), weight gain (Fig. 1, Panel C), non-cardiac pulmonary edema [32], and decreased renal perfusion [17]. Thus, the simultaneous decreases in peripheral vascular resistance, along with decreased circulating plasma volume combine to mediate reduced central venous pressure and marked drops in systolic and diastolic blood pressure [31]. These changes in cardiovascular function result in profound, but reversible organ hypoperfusion, as indicated by pre-renal pattern of rises in blood urea nitrogen > creatinine (Fig. 1, Panel D).

Alterations in myocardial function

In the face of decreasing intravascular volume and peripheral vascular resistance, other investigators have shown that compensatory increases in heart rate and cardiac index are usually seen [33, 34]. Paradoxically, left ventricular function may decrease during IL-2 therapy, as evidenced by decreased left ventricular stroke work index and left ventricular ejection fraction. Increased left ventricular end diastolic volume functions to maintain cardiac output [33]. These changes in myocardial performance may be related to increased TNFα, IL-6 or IL-1 levels, as these cytokines (but not IL-2) decrease myocardial contractile function *in vitro* [35]. The overall pattern of hypotension, vascular leak and myocardial depression following IL-2 therapy appears similar to the cardiovascular manifestations of septic shock [31]. One major difference between IL-2 induced cardiovascular toxicity and other shock syndromes (e.g. septic shock) is the reversibility of renal dysfunction. This is in strong contrast to the high incidence of acute tubular necrosis observed in other shock syndromes, such as septic shock.

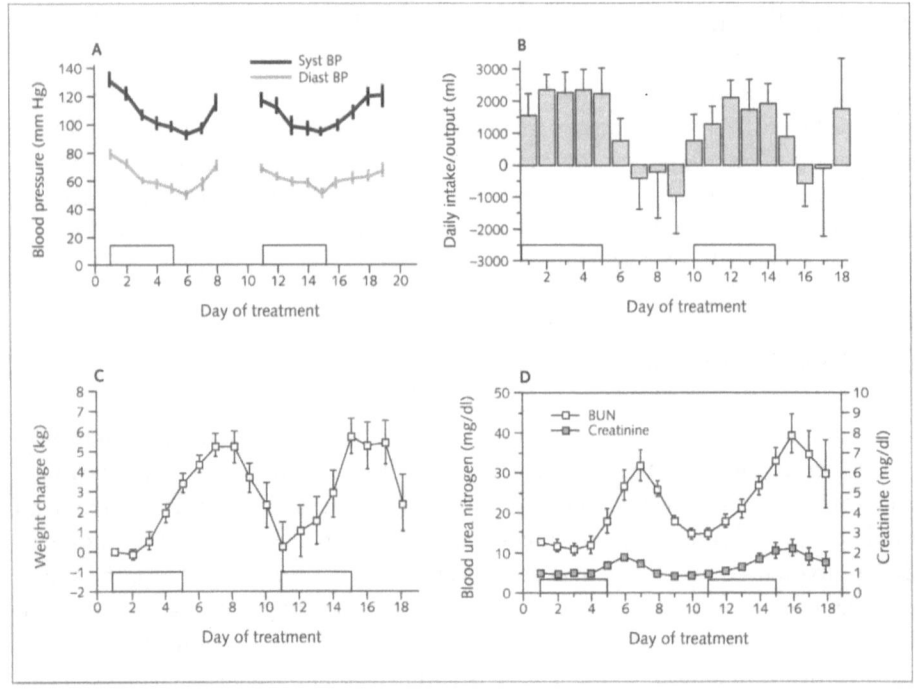

Figure 1
Development of hypotension and vascular leak in patients treated with high-dose IL-2.
Panel A: Systolic and diastolic blood pressure was measured at least every 4 h during high dose
i.v. bolus IL-2 therapy. The lowest daily blood pressure of the first 13 patients treated with IL-2 at the University of Utah is shown (mean ± SEM). The bars indicate the periods of IL-2 treatment (600 000 IU/kg every 8 h on days 1–5 and 11–15). It should be noted that blood pressure changes were aggressively managed with fluids, albumin, and pressor administration to maintain a systolic BP ≥ 90 mm Hg. Doses of IL-2 were omitted if maintenance of this lower limit could not be maintained on less than 4 μg/kg/min dopamine. Panel B: Fluid retention induced by IL-2 treatment. Complete daily fluid intake and urine output were measured in IL-2 treated patients (mean ± SEM). Panel C: Weight gain during IL-2 treatment of patients. Data is shown as change in daily weight from baseline (mean ± SEM). Panel D: Development of pre-renal azotemia in IL-2 treated patients. Daily serum samples were analyzed for urea nitrogen (BUN) and creatinine. Results by treatment day are shown as mean ± SEM.

Clinical management of hypotension and VLS

Patients at the University of Utah treated with IL-2 undergo close hemodynamic monitoring, and fluid (100–150 ml isotonic saline/h), colloids (albumin) and pressors (dopamine and neosynephrine) are administered to counteract hypotension and to improve oliguria [28]. Once patients require ≥ 4 µg/kg/min dopamine or addition of other pressor agents, such as neosynephrine, further doses of IL-2 are held. The patients described above (Fig. 1) received 12.9 ± 1.1 and 6.8 ± 4.2 doses out of 14 planned doses of IL-2 during each half of the treatment course. Overall, our experience is that one-third to one-half of planned IL-2 doses are omitted due to hypotension or other toxicities (in > 150 patients treated with high dose i.v. IL-2 regimens). In every patient, IL-2 induced hypotension has resolved rapidly (8–24 h) after IL-2 administration ceased.

Possible mediators of IL-2 induced vascular toxicity

Nitric oxide (NO) is known to be a major regulatory factor controlling resting vasomotor tone (reviewed in [36, 37]). Endogenous low levels of NO synthesis (produced by the endothelial NOS isoform) plays an important role in the physiologic regulation of vasomotor tone [38, 39]. Stimuli, such as histamine, bradykinin, serotonin or shear stress, signal endothelial cells to synthesize small increments of NO [36]. It should be noted that the mechanism of action of most pharmacologically useful vasodilators also involves either direct release of NO (e.g., sodium nitroprusside) or indirect metabolism of nitrates to NO (e.g., nitroglycerin, isosorbide dinitrate) [40]. NO generated from endothelial cells or pharmacologic donors diffuses to vascular smooth muscle cells and induces vasodilation and increased blood flow. The mechanism for NO induced vasodilation is mediated *via* interaction with a heme-prosthetic group of soluble guanylate cyclase (sGC), resulting in a structural change that displaces the iron from the plane of the heme molecule [41]. Interaction of NO with sGC activates the enzyme, resulting in increased intracellular cGMP synthesis [42]. Intracellular levels of cGMP are further regulated by GMP-specific phosphodiesterases [43]. Subsequent events include the activation of cGMP-dependent protein kinases (PKG) [44], activation of Ca^{2+} activated K^+ channels [45], and decreases in cytosolic calcium concentration in endothelial and cardiac muscle cells *via* alterations in calcium transporter function [46–48]. It is thought that an end-product of these interactions may be decreased myosin phosphorylation, resulting in cellular relaxation [49].

Evidence that NO synthesis is activated by IL-2 treatment

Since IL-2 triggers release of inflammatory cytokines (IFNγ, TNFα and IL-1β) from LAK cells which activate the inducible L-arginine:NO synthesis pathway in rodents [29], we hypothesized that NO synthesis was induced in IL-2 treated patients and acted as a mediator of hypotension and vascular leak. It should be noted that at the time we performed our initial experiments in patients receiving high-dose IL-2 for renal carcinoma or melanoma, it was not yet possible to induce this pathway in human cells *in vitro*. Our study demonstrated that high levels of NO synthesis were induced in patients during IL-2 treatment [50]. Measurement of urine nitrate (NO_3^-) excretion (a metabolite of NO) revealed 6–10-fold increases on days 5–7 following a 5-day course of IL-2 treatment in patients with kidney cancer or melanoma (Fig. 2). We attributed the greater rise during the first half of the treatment course to the fact that these patients received about twice as many doses of IL-2. The derivation of the urinary NO_3^- from the L-arginine dependent pathway of NO synthesis (rather than *via* the enzyme arginase in the urea cycle) was confirmed by metabolic tracer studies using guanidino-^{15}N-labeled L-arginine.

Development of murine models of IL-2 treatment

In order to further study mechanisms of IL-2 induced hypotension and vascular leak, we felt that a murine model of IL-2 treatment would be helpful. Groups of normal C3H/HeN mice (four mice per cage) were acclimated to a nitrate/nitrite-free diet in metabolic cages. Sequential 24 h collections of all urine excreted by the mice were used to quantify NO synthesis. At the onset of the experiment, mice were injected with 10^6 RD-995 tumor cells subcutaneously. On day 10, when tumors had grown to approximately 5 mm diameter, mice were begun on twice daily IL-2 treatment at doses shown for 5 days (Fig. 3). The RD995 tumor is a UV light induced "fibrosarcoma" which grows progressively in non-immunosuppressed syngeneic mice, and is thus termed a "progressor" tumor [51]. Progressive subcutaneous growth of this tumor (without IL-2 treatment) results in induction of intratumoral NO synthesis due to the host immune response [52].

This experiment demonstrated that IL-2 produced a dose-dependent induction of NO synthesis in mice (Panel A). Excretion of NO_2^-/NO_3^- peaked on days 5–8 of the treatment protocol. We have previously established that the Griess reaction is a reliable technique for analyzing NO synthesis *in vivo*, as long as exogenous dietary intake of NO_2^-/NO_3^- is minimized and bacterial contamination of urine specimens is avoided. A dose-dependent reduction in tumor growth was also observed, compared to controls (Panel B). This antitumor response proved transient, however, since tumor growth rates returned to baseline levels within 7–10 days of IL-2 treatment, similar to a response pattern seen in many IL-2 treated patients.

Differences in NO synthesis in mouse strains

When we attempted to treat C3H/HeN mice at doses of IL-2 published by other investigators in C57/Bl6 mice [10–12], we noted nearly 100% mortality. This obser-

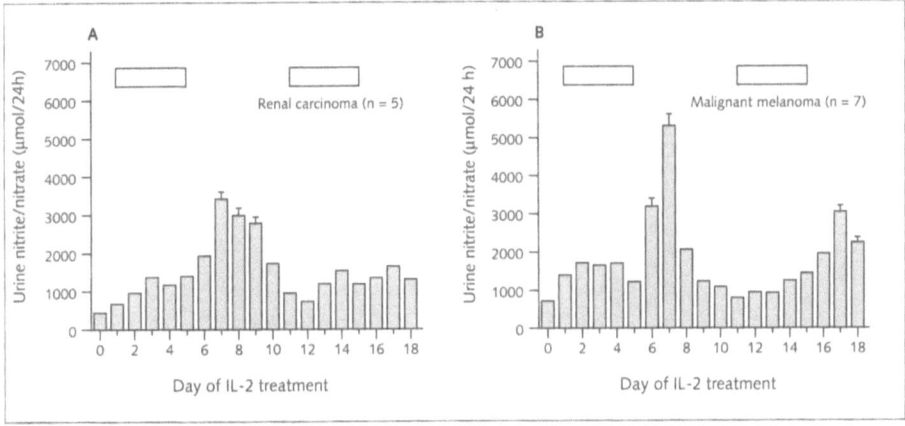

Figure 2

Urinary nitrite/nitrate excretion in IL-2 treated patients. Activity of the L-arginine dependent pathway was assessed by measuring urine nitrite/nitrate (stable degradation products of NO during IL-2 therapy. Patients were maintained on a fixed low nitrate intake during the experiment. All daily urine excretion was collected and analyzed for total nitrite/nitrate excretion. The bars indicate the periods of IL-2 treatment (600 000 IU/kg every 8 h on days 1–5 and 11–15). The pattern of IL-2 induced changes in urinary NO metabolite excretion in melanoma (panel A) and renal cell carcinoma patients (panel B) is shown.

vation suggested substantial differences in IL-2 induced NO synthesis between mouse strains. This possibility was evaluated by performing dose response experiments in BALB/c, C3H/HeN and C57/Bl6 mice. Our experiments showed that levels of NO synthesis induced in these strains in response to a 5-day course of IL-2 treatment differed substantially, with C3H/HeN mice being the most sensitive (maximum tolerated dose of IL-2 200 000 IU bid for 5 days). In contrast, BALB/c mice tolerated a far greater dose of IL-2 (400 000 IU IL-2 bid for 5 days). These findings correlated with greater induction of NO synthesis in C3H/HeN mice (peak urinary nitrite/nitrate excretion 3.3 µmol/mouse per day *versus* 2.0 µmol/mice/day in BALB/c animals). These findings agree with observations by Mills et al. who found that macrophages from C57BL/6 mice were more easily activated to synthesize NO by LPS/IFNγ, than those from BALB/c and DBA/2 strains [53].

Inhibition of IL-2 induced NO synthesis in mice

Studies by Hibbs and colleagues that originally identified the L-arginine:NO pathway suggested that L-arginine analogues had the potential to block NO synthesis *in*

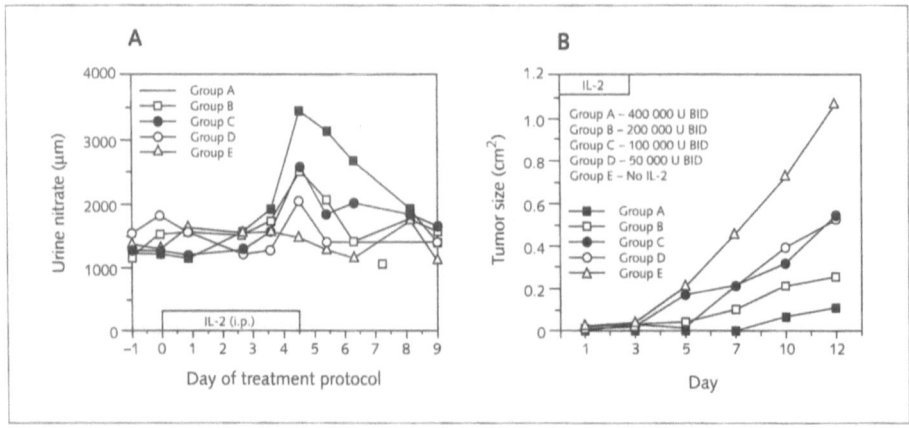

Figure 3
The effect of increasing IL-2 doses on NO synthesis and tumor response.
To test for a possible relationship between IL-2 dose and NO synthesis, mice were implanted with 10^6 RD-995 fibrosarcoma cells and acclimated to metabolic cages for 7 days. Mice were then treated with increasing concentrations of IL-2 (0, 50 000, 100 000, 200 000 and 400 000 IU IL-2 injected subcutaneously twice daily for 5 days). Panel A: Sequential 24 h collections of pooled urine from groups of four mice were used to quantify IL-2 induced NO metabolite excretion. Panel B: Cross-sectional tumor area (maximum dimension × perpendicular measurement) was measured every other day starting 24 h following the onset of IL-2 treatment (day 1) and is plotted as change from baseline (mean ± SD).

vitro [54]. We evaluated whether chronic N^G-monomethyl-L-arginine (NMMA) administration to mice could be used as a pharmacologic inhibitor of NO synthesis in our murine model [55]. These experiments demonstrated that continuous s.c. infusion of NMMA (28 µl/day of a 3.38 M solution-the maximum solubility of NMMA in PBS) *via* osmotic minipumps blocked NO synthesis induced by i.p. BCG infection. After stabilization of mice on a NO_2^-/NO_3^- free diet in metabolic cages, BCG infected mice excreted approximately 6.0 µmol/mouse/day NO_2^-/NO_3^-. NMMA administration decreased urinary NO_2^-/NO_3^- excretion to baseline (~ 1.0 µmol/mouse/day, 83% reduction) within 24 h following pump implantation. This effect lasted 8–9 days.

To test the effect of NMMA on NO synthesis in normal and IL-2 treated mice, C3H/HeN mice (four mice per cage) were acclimated to a nitrate/nitrite-free diet and metabolic cages for 7 days. Weight, food and water intake, as well as urine output per group were recorded daily. At the onset of the experiment, mice were injected with 10^6 RD-995 tumor cells s.q. (first arrow). On day 10, when tumors had grown to approximately 5 mm diameter, mice were implanted subcutaneously with

Alzet continuous infusion pumps (Model 2001), containing 225 µl of 3.38 M NMMA (second arrow). Control mice underwent sham pump implantation. Beginning on day 3, IL-2 treated mice received a 5-day course (180 000 IU i.p. every 12 h for 5 days), with LAK cells given i.v. on days 3 and 6 of the experiment (10^8 cells each day) (Fig. 4).

IL-2 treatment increased NO production three-fold over baseline. Peak NO_2^-/NO_3^- excretion was again seen on days 6–9 following a 5-day course of IL-2. This increase was completely blocked by NMMA infusion, demonstrating that the source of NO was from nitric oxide synthase. These experiments also demonstrated that chronic NMMA infusion was well tolerated in mice. Control and experimental animals had similar water and food intake, urine output and weight. Significant changes in blood counts and serum chemistries were not observed, although there was a trend toward increasing prerenal azotemia in NMMA treated groups. NMMA did not appear to affect LAK cell induction *in vitro* or *in vivo*. Tumor growth was transiently inhibited, as shown above. Subsequent experiments have shown that the major source of NO in IL-2 treated mice is derived from the inducible nitric oxide synthase (iNOS) enzyme isoform. This conclusion is based on the detection of iNOS mRNA in tissues of mice treated with IL-2 (Fig. 5) by RT-PCR. A 345 bp iNOS cDNA product was demonstrated in spleen, liver, kidney, skeletal muscle and tumor. In an untreated control mouse, only kidney expression of iNOS mRNA was seen (not shown). Further studies have also demonstrated iNOS protein expression by Western blot or flow cytometry (not shown). Additional proof that the iNOS enzyme is the source of IL-2 induced NO is derived from studies in iNOS knockout mice (generous gift from Dr. Victor Laubach). These mice fail to increase urinary NO_2^-/NO_3^- excretion following IL-2 treatment (manuscript in preparation).

Evaluation of hypotension and VLS following IL-2 treatment of mice

Using pharmacologic inhibitors of NOS enzymes, Kilbourn recently proved that NO plays an important role in mediating TNF, and subsequently IL-2-induced hypotension in a dog model [56, 57]. We subsequently developed techniques to quantify hypotension and vascular leak in IL-2 treated mice. Mice (groups of four animals) were treated with 180 000 IU/kg IL-2 i.p. for 5 days (10 doses). Parallel groups of mice were treated with NMMA, to block NO synthesis [55]. 2 h after the last dose of IL-2, systolic blood pressure was measured *via* tail cuff (Stoelting, Wood Dell, IL) and using a PowerLab digital signal transducer (AD instruments, Mountain View, CA). Analysis was performed using Chart 3.6.1 software (AD instruments). Data is expressed as mean of triplicate measurements ± SD (Fig. 6, Panel A). Immediately prior to blood pressure measurements, mice were also infused with 0.1 ml [^{125}I]-albumin solution (approximately 125 000 cpm) i.v. 2 h after this injection, mice

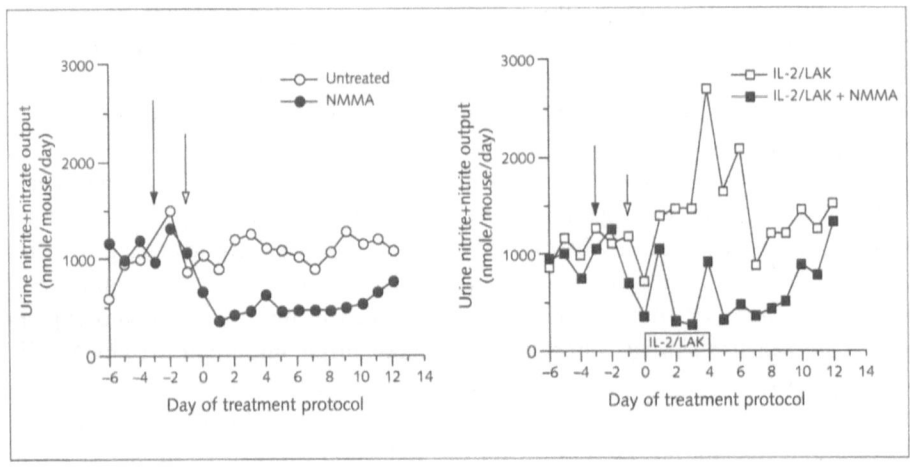

Figure 4

Inhibition of NO synthesis in a murine IL-2 treatment model by NMMA. Four groups of normal C3H/HeN mice (four mice per cage) were acclimated to a nitrate/nitrite-free diet and metabolic cages for 7 days. Weight, food and water intake, as well as urine output per group were recorded daily. At the onset of the experiment, mice were injected with 10^6 RD-995 tumor cells s.q (first arrow). On day 10, when tumors had grown to approximately 5 mm diameter, mice were implanted subcutaneously with Alzet continuous infusion pumps (Model 2001), containing 225 µl of 3.38 M NMMA (second arrow). Control mice underwent sham pump implantation. Beginning on day 3, mice received a 5-day course of IL-2 (180 000 IU i.p. every 12 h for 5 days), with LAK cells given i.v. on days 3 and 6 (10^8 cells each day) (Fig. 1). Tumors size and and urine nitrate excretion (shown above) were evaluated daily. Panel A: Urinary NO metabolite excretion in groups of normal or NMMA treated normal mice. Panel B: NO metabolite excretion in groups of IL-2 treated mice with or without NMMA infusion.

were sacrificed. Organ wet weight and [125I]-albumin retention was quantified (Fig. 6, Panel B) [58].

This experiment demonstrated that IL-2 administration to mice induced marked hypotension (> 40 mm Hg drop in systolic blood pressure). NMMA administration partially reversed the hypotension. Since IL-2 was administered i.p., the greatest VLS was observed in abdominal organs, due to prolonged retention of IL-2 in the peritoneum. Substantial evidence for vascular leak was seen in the liver, spleen and intestines. As an example, the percentage of radiolabel retained in the liver compared to the remainder of the animal is shown (mean ± SD). NMMA administration appeared to decrease the vascular pool within the organs of non-IL-2 treated con-

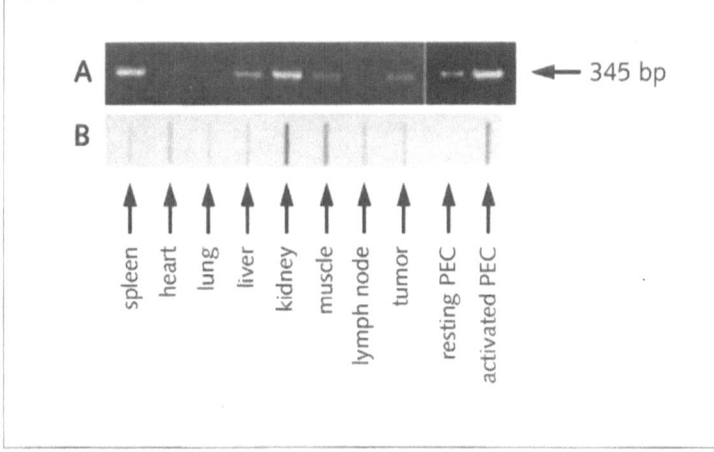

Figure 5

Expression of iNOS mRNA following IL-2 treatment of mice. Detection of tissue iNOS mRNA expression in IL-2 treated mice: RD-995 tumor bearing mice were treated with a 5-day course of IL-2. Mice were sacrificed 2 h following the final dose of IL-2, and mRNA was isolated from biopsies of various tissues. RT-PCR for iNOS was performed (30 cycles; 15 s at 94 °C, 15 s at 60 °C and 30 s at 72 °C). Primers used for iNOS detection were: upstream 5'-AGGCCACATCGGATTTCAC-3'; downstream 5'-TACAGTTCCGAGCGTCAAAGA-3'. RT-PCR for β-actin was performed on all samples to verify equivalent PCR amplification and gel loading (not shown). Resting and cytokine activated peritoneal exudate cells served as negative and positive controls.

trol mice (perhaps by blocking constitutive endothelial NO synthesis). Concomitant administration of NMMA (at its maximum solubility) with IL-2 was only partially able to reverse IL-2 induced hypotension, but appeared to almost completely inhibit vascular leak. Thus NO appears to be an important mediator of both hypotension and VLS. This model has proven useful in evaluating potential inhibitors of IL-2 induced cardiovascular toxicity.

For example, we have attempted to perform a IL-2 dose escalation experiment, using continuous infusions of NMMA to block NO synthesis. To our surprise, only a 10–20% escalation of IL-2 dose was feasible (data not shown). We believe that there are two possible explanations for this observation: either additional mechanisms contribute to IL-2 induced hypotension and vascular leak that are not mediated by NO, or alternatively other non-cardiovascular dose-limiting toxicities are induced by the escalated doses of IL-2. We are currently investigating these possibilities.

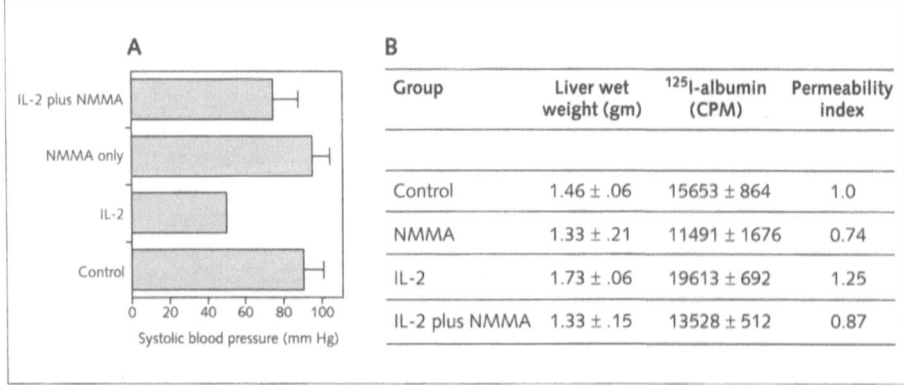

A (chart) — Systolic blood pressure (mm Hg) for groups: IL-2 plus NMMA, NMMA only, IL-2, Control

B

Group	Liver wet weight (gm)	^{125}I-albumin (CPM)	Permeability index
Control	1.46 ± .06	15653 ± 864	1.0
NMMA	1.33 ± .21	11491 ± 1676	0.74
IL-2	1.73 ± .06	19613 ± 692	1.25
IL-2 plus NMMA	1.33 ± .15	13528 ± 512	0.87

Figure 6

Evaluation of hypotension and vascular leak in IL-2 treated mice. Mice (groups of four animals) were treated with 180 000 IU/kg IL-2 i.p. for 5 days (10 doses). Parallel groups of mice were treated with NMMA (18.5 mg N^G-monomethyl-L-arginine/mouse/day via subcutaneous infusion pump), to block NO synthesis. Panel A: 2 h after the last dose of IL-2, systolic blood pressure was measured via tail cuff (Stoelting, Wood Dell, IL) and using a PowerLab digital signal transducer (AD instruments, Mountain View, CA). Analysis was performed using Chart 3.6.1 software (AD instruments), showing substantial drops in blood pressure in IL-2 treated mice, and partial reversal with NMMA. Data is expressed as mean ± SD. Panel B: Immediately before blood pressure measurements, mice were infused with 0.1 ml [^{125}I]-albumin solution (approximately 125 000 cpm) i.v. After 2 h, mice were sacrificed. Organ wet weight and [^{125}I]-albumin retention was quantified. Data from liver retention of radioalbumin are shown. The following p values were observed for liver [^{125}I]-albumin accumulation (cpm): control versus IL-2, p = 0.0014; control versus IL-2 + NMMA, p > 0.05; IL-2 versus NMMA + IL-2, p = 0.0014, NMMA versus IL-2 + NMMA, p > 0.05. Differences in organ weight between groups did not achieve statistical significance at the p < 0.05 level by paired t-test.

Anticancer effects mediated by IL-2 induced NO synthesis

Macrophage anticancer mechanisms

Murine macrophages acquire potent antitumor potential when activated by cytokines produced during a cell mediated immune response. Activation signals include the lymphokine interferon γ (IFNγ) and the monokine, tumor necrosis factor (TNFα) [59, 60]. Cytotoxic macrophages have a variety of effects on tumor cells, including release of intracellular iron, as well as inhibition of mitochondrial respiration, DNA synthesis and cellular proliferation [61, 62]. In 1987, Hibbs and coworkers reported that the induction of macrophage cytotoxicity was dependent on the amino acid L-arginine [54]. Subsequently the effector molecule responsible for L-arginine dependent cytotoxicity was shown to be NO [63, 64]. Discovery of the cytokine induced L-arginine: NO pathway explained many of the observed biochemical changes in target cells. Major intracellular targets of NO appear to be intracellular iron-sulfur [4Fe-4S] prosthetic groups of Complex I and Complex II of the mitochondrial electron transport system and the citric acid cycle enzyme aconitase, as well as non-heme iron in ribonucleotide reductase [65–67]. Identification of iron-nitrosyl-sulfur complexes by electron paramagnetic resonance (EPR) spectroscopy linked metabolic inhibition of enzymes with [4Fe-4S] prosthetic groups with NO synthesis by activated macrophages [68].

Additional NO interactions that contribute to anticancer activity

NO can interact with a number of other cellular targets to yield products which initiate cytotoxic activity against cancer cells [69]. In the presence of superoxide, NO is converted to peroxynitrite which in turn induces protein tyrosine nitration [70, 71]. Formation of nitrotyrosine can affect the function of proteins and modify the growth characteristic of cells [70, 71]. Indeed, peroxynitrite has been shown to induce apoptosis in HL-60 cells [72]. NO can also affect protein function and cell growth through the nitrosylation of thiol residues [73]. For example, S-nitrosylation of glyceraldehyde phosphate dehydrogenase by NO has been extensively studied, although the role played by NO is the subject of controversy [74]. Another mechanism by which NO could affect intracellular protein function and therefore growth is by activating ADP ribosyl transferase, resulting in protein ADP-ribosylation [75]. NO has also been shown to induce DNA damage by causing DNA strand breaks, *via* deamination of purine bases [76]. The net effect of metabolic changes induced by NO in tumor and normal cells may be to induce apoptosis [77, 78].

Evaluation of NO as an IL-2 induced anticancer mechanism in mice

We have previously shown that LAK cell mediated antitumor mechanisms do not appear to be inhibited by NO *in vivo* [55]. Paradoxically, subsequent studies in this laboratory have shown that high concentrations of NO appear to inhibit activation of LAK cell precursors by IL-2 by triggering apoptosis of these lymphocytes [79]. In order to test whether IL-2 induced NO synthesis was beneficial or detrimental in murine models, we needed to devise a way to dissociate LAK cell and NO mediated mechanisms. This opportunity was provided by the discovery that Meth A, a well characterized methylcholanthrene induced fibrosarcoma tumor cell line (obtained from Lloyd Old, MSKCC) [80], was resistant to LAK cell mediated cytolysis [81]. This property allowed us to test the role of IL-2 induced NO synthesis in IL-2 treatment responses. Our experiments demonstrated that NO synthesis in Meth A malignant ascites was not active in control mice, but was induced by subcutaneous IL-2 treatment. NO production was inhibited by coculture of cells with 1 mM NMMA. EPR spectroscopy provided evidence of NO induced injury to tumor cells derived from the IL-2 treated, but not control mice. NO production in malignant ascites correlated in an inverse fashion with tumor cell proliferation. Immunomagnetic depletion of macrophages using MAC-1 (CD11b) MAb suggested that both macrophages and tumor cells were involved in IL-2-induced NO synthesis (see below). Flow cytometric analysis revealed that IL-2 treatment of mice increased CD4 and CD8 lymphocyte and macrophage recruitment into malignant ascites, as well as increased iNOS expression in macrophages.

IL-2 treatment of mice bearing Meth A ascites resulted in substantial reductions in the intraperitoneal tumor burden and significantly prolonged survival of mice with advanced tumors (mean 23 vs. 16 days, $p < 0.0001$), with ~ 10% long term disease-free survival (Fig. 7). This survival advantage was blocked by co-administration of NMMA, strongly suggesting that NO mediated the antitumor response. Subsequent experiments established that earlier initiation of IL-2 therapy (day 3 vs. day 7 following tumor implantation) markedly increased the frequency of complete responses. These experiments confirmed that IL-2 induced NO synthesis can mediate beneficial anticancer effects *in vivo*.

Induction of tumor cell apoptosis by NO

The apparent reduction of tumor cell burden in IL-2 treated mice bearing Meth A ascites was not fully explained by known antitumor mechanisms mediated by NO, which are predominantly cytostatic. Evaluation of Wright-stained cytocentrifuge slides of ascites cells during IL-2 therapy showed macrophages adherent to tumor cells, which exhibited marked nuclear chromatin condensation and cytoplasmic blebbing in IL-2 treated mice, but not controls. Since these findings were suggestive of tumor cell apoptosis, we evaluated whether NO could induce this process in Meth A cells [82]. Meth A tumor cells were exposed to pure NO gas, to avoid other agonists that could be induced by IL-2 treatment within malignant ascites. NO exposed Meth A demonstrated DNA fragmentation characteristic of apoptosis (Fig. 8). Similar DNA fragmentation was observed when activated macrophages or pharmacologic NO donors were added to tumor cells, suggesting that physiologic concentrations of NO also are capable of inducing apoptosis.

We subsequently tested whether additional tumor cell lines were susceptible to NO induced apoptosis. Murine RD-995 fibrosarcomas and B-16 melanoma cells also proved susceptible. Human DLD-1 colon cancer cells and HL-60, U937 and

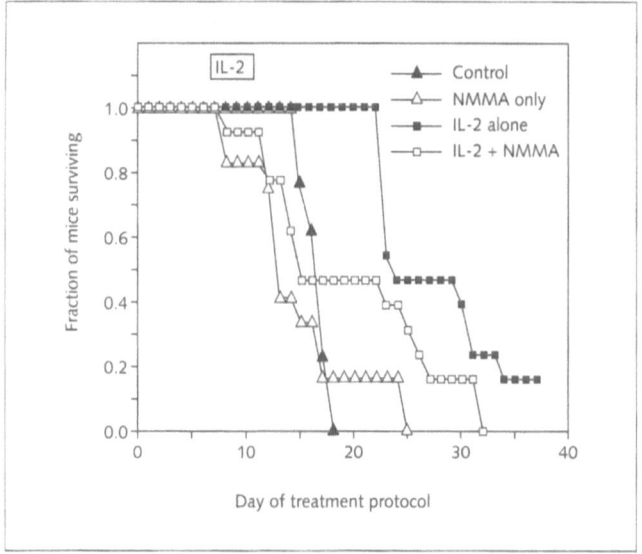

Figure 7
Survival in Meth A ascites tumor-bearing mice treated with IL-2. Mice received intraperi-
toneal injections of 2×10^6 Meth A tumor cells at the onset of the experiment (termed day
0). On day 5, groups receiving NMMA therapy were implanted subcutaneously with Alzet
continuous infusion pumps as described. The other groups of mice underwent sham pump
implantation. On day 6, IL-2 therapy was begun in the appropriate groups. Survival of the
mice was evaluated daily. Median survival of IL-2 treated animals (23 days) was significant-
ly different from controls (16 days; p = 0.0001 by stratified Wilcoxon test). NMMA admin-
istration resulted in decreased survival of IL-2 treated mice (median, 14 days, p = 0.04) ver-
sus mice receiving IL-2 alone.

K562 leukemia cells also were triggered to undergo apoptosis following exposure to either NO gas or soluble NO donors (e.g. S-nitroso-acetyl D-penicillamine).

Induction of endogenous NO synthesis in tumor cells by LAK cell cytokines

IL-2 activated lymphocytes (termed lymphokine activated killer or LAK cells) secrete inflammatory cytokines such as IFNγ and TNFα. Since these cytokines can induce NO synthesis in some human cells, such as hepatocytes, we evaluated whether LAK cells could activate this signaling pathway in human DLD-1 colon cancer cells [83]. Neither LAK cells nor DLD-1 cells produced significant nitrite (< 3 μM), a stable metabolite of NO, during a 3-day exposure to IL-2 (6000 IU/ml)

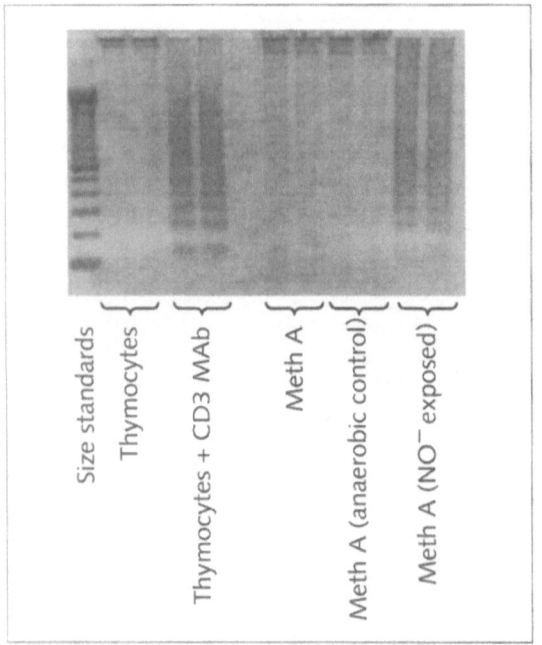

Figure 8

Induction of apoptosis in Meth A fibrosarcoma cells by NO. Meth A tumor cells were placed into a glass Petri dish at 10^8 cells per ml in a minimal volume of RPMI 1640 containing 0.1 mM HEPES. Petri dishes was depleted of oxygen in a hypobaric chamber by flushing with pure nitrogen gas for 15 min. This procedure is necessary to avoid the formation of highly toxic NO_2 from reaction of NO with O_2. Following degassing, tumor cells were exposed to 100% NO gas for 30 min. Following a second degassing in a nitrogen atmosphere, cells were placed into cell culture for 18 h and DNA isolated. Samples were evaluated for DNA fragmentation by electrophoresis on 1% agarose. Controls for this experiment included DNA from untreated Meth A tumor cells, and DNA from cells that were placed in the anaerobic environment for the same length of time as the NO exposed cells, but without exposure to NO gas. Positive and negative controls for this experiment were untreated murine thymocytes as well as thymocytes activated with CD3 MAb (known to undergo apoptosis).

in vitro. In contrast, coculture of DLD-1 cells with A 1:2 dilution of LAK cell supernatant in fresh medium induced substantial nitrite production (40.7 ± 1.8 μM) (Fig. 9A). We showed that tumor cell NO synthesis was mediated *via* LAK cell cytokines, as NO synthesis was blocked by anti-IFNγ MAb, but not TNFα MAb (5–10 μg/ml, R&D Systems) (Fig. 9B). Similar findings could be induced by adding

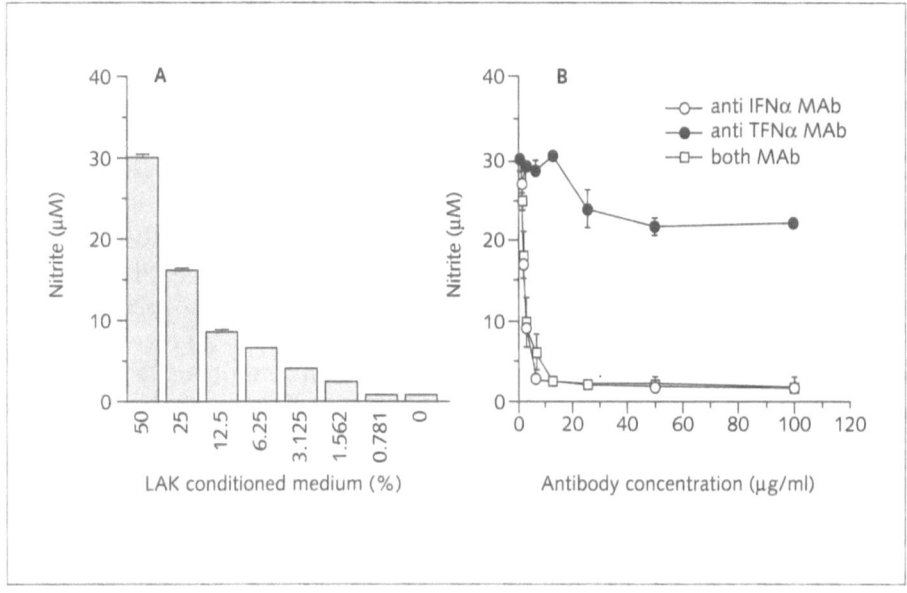

Figure 9
Induction of endogenous NO synthesis in tumor cells by LAK cell cytokines.
Panel A: Induction of NO synthesis in DLD-1 cells by LAK cell conditioned medium. Human peripheral blood lymphocytes (PBL) were isolated on Ficoll-Hypaque. Conditioned medium was prepared by harvesting supernatants from LAK cells cultured with 6000 IU/ml recombinant human IL-2 for 72 h in bulk cell cultures. Serial dilutions (0–50% v:v) of conditioned medium in fresh RPMI 1640 medium (with 5% FCS) were added to DLD-1 cells (2 × 10^6 cells/ml) in microtiter wells. After a 3-day culture (37 °C; 5% CO_2), nitrite accumulation was measured in 50 μl culture supernatants by colorimetric microtiter assay. The result is expressed as mean ± SD of triplicate wells. Panel B: Inhibition of NO synthesis by anti-IFNγ MAb. DLD-1 colon cancer cells (2 × 10^6 cells/ml) were cultured in the presence of 50% LAK conditioned medium (from 72 h LAK cultures). Serial dilutions of blocking MAb directed against human IFNγ or TNFα were added to parallel microtiter wells. Maximum antibody concentrations were 100 μg/ml. At 48 h, nitrite was measured by colorimetric microtiter assay (mean ± SD of triplicate wells).

exogenous recombinant cytokines to DLD-1 cultures. Endogenous NO synthesis inhibited tumor cell proliferation and induced programmed cell death. We therefore have identified an additional non-contact mediated mechanism for LAK cell killing of tumor cells, involving induction of NO synthesis within tumor cells by physiologically achievable concentrations of cytokines.

Is NO predominantly a mediator of toxicity or mechanism of IL-2 induced anticancer responses?

Current evidence suggests that nitric oxide (NO) is an important mediator involved in the physiologic regulation of systemic vasomotor tone. We and other investigators have shown that NO contributes to the pathogenesis of VLS, hypotension and myocardial depression, which are observed as dose-limiting toxicities following administration of a number of cytokines (including IL-1, IL-2, IL-12 and TNFα. NO can also inhibit LAK cell induction by IL-2 [79], as well as other immunologic functions [84–86]. On the other hand, NO also can inhibit cellular respiration and DNA synthesis in tumor cells, triggering programmed cell death. Our experiments have shown that NO can contribute to anticancer responses in murine models of IL-2 treatment [81]. An anti-cancer effect of NO in humans is suggested by recent studies by Anderson et al. which showed a correlation of clinical responses to IL-2 based CVD-biochemotherapy and indicators of macrophage activation and NO synthesis [87]. These apparently paradoxical observations remain to be reconciled. A better understanding of these possibilities seem important, since pharmacologic interventions can now be designed to either block NO synthesis or to enhance NO or perhaps more selectively target NO synthesis within tumors (e.g. *via* gene therapy approaches). It also appears to be feasible to inhibit intermediate signaling pathways activated by NO to signal vasodilatation, *via* inhibitors of guanylate cyclase (which might dissociate hypotension and anticancer activity) and other agents. Until the role of IL-2 induced NO synthesis is better understood, we have been reluctant to employ pharmacologic inhibitors of NO synthases to counteract IL-2 induced hypotension and VLS. We are focusing instead on the development and testing of novel agents to dissociate IL-2 induced cardiovascular toxicity from potential anticancer mechanisms mediated by NO.

Acknowledgements
These studies were funded by grants from the National Institutes of Health (U01 CA58248; R01 CA67404), and the Huntsman Cancer Institute. I would like to acknowledge the contributions of numerous individuals to clinical and basic science studies of IL-2 induced NO synthesis. Clinical collaborators included John H. Ward, John B. Hibbs Jr., Christof Westenfelder and the Huntsman General Clinical Research Center (Dr. James Kushner, director; Carol Bowcutt, Head Nurse). Laboratory studies were aided by Chang-Yeol Yim, John McGregor, Shane Gonzales, Ryan Peterson, Julie Smith, Oh-Deog Kwon, Neil Bastian, Heinz-Josef Lenz, John B. Hibbs Jr., and others.

References

1   Sana TR, Wu Z, Smith KA, Ciardelli TL (1994) Expression and ligand binding charac-terization of the beta-subunit (p75) ectodomain of the interleukin-2 receptor. *Biochem* 33: 5838–5845

2   Nakarai T, Robertson MJ, Streuli M, Wu Z, Ciardelli TL, Smith KA, Ritz J (1994) Inter-leukin 2 receptor gamma chain expression on resting and activated lymphoid cells. *J Exp Med* 180: 241–251

3   Mertelsmann R, Welte K (1986) Human interleukin-2 molecular biology, physiology and clinical possibilities. *Immunobiol* 172: 400–419

4   Weiss A (1993) T lymphocyte activation. In: WE Paul (ed): *Fundamental immunology*. Raven Press, New York, 467–504

5   Lotze MT, Grimm EA, Mazumder A, Strausser JL, Rosenberg SA (1981) Lysis of fresh and cultured autologous tumor by human lymphocytes cultured in T-cell growth factor. *Cancer Res* 41: 4420–4425

6   Rayner AA, Grimm EA, Lotze MT, Wilson DJ, Rosenberg SA (1985) Lymphokine-acti-vated killer (LAK) cell phenomenon. IV. Lysis by LAK cell clones of fresh human tumor cells from autologous and multiple allogeneic tumors. *J Natl Cancer Inst* 75: 67–75

7   Hank JA, Kohler PC, Weil-Hillman G, Rosenthal N, Moore KH, Storer B, Minkoff D, Bradshaw J, Bechhofer R, Sondel PM (1988) *In vivo* induction of the lymphokine-acti-vated killer phenomenon: IL-2-dependent human non-major histocompatibility com-plex-restricted cytotoxicity generated *in vivo* during administration of human recombi-nant interleukin-2. *Cancer Res* 48: 1965–1971

8   Lanier LL, Le AM, Civin CI, Loken MR, Phillips JH (1986) The relationship of CD16 (Leu-11) and Leu-19 (NKH-1) antigen expression on human peripheral blood NK cells and cytotoxic T lymphocytes. *J Immunol* 136: 4480–4486

9   Harker WG, Tom C, McGregor JR, Slade L, Samlowski WE (1990) Human tumor cell line resistance to chemotherapeutic agents does not predict resistance to natural killer or lymphokine-activated killer cell-mediated cytolysis. *Cancer Res* 50: 5931–5936

10 Papa MZ, Mulé JJ, Rosenberg SA (1986) Antitumor efficacy of lymphokine-activated killer cells and recombinant interleukin 2 *in vivo*: successful immunotherapy of estab-lished pulmonary metastases from weakly immunogenic and nonimmunogenic murine tumors of three district histological types. *Cancer Res* 46: 4973–4978

11 Lafreniere R, Rosenberg SA (1985) Successful immunotherapy of murine experimental hepatic metastases with lymphokine-activated killer cells and recombinant interleukin 2. *Cancer Res* 45: 3735–3741

12 Mulé JJ, Shu S, Rosenberg SA (1985) The anti-tumor efficacy of lymphokine-activated killer cells and recombinant interleukin 2 *in vivo*. *J Immunol* 135: 646–652

13 Eberlein TJ, Rosenstein M, Rosenberg SA (1982) Regression of a disseminated syn-geneic solid tumor by systemic transfer of lymphoid cells expanded in interleukin-2. *J Exp Med* 156: 385–397

14 Rosenberg SA, Mulé JJ, Spiess PJ, Reichert CM, Schwarz SL (1985) Regression of estab-

lished pulmonary metastases and subcutaneous tumor mediated by the systemic administration of high-dose recombinant interleukin 2. *J Exp Med* 161: 1169–1188

15 Ettinghausen SE, Rosenberg SA (1986) Immunotherapy of murine sarcomas using lymphokine activated killer cells: optimization of the schedule and route of administration of recombinant interleukin-2. *Cancer Res* 46: 2784–2792

16 Ettinghausen SE, Puri RK, Rosenberg SA (1988) Increased vascular permeability in organs mediated by the systemic administration of lymphokine-activated killer cells and recombinant interleukin-2 in mice. *J Natl Cancer Inst* 80: 177–188

17 Rosenstein M, Ettinghausen SE, Rosenberg SA (1986) Extravasation of intravascular fluid mediated by the systemic administration of recombinant interleukin 2. *J Immunol* 137: 1735–1742

18 Rosenberg SA (1991) Adoptive cellular therapy in patients with advanced cancer: An update. *Biol Ther Cancer* 1: 1–15

19 Rosenberg SA, Yang JC, Topalian SL, Schwartzentruber DJ, Weber JS, Parkinson DR, Seipp CA, Einhorn JH, White DE (1994) Treatment of 283 consecutive patients with metastatic melanoma or renal cell cancer using high-dose bolus interleukin 2. *JAMA* 271: 907–913

20 Hawkins MJ (1989) IL-2/LAK: Current status and possible future directions. *Princip Pract Oncol* 3, 8: 1–14

21 Kim B, Louie AC (1992) Surgical resection following interleukin-2 therapy for metastatic renal cell carcinoma prolongs remission. *Arch Surg* 127: 1343–1349

22 Fisher RI, Rosenberg SA, Sznol M, Parkinson DR, Fyfe G (1997) High-dose aldesleukin in renal cell carcinoma: Long term survival update. *Cancer J* 3: S70–S72

23 Legha SS, Ring S, Eton O, Bedikian A, Plager C, Papadopoulos N (1997) Development and results of biochemotherapy in metastatic malignant melanoma: The University of Texas M.D. Anderson Cancer Center Experience. *Cancer J* 3: S9–S15

24 Legha SS (1997) Durable complete responses in metastatic melanoma treated with interleukin-2 in combination with interferon alpha and chemotherapy. *Semin Oncol* 24 (1 Suppl 4): S39–S43

25 Khatri VP, Fehniger TA, Baiocchi RA, Yu F, Shah MH, Schiller DS, Gould M, Gazzinelli RT, Bernstein ZP, Caligiuri MA (1998) Ultra low dose interleukin-2 therapy promotes a type 1 cytokine profile *in vivo* in patients with AIDS and AIDS-associated malignancies. *J Clin Invest* 101 (6): 1373–1378

26 Jacobson EL, Pilaro F, Smith KA (1996) Rational interleukin 2 therapy for HIV positive individuals: daily low doses enhance immune function without toxicity. *Proc Natl Acad Sci USA* 93 (19): 10405–10410

27 Siegel JP, Puri RK (1991) Interleukin-2 toxicity. *J Clin Oncol* 9: 694–704

28 Margolin KA, Rayner AA, Hawkins MA, Atkins MB, Dutcher JP, Fisher RI, Weiss GR, Doroshow JH, Jaffe HS, Roper M et al (1989) Interleukin-2 and lymphokine-activated killer cell therapy of solid tumors: Analysis of toxicity and management guidelines. *J Clin Oncol* 7: 486–498

29 Gemlo BT, Palladino MA, Jaffe HS, Espevik TP, Rayner AA (1988) Circulating

cytokines in patients with metastatic cancer treated with recombinant interleukin 2 and lymphokine-activated killer cells. *Cancer Res* 48: 5864–5867

30 Jablons DM, Mulé JJ, McIntosh JK, Sehgal PB, May LT, Huang CM, Rosenberg SA, Lotze MT (1989) IL-6/IFN-b-2 as a circulating hormone: Induction by cytokine administration in humans. *J Immunol* 142: 1542–1547

31 Ognibene FP, Rosenberg SA, Lotze M, Skibber J, Parker MM, Shelhamer JH, Parrillo JE (1988) Interleukin-2 administration causes reversible hemodynamic changes and left ventricular dysfunction similar to those seen in septic shock. *Chest* 94: 750–754

32 Mann H, Ward JH, Samlowski WE (1990) Vascular leak syndrome associated with interleukin-2: Chest radiographic manifestations. *Radiology* 176: 191–194

33 Lee RE, Lotze MT, Skibber JM, Tucker E, Bonow RO, Ognibene FP, Carrasquillo JA, Shelhamer JH, Parillo JE, Rosenberg SA (1989) Cardiorespiratory effects of immunotherapy with interleukin-2. *J Clin Oncol* 7: 7–20

34 Gaynor ER, Vitek L, Sticklin L, Creekmore SP, Ferraro ME, Thomas JXJr, Fisher SG, Fisher RI (1988) The hemodynamic effects of treatment with interleukin-2 and lymphokine-activated killer cells. *Ann Intern Med* 109: 953–958

35 Finkel MS, Oddis CV, Jacob TD, Watkins SC, Hattler BG, Simmons RL (1992) Negative inotropic effects of cytokines on the heart mediated by nitric oxide. *Science* 257: 387–389

36 Ignarro LJ (1996) Physiology and pathophysiology of nitric oxide. *Kidney Int* 55 (suppl): S2–S5

37 Moncada S, Palmer RMJ, Higgs EA (1991) NO: physiology, pathophysiology, and pharmacology. *Pharmacol Rev* 43: 109–142

38 Vallance P, Collier J, Moncada S (1989) Effects of endothelium-derived nitric oxide on peripheral arteriolar tone in man. *Lancet* 2: 997–1000

39 Brenner BM, Troy JL, Ballermann BJ (1989) Endothelium-dependent vascular responses. *J Clin Invest* 84: 1373–1378

40 Torfgard KE, Ahlner J (1994) Mechanisms of action of nitrates. Cardiovasc. *Drugs Ther* 8: 701–717

41 Ignarro LJ (1994) Regulation of cytosolic guanylyl cyclase by porphyrins and metalloporphyrins. *Adv Pharmacol* 26: 35–65

42 Drewett JG, Garbers DL (1994) The family of guanylyl cyclase receptors and their ligands. *Endocrine Rev* 15: 135–162

43 Delpy E, le Monnier de Gouville AC (1996) Cardiovascular effects of a novel, potent and selective phosphodiesterase 5 inhibitor, DMPPO: *in vitro* and *in vivo* characterization. *Br J Pharmacol* 118: 1377–1384

44 Francis SH, Corbin JD (1994) Progress in understanding the mechanism and function of cyclic GMP-dependent protein kinase. *Adv Pharmacol* 26: 115–170

45 Lincoln TM, Cornwell TL, Komalavilas P, Boerth N (1996) Cyclic GMP-dependent protein kinase in nitric oxide signalling. *Methods Enzymol* 269: 149–167

46 Hobbs AJ, Ignarro LJ (1996) Nitric oxide-cyclic GMP signal transduction system. *Methods Enzymol* 269: 134–148

47   Quignard JF, Frapier JM, Harricane MC, Albat B, Nargeot J, Richard S (1997) Voltage-gated calcium channel currents in human coronary myocytes. Regulation by cyclic GMP and nitric oxide. *J Clin Invest* 99: 185–193

48   Hirata M, Murad F (1994) Interrelationships of cyclic GMP, inositol phosphates and calcium. *Adv Pharmacol* 26: 195–216

49   Murad F (1994) Regulation of cytosolic guanylyl cyclase by nitric oxide: the NO-cyclic GMP signal transduction system. *Adv Pharmacol* 26: 19–33

50   Hibbs JBJr, Westenfelder C, Taintor R, Vavrin Z, Kablitz C, Baranowski RL, Ward JH, Menlove RL, McMurry MP, Kushner JP et al (1992) Evidence for cytokine inducible nitric oxide synthesis from L-arginine in patients receiving interleukin-2 therapy. *J Clin Invest* 89: 867–877

51   Kripke ML (1977) Latency, histology, and antigenicity of tumors induced by ultraviolet light in three inbred mouse strains. *Cancer Res* 37: 1395–1400

52   Yim C-Y, Bastian NR, Smith JC, Hibbs JBJr, Samlowski WE (1993) Macrophage nitric oxide synthesis delays progression of ultraviolet light induced murine skin cancers. *Cancer Res* 55: 5507–5511

53   Mills CD, Kincaid K, Alt JM, Heilman MJ, Hill AM (2000) M-1/M-2 macrophages and the Th1/Th2 paradigm. *J Immunol* 164 (12): 6166–6173

54   Hibbs JB Jr, Vavrin Z, Taintor RR (1987) L-arginine is required for expression of the activated macrophage effector mechanism causing selective metabolic inhibition in target cells. *J Immunol* 138: 550–565

55   Samlowski WE, Yim C-Y, McGregor JR, Kwon O-D, Gonzales S, Hibbs JB Jr (1995) Effectiveness and toxicity of protracted nitric oxide synthesis inhibition during IL-2 treatment of mice. *J Immunother* 18: 166–178

56   Kilbourn RG, Jubran A, Gross SS, Griffith OW, Levi R, Adams J, Lodato RF (1990) Reversal of endotoxin-mediated shock by N^G-methyl-L-arginine, an inhibitor of nitric oxide synthesis. *Biochem Biophys Res Commun* 172: 1132–1138

57   Kilbourn RG, Owen Schaub LB, Cromeens DM, Gross SS, Flaherty MJ, Santee SM, Alak AM, Griffith OW (1994) N^G-methyl-L-arginine, an inhibitor of nitric oxide formation, reverses IL-2-mediated hypotension in dogs. *J Appl Physiol* 76: 1130–1137

58   Gilliland G, Perrin S, Blanchard K, Bunn HF (1990) Analysis of cytokine mRNA and DNA: Detection and quantitation by competitive polymerase chain reaction. *Proc Natl Acad Sci USA* 87: 2725–2729

59   Drapier J-C, Wietzerbin J, Hibbs JB Jr (1988) Interferon-γ and tumor necrosis factor induce the L-arginine-dependent cytotoxic effector mechanism in murine macrophages. *Eur J Immunol* 18: 1587–1592

60   Ding AH, Nathan CF, Stuehr DJ (1988) Release of reactive nitrogen intermediates and reactive oxygen intermediates from mouse peritoneal macrophages. *J Immunol* 141: 2407–2412

61   Hibbs JB Jr, Taintor RR, Vavrin Z (1984) Iron depletion: possible cause of tumor cell cytotoxicity induced by activated macrophages. *Biochem Biophys Res Commun* 123: 716–723

62   Granger DL, Taintor RR, Cook JL, Hibbs JB Jr (1980) Injury of neoplastic cells by murine macrophages leads to inhibition of mitochondrial respiration. *J Clin Invest* 65: 357–370

63   Hibbs JB Jr, Taintor RR, Vavrin Z, Rachlin EM (1988) Nitric oxide: a cytotoxic activated macrophage effector molecule. *Biochem Biophys Res Commun* 157: 87–94

64   Stuehr DJ, Nathan CF (1989) Nitric oxide: A macrophage product responsible for cytostasis and respiratory inhibition in tumor target cells. *J Exp Med* 169: 1543–1555

65   Granger DL, Lehninger AL (1982) Sites of inhibition of mitochondrial electron transport in macrophage-injured neoplastic cells. *J Cell Biol* 95: 527–535

66   Drapier J-C, Hibbs JB Jr (1988) Differentiation of murine macrophages to express non-specific cytotoxicity for tumor cells results in L-arginine-dependent inhibition of mitochondrial iron-sulfur enzymes in the macrophage effector cells. *J Immunol* 140: 2829–2838

67   Lepoivre M, Fieschi F, Coves J, Thelander L, Fontecave M (1991) Inactivation of ribonucleotide reductase by nitric oxide. *Biochem Biophys Res Commun* 179: 442–448

68   Lancaster JRJr, Hibbs JBJr (1990) EPR demonstration of iron-nitrosyl complex formation by cytotoxic activated macrophages. *Proc Natl Acad Sci USA* 87: 1223–1227

69   Henry Y, Lepoivre M, Drapier JC, Ducrocz C, Boucher JL, Guissani A (1993) EPR characterization of molecular targets for NO in mammalian cells and organelles. *FASEB J* 7: 1124–1134

70   Gow AJ, Duran D, Malcolm S, Ischiropoulos H (1996) Effects of peroxynitrite-induced protein modifications on tyrosine phosphorylation and degradation. *FEBS Lett* 385: 63–66

71   Crow JP, Beckman JS (1995) The role of peroxynitrite in nitric oxide-mediated toxicity. *Curr Top Microbiol Immunol* 196: 57–73

72   Lin KT, Xue JY, Nomen M, Spur B, Wong PY (1995) Peroxynitrite-induced apoptosis in HL-60 cells. *J Biol Chem* 270: 16487–16490

73   Stamler JS (1994) Redox signaling: nitrosylation and related target interactions of nitric oxide. *Cell* 78: 931–936

74   Brüne B, Lapetina EG (1995) Glyceraldehyde-3-phosphate dehydrogenase: a target for nitric oxide signaling. *Adv Pharmacol* 34: 351–360

75   Brüne B, Lapetina EG (1989) Activation of a cytosolic ADP-ribosyltransferase by nitric oxide-generating agents. *J Biol Chem* 264: 8455–8458

76   Nguyen T, Brunson D, Crespi CL, Penman BW, Wishnok JS, Tannenbaum SR (1992) DNA damage and mutation in human cells exposed to nitric oxide *in vitro*. *Proc Natl Acad Sci USA* 89: 3030–3034

77   Geng YJ, Hellstrand K, Wennmalm A, Hansson GK (1996) Apoptotic death of human leukemic cells induced by vascular cells expressing nitric oxide synthase in response to gamma-interferon and tumor necrosis factor-alpha. *Cancer Res* 56: 866–874

78   Albina JE, Cui S, Mateo RB, Reichner JS (1993) Nitric oxide-mediated apoptosis in murine peritoneal macrophages. *J Immunol* 150: 5080–5085

79   Samlowski WE, Yim CY, McGregor JR (1998) Nitric oxide exposure inhibits induction

of lymphokine-activated killer cells by inducing precursor apoptosis. *Nitric Oxide* 2: 45–56

80 Borberg H, Oettgen HF, Choudry K, Beattie EJ (1972) Inhibition of established transplants of chemically induced sarcomas in syngeneic mice by lymphocytes from immunized donors. *Int J Cancer* 10: 539–547

81 Yim C-Y, McGregor JR, Kwon O-D, Bastian NR, Rees M, Mori M, Hibbs JB Jr, Samlowski WE (1995) Nitric oxide synthesis contributes to IL-2 induced antitumor responses against intraperitoneal Meth A tumor. *J Immunol* 155: 4382–4390

82 Samlowski WE, McGregor JR, Bastian NR, Kwon O-D, Yim C-Y (1996) Tumor cell apoptosis may represent a novel cytotoxic mechanism resulting from IL-2 induced nitric oxide (NO.) synthesis. In: JS Stamler, SS Gross, S Moncada (eds): *The biology of nitric oxide*. Portland Press, London, 164–165

83 Kwak J-Y, Han MK, Choi K-S, Park I-H, Park S-Y, Sohn M-H, Kim U-H, Mcgregor JR, Samlowski WE, Yim C-Y (2000) Cytokines secreted by lymphokine activated killer cells induce endogenous nitric oxide synthesis and apoptosis in DLD-1 colon cancer cells. *Cell Immunol* 203: 84–94 (Abstr)

84 Langrehr JM, Dull KE, Ochoa JB, Billiar TR, Ildstad ST, Schraut WH, Simmons RL, HoffmanRA (1992) Evidence that nitric oxide production by *in vivo* allosensitized cells inhibits the development of allospecific CTL. *Transplantation* 53: 632–640

85 Hoffman RA, Langrehr JM, Wren SM, Dull KE, Ildstad ST, McCarthy SA, Simmons RL (1993) Characterization of the immunosuppressive effects of nitric oxide in graft vs. host disease. *J Immunol* 151: 1508–1518

86 Mills CD (1991) Molecular basis of "suppressor" macrophages. Arginine metabolism *via* the nitric oxide synthetase pathway. *J Immunol* 146: 2719–2723

87 Anderson CM, Buzaid AC, Sussman J, Lee JJ, Ali Osman F, Braunschweiger PG, Plager C, Bedikian A, Papadopoulos N, Eton O et al (1998) Nitric oxide and neopterin levels and clinical response in stage III melanoma patients receiving concurrent biochemotherapy. *Melanoma Res* 8 (2): 149–155

Index

The PIR-Series
Progress in Inflammation Research

Homepage: http://www.birkhauser.ch

Up-to-date information on the latest developments in the pathology, mechanisms and therapy of inflammatory disease are provided in this monograph series. Areas covered include vascular responses, skin inflammation, pain, neuroinflammation, arthritis cartilage and bone, airways inflammation and asthma, allergy, cytokines and inflammatory mediators, cell signalling, and recent advances in drug therapy. Each volume is edited by acknowledged experts providing succinct overviews on specific topics intended to inform and explain. The series is of interest to academic and industrial biomedical researchers, drug development personnel and rheumatologists, allergists, pathologists, dermatologists and other clinicians requiring regular scientific updates.